PROVINGS
Volume I

How Understanding Provings
Offers An Essential Foundation
To Successful Patient Care

With a Proving of *Alcoholus*

Also by Paul Herscu, N.D.

*The Homeopathic Treatment of Children:
Pediatric Constitutional Types*

*Stramonium, With an Introduction to Analysis
using Cycles and Segments*

PROVINGS
Volume I

How Understanding Provings
Offers An Essential Foundation
To Successful Patient Care

With a Proving of *Alcoholus*

By **Paul Herscu, ND**

- with -
Frank Gruber, MD
Todd Hoover, MD
Amy Rothenberg, ND
Christopher Ryan, MD

Cornerstones of Homeopathy

PROVINGS
Volume I
With a Proving of *Alcoholus*

Copyright © 2002 by Paul Herscu, N.D.
ISBN 0-9654004-4-1
All rights reserved

Published by
The New England School of Homeopathy Press
356 Middle Street, Amherst, Massachusetts 01002

Cover Art by Amy Rothenberg
Index by S. Rosko Rossoff
Designed and Typeset by David Caputo, Positronic Design
Printing by Happy-Valley.com

Printed in The United States of America

Copyright © 2002 by Paul Herscu, N.D. All rights reserved. No part of this book may be reproduced or transmitted in any form or by any means, electronic or mechanical, including photocopying, recording, or by any information storage and retrieval system, or otherwise without permission in writing from the publisher.

This book is written as an educational resource for homeopathic physicians. It is not intended to replace appropriate diagnosis and / or treatment by a qualified physician. For information on the New England School of Homeopathy turn to page 321.

Published by
The New England School of Homeopathy Press
356 Middle Street • Amherst, Massachusetts 01002
www.NESH.com • info@nesh.com • 413.256.5949

Library of Congress Catalog Card Number: 2002110043
ISBN 0-9654004-4-1

*This book is dedicated with honor and respect to
homeopaths of the past, present and future:
truth in perception and skill in practice
should remain our highest goals.*

*This book is also dedicated to my son Jonah,
who continually teaches me that persevering at any endeavor,
getting back to the basics and practicing them,
is the necessary work which paves the road to excellence.*

Acknowledgments

For a project this important, let alone this large, I needed a tremendous amount of support and help. It seemed like just the right people were there at the right time. Friends and colleagues came with the only question of, "How can I help?" as each shared from his or her area of interest, skill or expertise. It is a pleasure to thank these people individually.

I would like to thank Amy Rothenberg, ND, my wife and partner. To say that I am the luckiest man alive to be married to Amy is an understatement. Any of you that know Amy would understand me when I say that I learn more about life, love and the power of a good heart from being around her every day. I often feel like a kid in a candy store because she is in my life.

Reluctantly drawn into this project, Amy felt it more important for me to continue writing my next *materia medica*. As the project developed, however, she came to be an enthusiastic and focused supporter. By the time the writing came to pass, she was the chief point person who read the entire manuscript. By this I mean that every part of this work was questioned from her perspective; I reworked whole sections at her suggestion. (I also learned to practice non-attachment, as I would watch ten pages edited down to two. She does this with a small glint in her eye. Believe me, *you* are the beneficiary there.) It was often her questions that led to the explanations that are within these pages and her choice of words which elucidate some delicate points.

I would also like to thank Frank Gruber, MD for his work on Chapter Two. He was well trained in a number of fields and expert in many. Over the course of years of discussions, we delved into many realms of this work. I asked him to help organize our lengthy discourses which he did, and by so doing prodded me with many pointed questions which enabled me to better articulate my thoughts and observations. His support of all of my work in the world of homeopathy has been incredibly valuable to me and his untimely death in the year 2000 cut short a collaborative relationship which I sorely miss. His gifts to this world were many; those who knew him benefited from his open nature, quiet intellect and loving presence.

I would like to thank Todd Hoover, MD for his work on Chapter Three. I spent many months organizing the language behind the theory of how provings related to the general concepts of *Stress* and *Strain* and to *Cycles* and *Segments* and as long of a time organizing a lecture that I would deliver over a span of some days on the subject. Todd sat through that lecture, typed it up and then added historical context to form the guts of Chapter Three. He understands this work inside and out and is a fine thinker, practitioner, writer, and the best of friends. There are many contributions to the field of homeopathy that will come from his concerted efforts and I look forward as his life and career unfold.

I also need to thank Christopher Ryan, MD for his work on Chapter Four. Chris and I discussed the whole realm of homeopathy so many times, over dinners, breakfasts, and even poker games. I grilled him for his perceptions which I greatly cherished and respected as well as for information about his discussions on homeopathy with his medical colleagues. It was a great frustration to him that the orthodox medical world could not appreciate the gifts that homeopathy brought to it. I asked him to enumerate those gifts and that is the work described in the end of Chapter Four. His keen insight as to the uses of proving as an adjunct to the current drug testing protocol is brilliant and I believe it will eventually be used. I especially think it is useful for us, as homeopaths, as it gives us an entry into the discussion of homeopathy with our medical colleagues, an angle that can not really be refused by any scientist. His early death a few years back was a tremendous loss to his family, the homeopathic community and especially to me.

I would like to thank Ed Shalts, MD, who works at Beth Israel Medical Center in New York City. He drove me further into a realm that is not my main interest, but one that is an essential piece of work to complement any study of provings. The question I posed in class was, "Can a trained homeopath tell if someone took a placebo versus a verum?" I then went on in a small experiment to demonstrate how it could be done. On the face of it the question is ridiculous and so simple it does not deserve a second glance. However, it was the discussion between us that brought home to me the point that I make to everyone else: Test your assumptions! You may find that they are correct, and yet by testing your ideas, at the same time find a new aspect that you did not appreciate. Or you may find that they are wrong and find ways of working with the new results.

Ed encouraged us to conduct a much larger study to test this hypothesis and then to publish it. We carried out a few pilot studies based on this question and the results were positive enough that a larger, multi-centered study is underway. This will go a long way to underscoring the efficacy of homeopathy.

In terms of Chapter Seven, I would like to thank three people.

Sam Mawn-Mahlau once again came through with expert and precise legal advice and gathered the material that formed the consent forms that we give to supervising homeopaths as well as to provers. Medical testing on people in this country is ruled by the concept of informed consent and medical safety. As a result, having a document such as this was invaluable to me.

I also would like to thank Jeenet Lawton. She typed up our notes for those documents and then edited them. The forms that the homeopaths and provers were using were very important and needed to be perfectly understood. I trust Jeenet to do such editing work and am never disappointed.

The last part of Chapter Seven is the documentation for the proving web site. I am not a technologically gifted person. However I do have a friend, Graham Hall, that is. He sat with a pen in hand and listened to what I was looking for. We ended up with many trials and errors on the project. But when it was said and done, it worked the way I wanted it to. We set up a website and then conducted a proving using it.

The idea is a simple one. One of the most difficult aspects of conducting a proving, once the philosophy and methodology is settled on, is entering and collating all the information we receive from our provers. I am not talking about deciding which symptoms to choose. That happens originally with each homeopath who is supervising each prover by him or herself. However, once the symptoms are decided upon, it can still be difficult to enter all the information. Once entered it becomes extremely time consuming to organize the material. I thought it would be a good idea if some of that work would be done in a more timely fashion. I also thought it would be interesting to have the primary investigator be able to look at the proving on a daily basis if he or she wanted to. In that way, the proving can be seen as it unfolds. Graham designed the program and it has worked well.

I would like to thank Jack Lawyer and Jane Ryan for providing much general support for this endeavor as well as for many other aspects of my work and my life.

I would like to thank Joan Rothenberg, Linda Smith and Kim McGuire for typing portions of this manuscript.

While I will thank the provers and the homeopaths who provided the 18 records listed in Part 2 of this volume, I am even more appreciative of the ones that had no symptoms to report. I especially want to mention Jack Lawyer and Jonathan Marchand, MD. I have never met two people who so dearly wanted to see the proving at work. They desperately wanted *something to happen* with their provers. And wouldn't you know it, while their provers did have symptoms, the symptoms did not rise to the level where they could clearly be attributed to having taken the remedy. In fact, there was no way to tell whether they took a remedy or not. I appreciated their feelings of disappointment, but at the same time I am very thankful for their work and honesty. It is by their work that I could tell our profession is moving forward. As you will see, a successful experiment is successful not by what is included but by what is left out. It is by the exclusion of information that we better focus the experiment. When these two people announced that there were no symptoms to be found during their part of the proving, mirrored by other provers during these few provings, it was a turning point, a proof, of my work; it formed one of the pillars of truth of my philosophy and methodology. Thank you very much.

Lastly, though no doubt, most importantly, I need to thank the hundreds of people in the past New England School of Homeopathy courses and seminars who participated in the heated discussions and debates that preceded any such monumental task such as conducting a proving. It was by the questions that my students and colleagues asked, that I discovered and refined what it was that I needed to articulate. By being pushed by their curiosity, differing understandings and fresh perspectives on the topic, I was forced to look both more broadly and with a finer eye to details than I would have on my own.

In addition, I want to thank all those who participated in the proving process itself. Clearly, this proving, this book, this *materia medica*, would never have happened without their willingness to see and experience first hand, the effects and process of the provings. I owe a huge debt to my students for many things, but most of all, I thank each person, for giving me the best job any man could ever hope to have: teaching something I love.

Paul Herscu
Amherst, Massachusetts
April 4, 2002

Author's Comments

Writing a book has never been so important for me. In my original studying days, I learned from the old homeopathic *materia medicas* and journals of the profession. Since that time, my patients have been my primary teachers. It is what happens to them in the course of my care that dictates the nature of my work.

For me, writing *materia medica* is basically a matter of understanding and synthesizing my experiences as a physician.

Over the years, writing *materia medica* has been a joy to me; it is increasingly rewarding when I hear from another homeopath that my thoughts and ideas about a remedy enabled him or her to prescribe it accurately. It is my hope that this book will similarly enhance the study and practice of homeopathy by laying forth a comprehensive understanding of provings and how they relate not only to the introduction of remedies to our pharmacy, but also, how having a working understanding of provings is an essential component to the practice of homeopathy.

Comprehending the applications of provings should never be relegated to first year homeopathic curriculum and then shelved for occasional reference. Keeping the vital knowledge of this cornerstone of our profession somewhere central in the homeopathic mind *will help practice outcomes from the initial prescription through the long term follow-up.* The reason for this is that day to day practice follows exactly the same rules, protocols and outcomes of provings. They are in fact the same process, as described below.

This work is presented in two volumes. Volume One has two parts. Part 1 is a series of chapters that I have published over the past few years on my theory and philosophy regarding provings. Part 2 is devoted to an example of the application of this theory, the proving of *Alcoholus*.

Volume Two is a compendium volume of articles and texts that incorporate much of our history as a profession as it relates to provings. It is the study of what our forebears went through on their way to understand how to improve this process. It is by presenting Volume Two of this proving work, that I hope to ease any future experimenter's work. They will be able to look at the history and see what those authors were contending with, to see how I ended up with my theory. Hopefully my theory can also explain their work in a new and more comprehensive light. It is by making these articles easily accessible for reading and studying, that the community can inform itself and move forward, away from rhetoric and towards pure science.

I hope this work provides the framework and language for the evolution of our work to a more perfect application; helping people deeply and carefully, which is above all, our highest calling.

Table of Contents

Acknowledgements vi
Author's Comments x

Part One: A Model of Homeopathic Provings

Introduction 3
Chapter 1: Basic Concepts... 5
Chapter 2: Why Provings Are Important to You 13
Chapter 3: Provings From the Models of
   Cycles and *Segments* as Well as *Stress* and *Strain*............. 23
Chapter 4: What Provings Add to the Medical Community 39
Chapter 5: What Provings Are Not 65
Chapter 6: What Provings Are or Great Exaptations............ 85
Chapter 7: Conducting a Proving–One Method, With Tools.... 107
Chapter 8: Conclusion 137

Part Two: The Proving of *Alcoholus*

Introduction 143
Chapter 9: Why Me? Why Prove the Substance Alcohol?
   How do You Prepare it? 147
Chapter 10: Alcohol and Humans: Why the Connection? 155
Chapter 11: Pathophysiology of Alcohol 159
Chapter 12: Materia Medica of *Alcoholus*..................... 167
Chapter 13: A Short Case 183
Chapter 14: The Rubrics of *Alcoholus*........................ 187
Chapter 15: The Proving Journals 203

New England School of Homeopathy 321
Index... 323

Part One
A Model of Homeopathic Provings

Introduction

The first part of this book is dedicated to the model of provings from the physiologic perspective of *Stress* and *Strain*. It focuses, for the first time in homeopathy on a theory of what actually occurs during a proving, and then goes on to the application of that model. This part is organized into the following chapters:

Chapter 1 describes the basic concepts of *Stress* and *Strain* as well as *Cycles* and *Segments*.

Chapter 2 is devoted to why you, the homeopath should be interested in this topic, even if you are solely a clinician.

Chapter 3 represents the model of what happens in a proving. This is new to homeopathy and lays a foundation for the understanding of provings.

Chapter 4 describes why the concept and history of provings is important to the homeopath but equally important to the greater medical world.

Chapter 5 illustrates the different methods of provings that are currently in vogue and discusses some of their shortfalls.

Chapter 6 offers the reasoning behind why certain instruments of measurement are used in the proving; as well as the logic behind how to conduct a proving.

Chapter 7 is devoted to the actual tools, resources and handouts used in conducting a proving.

— Chapter 1 —
Basic Concepts

I would like to define some basic principles in this short chapter. A point to keep in mind is that all of these concepts are thoroughly explained elsewhere. The main goal in this book is to focus on provings and that is where I will keep it. That said, it will be helpful to understand some basic underpinning of a model of health, disease, and homeopathy as I see it.

Stress and *Strain*

The main point here is one that is agreed upon by biologists and scientists, which places homeopathy not on the outside of science but right in the middle of it. Let's look at the illustration below:

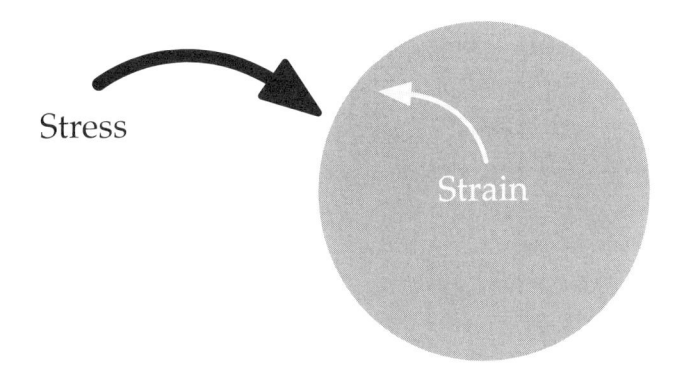

The basic concept is that given a certain predisposition, a person will experience a substance as a *Stress*. By the word *Stress* I am not placing a connotation on it; it is not a good thing or a bad thing. Rather, I am saying that the substance, because of the individual's predisposition, shows up as a *Stress*.

As a result of experiencing this *Stress* the individual must respond. That response is what we call *Straining*. It is the reaction of the body to experiencing that particular *Stress*. Using this language, we can say that symptoms produced are due to the person *Straining* against the *Stress* that is felt due to a person's predisposition. All living systems work this way. For example, when a woman exercises, the exertion is the *Stress* and the building up of muscles of the legs and of the heart is the response, the *Strain*. Another example is when a child develops a fever; the bacteria is the *Stress*, the body attempting to burn it out is the *Strain*, by raising the temperature so that the immune system functions more efficiently.

With this model of *Stress* and *Strain* in hand we can refine the definition of provings altogether, thereby shifting the very basis of homeopathy to become more precise.

Provings Explained Through the Language of *Stress* and *Strain*

What is a proving? We have a potentized substance. To use this substance as a medicine, we need to find the type of person who will be cured by it. In order to do that, we give it to people as a test. This is the basis of a proving. Ideally, a person to whom we give the substance would be cured of *all* of their symptoms by taking the remedy in question. Ideally, if we found several such people who took the remedy and were cured by it, then wrote down their cured symptoms, that would be the end of the proving as the description became elucidated. This happens only rarely, but let's look at the possibility using the language of *Stress* and *Strain*.

We can understand that in such a prover, the individual predisposition was such that the *Stress* (the remedy given*)* had to be responded to. When they *Strained* against this *Stress*, the overall pattern of their response was similar to the chronic pattern of their response towards all the *Stresses* of life. Once the remedy was given, it was at this more efficient level of response that the person was cured of their chronic problems. Finding out who these people are and the symptoms that are cured is the primary focus of a proving. Writing down the symptoms of the person's chronic *Straining* pattern, that which went away, is very important.

As you will read in the following chapters, the above scenario is usually *not* the outcome. Some people that are taking the potentized substance are somewhat sensitive to it, but are not cured by it. In fact, these people definitely experience the substance as noxious, as a *Stress*, and are therefore forced to *Strain* against it. However, the pattern of *Strain* that they produce is not the same as the pattern they normally produce towards the *Stresses* of the outside world. As a result, they *Strain* against the remedy in a new way and by doing so they produce new symptoms.

This too is looked for in a proving. Why? Because, as you will read in chapter Two, the fact that the person *Strains* against this substance means that this person has some sensitivity to it, not as much as the person who was cured by it, but still, some sensitivity.

It was this discovery that led to the fuller understanding of provings and homeopathy. While the best description is one that describes the cured person, during a proving, the *next* best thing is to describe the way this one agent interacted with all sorts of people. We are not only interested in the people who are extremely sensitive to the remedy but those who are somewhat sensitive as well. We want to find out how people respond to the substance.

In a regular proving, there are many more people that have a lower level of similarity with the substance being tested than people who have such a perfect similarity that it will be their curative remedy. As a result, more people *develop* symptoms than *lose* symptoms. It can now be understood that in this process of developing symptoms to write down, in this process where the remedy symptoms are developing in our provers –rather than going away–that the definition of homeopathy came to be. We are going to treat by a substance that causes similar symptoms.

Origins

Originally this was a much easier task. The substances chosen were often toxic, though the tests were run with sub-toxic doses. Often, with the noxious dose, the prover was forced to respond with symptoms that showed a poisoning at worst, or at the least, some sort of a *Strain*, some sort of reaction. *By collecting **all** the symptoms of **all** the different **sensitive** provers, we were able to garner the **general qualities** and the **specific complaints** of someone who would be the perfect candidate for needing this remedy.*

As a result, the perfect outcome of a proving would be to give the remedy to a few people and have some become cured, and have others develop symptoms that are essentially similar to the ones that were cured in their colleagues.

Thinking of it in this manner, several points become clear. Understanding the concept of *Stress* and *Strain* makes all concepts of homeopathy more logical and easily understood.

It becomes easier to see why the process of provings makes sense.

It becomes easier to see why, by the diminishing of the toxic dose, we have less toxic symptoms.

Understanding these points will illustrate why, without a solid foundation in what provings mean, we develop many misconceptions within our profession of what it is that we do. These same misconceptions will follow you whether you are conducting or analyzing a proving, or in the follow-up analysis in your practice.

Essentially the process of provings, in the most perfect world, would be the same as the process of practicing homeopathy. During the practice of homeopathy you *treat* someone who is *ill* by giving them a *remedy* that you hope will *cure* them based on the symptom list. In a proving, with all the luck in the world, you would *dispense* a potentized *substance* to a person and coincidentally find that his or her *symptoms* disappear. You write down their description and that is that. The problem is that most people will not need the substance. The good fortune is that by dispensing a substance that the person is *somewhat* sensitive to, they will *Strain* anyway and, this time, produce symptom changes. Those symptom changes are what we write down to describe the general sphere of the remedy.

Provings as a First Step

So writing down the symptoms that were changed in the people that are sensitive to a substance is the first step towards understanding the full sphere of the remedy. But it does not end there; it only begins there. Where it *does* end is by describing how it is that the remedy acts in practice. We need to describe the effect of this substance upon a person who is totally and absolutely sensitive to it. The pattern of their *Strain* is the same as the pattern of the *Strain* described by the symptoms of this remedy by others who were only partially sensitive to it. Or to put it differently, the description of the medical use of the remedy in practice is the same as if you gave the substance to a person during the proving who absolutely needed the remedy. It would not be symptoms that he or she developed that you would have written down, but symptoms that disappeared by its use.

The process of provings is just like the practice of homeopathy with a substance that we do not yet know.

The process of writing provings where the remedy was curative is the actual writing of the *materia medica* of the remedy.

The process of homeopathic practice is the process of conducting a proving upon a person whom we hope is sensitive to a substance, and we choose that substance based on the symptoms listed in the proving books. The process of proving and the process of practice is at the same time a mirror image of itself and a continuation of one to the other.

Once this is understood, then a great deal of practice management, dosage, follow-up, and case analysis become easier to comprehend.

You can also see why I wrote the kind of *materia medica* I wrote. (*The Homeopathic Treatment of Children: Pediatric Constitutional Types* and *Stramonium with an Introduction to Analysis Using Cycles and Segments*) By focusing on the clinic, by focusing on what the cured patients looked like, and which symptoms went away, I attempted to move the process of *materia medica* writing and study one major step forward. It was the first *materia medica* written based on practice and not based on the provings or previous writing, i.e. based on the patients and not based on the books. It is the very nature of the work begun by provings, begun by Hahnemann and continuing in one long line until today.

Once you can see this connection, once you can understand the similarity between proving and practice–that it is the same exact process–then many of the arguments that have arisen in our profession in the last decades fall away. Once you understand that it is the same process, then your overall homeopathic understanding improves, not just your prescribing. The overall way you view your work improves as well.

These points have not been discussed or described in the past. As a result there are conflicts about *how* to conduct a proving and what the results mean. That conflict can never be resolved by focusing on the methodology alone. Rather, we need to look more closely at the underpinnings, at *what informs and guides* the methodology in order to reach an understanding of what a proving is: throughout this book we will do just that.

The Problem

I would like to illustrate the problem that exists currently, as it relates to provings. One question to the homeopathic community is, "Can you tell the difference between someone who took a remedy and someone who took a placebo?" This is the most basic of questions that underlies all of homeopathy. It forms the first pillar that homeopathic theory stands upon. If you can not tell the difference, then the concept of a homeopathic proving is completely false. Essentially, this has never been tested successfully with modern methods on a large scale. Edward Shalts, MD and I set up a few pilot studies to test just this.

After thinking about the different possible remedies to prove, I chose *Belladonna*. The pilot worked well in demonstrating where cutoffs should exist for this type of study: after how much time should you continue to accept symptoms and which symptoms should be taken. We got enough information to lead us to be sure that a large-scale study should proceed. It was a great study, to be discussed after the large-scale study is complete. I only want to share one experience that I had, which occurred at the same time as the study.

Before the experiment, I opened Kent's Repertory and put my finger down on the type. I looked to see which remedies I pointed to. I landed on six different remedies. Interestingly enough, during the pilot proving, major keynotes of all six remedies came up, in both the provers and the people who took the placebo.

Now here is the problem. Some of the people who took the *Belladonna* did not produce any symptoms at all. Other people who did not take the remedy developed symptoms of *Belladonna*. And yet other people developed symptoms, big keynotes of the remedies I had haphazardly pointed to. That is the reality of it. Designed poorly, there would be no way to determine which symptoms should be included. It is this very basic question, this confusion, that has led to so much conflict and inaccuracy in the field of provings. It is this confusion that has led people to include symptoms of people who did not even take the proving substance. It is the purpose of this book to lay out a clear philosophy as well as design for provings which will give us usable and accurate information.

As a result of the current confusion found in our profession, people have come up with questions and comments such as:

"Why do all the people, including the placebo group, get symptoms?"

"I wonder if it is because the people are so close together."

"I wonder if the remedies, being bundled together in a package, the placebo got the essence of the remedy that it was next to."

The theories expand daily. This confusion shows a total divorce of the proving from our clinical experience.

The Solution

There are so many reasons and so many ways that people are explaining how it is that the proving is showing symptoms in all the provers: people that got the remedy and people that did not. Chapters Five and Six delve deeply into these aspects and show that the old rules still apply and apply well. The old rules did not get repealed. The old rules are not out of fashion. Rather, what I hope to show is that there is a better and easier way to explain these phenomena.

The solution is to recall that the proving and the clinic are one and the same. They are mirror images, and the rules of one are the rules of the other. All homeopaths and all pharmacies have kept remedies near each other from the beginning of homeopathy and they have maintained their integrity. That has not changed. Many times a patient gets the wrong remedy and nothing happens. That has not changed. When we give a remedy, all the other people around are not proving it and having the remedies act upon them. The rules of one side of our work are mirrored in the other.

The work I present before you reconciles these two sides. It lays a theoretical foundation for the first time on what a proving is, and only after that, discusses the methodology.

Part 2 of this volume then exemplifies the work through a series of provings conducted over the past 5 years. By those provings I can say that the old rules apply. There is nothing unusual about the proving that does not occur in practice and that is not accounted for in this method. The results? There were many provers that did not respond to the remedy at all. Many people who participated did not get symptoms from the remedy and yet many people did get symptoms. A few other provers had cured symptoms.

It is by the work described in these pages of Part 1 that you will see why it was that our provings offered a few hundred symptoms. This is in contradistinction to many current provings which have many times more symptoms, even thousands of symptoms. Just like haphazardly choosing remedies out of rubrics, like I did when I opened the repertory and put my finger down on the type, the magical "effect" of a proving that seems to effect so many, so profoundly, can now be easily explained away by revealing inaccuracies in study designs.

I want to end with the following point. There is no body of people or political board that has tackled this issue well. Whenever people, good people, have attempted to contend with the topic, conflicts erupt and confusion reigns. I believe the reason is that these well-intentioned homeopaths have begun at the point of attempting to define a methodology without the steps preceding it, the theory underlying.

As a result many people, friends of mine, have delved into approaches that have led both their provings and their practices astray. What I attempt to do in these books is to describe and demonstrate a complete method of homeopathy. In this volume the topic is provings. It follows with the same rules and the same cosmology as the rest of homeopathy. I offer it as only a beginning place for a method that incorporates all of the best of our forebears. It is a place from which to begin a dialog, a place to build from. Just as happens in every field of science, once a glaring oversight is described, there is then a flood of innovations that develop from the whole field. I expect to see that flood happen here, in regards to what a proving is. It is a place to study, analyze, criticize and improve upon. Good science is cumulative, as it builds upon the past without throwing out previous accurate observations made. It is cumulative in that it incorporates new observations into a model that can explain things better than the past. This is my model as related to provings.

— Chapter 2 —
Why Provings Are Important to You

In this book, we begin to describe the issues involved in provings. Many homeopaths do not give enough import to this topic. They say either, "I know all I need to know about this topic," or, "I am a practitioner. I leave the provings up to others. I just want to practice." These belief systems are both short-sighted and dangerous to the practitioner. They show that there is 'something' missing from the understanding of the practitioner. That 'something' that is missing will translate to their practice in terms of patients not receiving the correct remedy. More than that, it shows that there is still a fragmented image of this work in the practitioner's mind. That makes practice less enjoyable, not just less effective. In this chapter, I will address many reasons why you should care about provings. I will also address many reasons of how it fits into the larger scheme of practice.

Let me be clear about this topic in one sentence. Understanding the mechanisms and philosophy behind provings will help your understanding of homeopathy and your practice immeasurably; more patients will get better!

So here is the interesting part. In the over 200 years of homeopathy, when speaking about provings, we have never developed a clear understanding of *what they are*. In over 200 years of homeopathy, we have spoken, agreed, and argued about how to do them but not what they are. As a result, there has been a mass of confusion about what symptoms to include during a proving. Currently, during this renaissance of provings, the conflicts have become so rancorous that divisions are being drawn and battles have begun. What these good meaning people miss, is they are arguing about **how to do a proving, not about what a proving is**. As such they will never agree.

This is not a new problem. In the last 20 years several societies have met to discuss what provings are. The disagreements were so great that the outcome was either nothing or only a weak description. Now these were not uninformed people who were thinking about this topic. They were some of the best minds in our profession. What was missing, however, was a model that could explain provings and at the same time fit them into the larger homeopathic theory. Without a model we could not develop a language to describe what happens. We were closed out of the full understanding.

Several books were written in the last few years about provings. In general, they are well written and great on the topic. They only lacked one thing. Even though the books were on provings, the only thing missing was *what* they were!!! This is a glaring absence.

The absence of an understanding of what provings are has led to the current confusions, inaccuracies and infighting that characterizes our profession at this time. So let's talk about all the reasons why you should know this aspect of homeopathy better. In the next chapters, we will discuss the philosophic foundations of provings from a model that describes it very well-the model I have been developing with many of you over the past 14 years. The following discussion is a collaboration between my work and thought, in an iterative process with Dr. Frank Gruber, one of my best friends and a great teacher. I am using his writing throughout the remainder of this chapter, until the summary, as he well represents my ideas and especially because it is light and friendly. I think in discussing a heady topic such as this, Frank's writing is a perfect counterpoint.

Why would you want to read a book about provings?

Homeopathy has been around for about 200 years but is just recently enjoying a renaissance in the United States, Europe and, in fact, the world. People are again becoming interested in how to use the remedies and how to arrive at the correct remedy in a specific patient. From parents to seasoned professional homeopaths, everyone seems eager to increase his or her skill level in prescribing.

How can this improve your case taking skills?

Let's look generally at what a proving is. A *Stress* pushes on a patient. His system *Strains* back in response by creating symptoms in order to adapt to the *Stress*. When a person is subjected to a *Stress* and symptoms are produced, that is a proving.

More specifically, when you conduct a proving, you give a person a substance (usually a potentized substance, these days) and notice what symptoms are produced from that experiment. The person may have none, a few, dozens or even hundreds of symptoms that are a result of taking that substance. This is his system's response to the *Stress* you have induced by giving him the substance. Which symptoms should you pay attention to? Which symptoms are important?

Now, what about case taking? When you interview a sick person, that patient may have dozens or hundreds of symptoms. Which symptoms do you pay attention to? Which symptoms are important? *The issues in both case taking and provings are the same. Not only are they the same, they are identical. When you understand the process involved in provings you come to a deeper understanding of case taking. Learning about the mechanics of a proving actually improves your case taking abilities.*

In this book we delve into the issues of how we decide which symptoms to take into consideration for the proving. Essentially, we will show that, from our model, we can understand this in the same way as we can understand which symptoms to take in the case analysis. It is a step by step process that is clearly spelled out. *Learning which symptoms to include in a proving enhances your ability to do the same thing in your case taking.*

Need to improve how you analyze a case?

So you have taken a case. You have a myriad of symptoms from the patient. How do you make sense of those symptoms? How do you put them together into a coherent package that somehow represents the patient and his or her problem?

There are as many ways to analyze a case as there are expert homeopaths. Everyone has his or her method. Here we are trying to present **one method that works very well in all cases.**

Frank continues: There are other good methods, some better in one type of situation than others. I remember sitting in a homeopathy class with a very good homeopath who was teaching his method of case analysis. It took one whole day to teach us the method, but by the end of the 8 hours I more or less understood the process. The next day he took a case and at the end of the case proceeded to use another method of analysis. He said that his method was not useful in this type of case. I was, needless to say, rather surprised.

However, the case analysis method presented in these chapters has been thoroughly tested for all types of cases. It is the *Cycles* and *Segment* **method.**

Taking a case and analyzing it is no different than analyzing the results of a proving. During the analysis of the proving, you are trying to make sense of the data so that you can shape it into a coherent picture of *materia medica*. In case analysis, you are trying to make sense of the data you elicited from the patient, shaping it into a picture that you match with remedies listed in the *materia medica*. In the next few chapters you will find the exact same method of analysis for the proving symptoms.

Need some help in learning how to find rubrics in the repertory?

After you analyze a case and decide what symptoms you are going to use to repertorize, you still have the sometimes daunting task of translating the symptoms into the language of the repertory. You have exactly the same problem when you are doing a proving. You have a group of symptoms that have arisen in your prover as a result of the administration of a remedy. You have analyzed the symptoms and decided which ones to use, but you have the same task of translating these symptoms into the language of the repertory.

One of the reasons for conducting a proving in the first place is to come up with a series of symptoms which you can submit to repertory publishers so they can include them in the repertory. You want to have these symptoms inserted into the repertory so that it serves as a useful tool for others to be able to prescribe that remedy. But which rubrics should the remedy be listed in? That is where you have to decide which rubrics are best described by the symptoms–the same issue you have when you are taking a case.

In these chapters you will find descriptions of how to choose the correct rubric, **so you will learn to increase your skill in finding rubrics in the repertory.**

Is your *materia medica* knowledge of the *remedies* just a long list of symptoms or does it make sense to you?

No one can really remember a long list of unrelated symptoms. That's why so few people actually use Hahnemann's *Materia Medica Pura*. It is the seminal text for our science, yet the way the symptoms are listed is not "user friendly." There is just no way to tie all these symptoms together **unless** you have a system for organizing them. This is again where the idea of *Cycles* and *Segments* come to our rescue.

Instead of making a laundry list of symptoms, the symptoms are listed according to the *Segment* of the *Cycle* that they represent. The symptoms are not altered or changed. Rather, we put the symptoms into context.

It is like the leaves on a tree which are organized onto branches and then the branches are organized onto a trunk. The *Segments* are the branches of the remedy and the *Cycle* is the trunk. In this way, all the pieces are tied together into an understandable unit. When listed in this way, you can not only understand why symptoms occur in a remedy, but can literally predict which other symptoms would be likely to occur.

In part 2 of this book, you will follow along as we take the symptoms of the remedy *Alcoholus* and extract from the raw data of our proving, how they fit into *Segments* and then ultimately how this comes together into the *Cycle* of the remedy. Every symptom of the remedy fits into one of the *Segments*. This is the exact same process that you follow for case analysis: organizing the symptoms into *Segments* and then putting the *Segments* together into a *Cycle*. You can use these skills to organize and analyze your case and then you can learn to organize and analyze less "user friendly" *materia medicas* so that they become easily usable when organized by *Cycles* and *Segments*.

How can reading a book on provings improve your ability at remedy selection?

Once you have your case organized by *Cycles* and *Segments* and you have your remedies organized by *Cycles* and *Segments*, your remedy selection process is very much enhanced. Since all of homeopathy is a matching process, the difficulty comes in deciding what you should match. Many less experienced homeopaths get trapped in matching poor keynotes. The patient says a few keynotes of the remedy *Lycopodium* and they are off prescribing *Lycopodium*. Ultimately they may need *Lycopodium*, but maybe not just now. Maybe there are other remedies to give before the *Lycopodium* but none the less, the patient already has these keynotes.

Instead of keynotes, **what you match in this system is the *Cycle* made of *Segments*, the totality of the patient**. When you have four or five *Segments* in a *Cycle*, it is not only the *Segments* but also the order of the *Segments* that allows you to match the *Cycle* of the patient to the *Cycle* of the correct remedy. Many remedies have similar *Segments*. That is why they share so many symptoms. However, the order in which the *Segments* are arranged in the *Cycle* of each remedy is different for each remedy. That's how you tell one remedy from the next. You simply match the *Cycle* of the patient to the *Cycle* of the closest remedy.

As you will see in the proving of *Alcoholus*, the *Segments* form into a coherent *Cycle*, which represents the remedy nicely. This serves as an example for your case taking. As you learn to create *Segments* and a *Cycle* for each case, you will be able to match these *Cycles* with the *Cycles* and *Segments* of the remedies. Since the provings were written as a laundry list of symptoms, understanding how to do this process will allow you to develop a fuller understanding of the remedy.

How about improving skills during a follow-up of a patient after giving a remedy?

In a proving you give the patient a remedy and try to assess what happened to him or her. What symptoms arose as a result of the action of the remedy? Or on the other hand, which of their symptoms went away as a result of the remedy? Or were there outside forces that acted to create symptoms that had no relationship to the remedy at all?

As an interesting example, what if you were doing a proving of the remedy *Arnica*. *Arnica* as a remedy is used in the treatment of injuries. Suppose that after you gave the provers a dose of *Arnica*, a number of them had an injury. Now you must decide whether those injuries were indeed accidental, that is, with no relationship to the remedy at all, or whether in proving the remedy these provers became more clumsy than usual, thus leading to the accidents. In that case did the remedy actually have an effect of creating clumsiness in the provers? You must decide then whether to take these symptoms as part of the proving or whether they were completely unrelated. But how do you decide?

In following up with a patient who has received a remedy, the issues are identical. Some of the patient's symptoms may get better, some may get worse, some may remain unchanged, and there may be some new symptoms. You have to decide what happened. Did the remedy influence the patient in a positive way? Did those symptoms that went away do so because of the remedy? Did new symptoms come up because of the remedy? Or were new symptoms unrelated to the remedy? Ultimately you have three choices to make: Wait and not prescribe, repeat the same remedy, or change remedies. However, these three choices are based on your assessment of the response of the patient's symptoms as above.

One of the biggest issues we hear often from homeopaths is: "How can I tell if a symptom change occurred because of the remedy versus because of the drug or herb they took, or the acupuncture they received?" Events occur in the course of treating people. We have to be able to understand what the remedy is doing and what the remedy is not doing. We need to learn how to attribute the appropriate effect to the remedy taken.

As you begin to understand the process for deciphering which symptoms in a proving are a result of the remedy and which symptoms most probably are not, you come to a better understanding of how to treat patients in follow-up as well. You learn to decide when you must wait and not prescribe, when you should represcribe the same remedy and when you should choose a new remedy.

Summary

In short, all of the skills involved in taking, analyzing, and repertorizing a case as well as understanding *materia medica*, remedy selection, and follow-up are involved in the process of conducting a proving. These skills are described in this book, first applying them to the proving and then indicating how the same skills are useful in working to find a remedy for a patient. **It is important for you, the practitioner, because as you grow in the understanding of the process of the proving you sharpen your skills for clinical practice, more patients will get better.**

Why would I, with the help of friends and colleagues write a book about provings?

Our Purpose

It is my intention to lay out, over a series of books, successful strategies for addressing all aspects of homeopathic practice to show that there is one model that can inform all of our decisions. I do not presume that each reader will agree with all aspects of what I do. What I plan, however, is to lay out one coherent approach to homeopathy. It remains for our readers to try these strategies, to evaluate this work based on how well it succeeds in their practice, and ultimately to help evolve the work to the next level.

In this and future books I plan to set forth a complete definition, philosophy, methodology and interpretation of provings, as well as demonstrate how provings ultimately relate to all other areas of homeopathy: case taking, case analysis, repertorization, *materia medica*, remedy selection, and follow-ups. I will show, in this and future books, how learning about provings ultimately improves performance in all these clinical areas of homeopathy.

The proving is the basic science of Homeopathy

Homeopathy is based on provings. Samuel Hahnemann utilized the hypothesis that "Like cures like." In order to prove that, he set up a series of individual experiments called provings.

In order for us to create an understanding of the entire process of Homeopathy in the mind of the reader, we have to begin at the beginning –the proving. We plan to demonstrate how the proving is related to and is the basis for all the other processes in Homeopathy.

Lack of agreement—defining our terms

The homeopathic community has held several large meetings in the last 20 years with the intention of deciding the best way to conduct a proving. The meetings have all terminated without a definitive document on provings because the participants have disagreed on some very fundamental issues.

First, as a community, we have not been able to agree on a model for Health and Disease. How do we define when a person is sick and when they are well? This may seem self evident but when you try to narrowly define these concepts, there is disagreement to the point that nothing ever gets resolved. So we discuss how our group defines Health and Disease.

Second, homeopathy itself is different things to different homeopaths. What is homeopathy? Each of the tenets of homeopathy has been subject to multitudes of interpretations. These books define one complete view of homeopathy.

Third, as a community, we can't reach an agreement on what a proving really is. There is no consensus on the definition. This lack of definition has led to considerable confusion in the homeopathic community. I want to delineate my definition of proving. This is why we don't describe just the methodology of provings but rather start from the beginning: our model of Health and Disease, our definition of homeopathy, and our definition of proving.

Repertory additions

We are concerned about the rapid number of additions which are being made to the repertory. Current technology is so powerful that we can make changes to the repertory very rapidly. How do you decide what to put in the repertory?

Once you conduct a proving there is disagreement on how many of the symptoms to take for the purpose of including in the repertory. For example, if you conduct a new proving on a substance, let's say "marsh grass", and the provers experience 5,000 total symptoms, should you place all of those symptoms in the repertory? If so, then there would be more symptoms in the repertory for "marsh grass" than there are for *Staphysagria* for example. Then it would be easier to come up with "marsh grass" when you are repertorizing as it would to come up with *Staphysagria*. This has happened already. There are new remedies that are listed in many more rubrics then remedies that we have used for one hundred years!

We fear that the rubrics of the repertory are expanding so rapidly that soon every remedy will be in every rubric. This will literally ruin the usefulness of the repertory as a tool. You won't be able to differentiate between frequently used remedies and very rare remedies, which come up frequently, due to the large number of symptoms taken into the repertory because of new provings.

In Hahnemann's provings, less than 200 symptoms were taken for some of the major polychrests. So, should we pay attention to only this symptom or that symptom? If so, then *which* symptoms should we pay attention to? These are difficult questions but there are rational solutions for all of these issues and all are addressed in this book.

Providing a model for provings to come

There are people who are interested in provings who do not know how to go about doing them, since there has been no agreed upon philosophy, theory, or method. I include my methodology and reasons behind it.

Again, our readers might disagree, and if so, I encourage them to publish their own work. However in so doing, we also encourage them to follow a model that is inclusive of the areas we have outlined. So, these books may serve as a model for others who wish to set up a model of their own. If they do, the hope is that this model serves as a baseline; I create an orientation to the process for what to include in other models. I, with help from my friends, establish a starting point.

This means that there are two types of models presented in this one book: The model of how to conduct a proving as well as the model of what should be included in any future efforts of creating a model for provings. There are still important substances which need to be proven. It is my hope that the model we provide will create a structure for the basis of such future provings. Again, we don't presume that our way is the only way. **We just encourage others to set forth a complete definition, philosophy, methodology and interpretation in their provings. Sometimes by articulating an example, by asking questions, it makes our blind spots come into view. It is at that point that many solutions become possible.**

Summary

I want to put forward a model of provings that fits into a greater model of homeopathy, which fits into an even greater model of Health and Disease. There is a great deal of confusion in homeopathy as exemplified by a general lack of consistently good results in practice. I want to present one model of a workable system of homeopathy. Our readers may not choose to use it but they will nevertheless find it a usable and extremely efficient model for practicing homeopathy.

In this book, we set forth a complete definition, philosophy, methodology and interpretation of provings, as well as demonstrate how provings ultimately relate to all areas of homeopathy. Everything in homeopathy is connected, just as every symptom of the patient is connected. As Dr. Gruber elucidated, learning about provings improves performance in all other areas of homeopathy.

The next chapter focuses on the philosophical model of what a proving is. This is the first time this has been done in homeopathy. We believe that this model will answer several important questions that persist in our community, not just about provings, but about case analysis, as well.

— Chapter 3 —
Provings From the Models of *Cycles* and *Segments* as Well as *Stress* and *Strain*

The 200 years following the initial provings by Hahnemann has brought considerable debate regarding exactly how provings should be conducted. Even to this day, learned homeopaths cannot agree on the exact methodology or even the definition of a proving. Before we tackle the question of methodology, we can first try to define the essence of the proving. What exactly is a proving? And how do provings fit within the context of homeopathy as a whole? The answers to these questions should not only form the basic framework for the methodology of provings, but should elucidate important aspects of our daily clinical practice. The methodology followed in our proving should reflect our entire philosophy of homeopathy. Complete consistency of philosophy from the definition of a drug, to the application of those curative agents, is essential if we are indeed practicing a science.

In this chapter, I begin to describe some of the historical aspects of provings. More importantly, I want to establish a philosophical model that explains what provings are. By understanding this, I believe that the fragmented image of our work will be one step closer to being mended; provings will take their rightful place in the natural order of a homeopath's understanding.

My observation is that our community has missed the most important consideration of provings which is as follows. Every time we give a remedy and the patient returns, if it was the wrong remedy, they have actually taken part in a test. In a way, every prescription of a potentized drug *is* a proving. Yes, it is a proving of a *known* drug, but still it is a proving, a test to see its effect. Without understanding this crucial point, I can see why some may have little interest in this aspect of our practice.

Once you understand the concepts behind provings, you will see that it relates specifically to all your follow-up theory and practice. As I mentioned in the first chapters, the problem is that we have not described what a proving is. Thus far, our community has only described how to conduct one. Without a theoretical basis of discussion, many complications arise that have led to a fragmentation of our profession and a lack of clear assessment of our case management.

As I also mentioned in the last chapter, the lack of a theoretical basis of what a proving is has led to the conflicts within our profession. It has led to our great societies not defining our most important test. It has led to great books written on the topic that are being misused because they only describe technique, not knowing that the description of the *'why it happens'* was missing.

What boggles my mind though is this last point. By not understanding a model of what a proving is and why it exists, we are methodically entering inaccuracies into our *materia medica*. The irony of this point is so striking, I don't know whether to laugh or weep. *By not understanding provings, we have created mistakes that Hahnemann was attempting to rid us of by creating a more perfect or pure materia medica of the drugs via the provings. We are nullifying his work and the very purpose of provings in the first place.*

In this chapter, we will discuss the philosophical underpinnings of provings from a model that describes it very well–the model I have been developing over the past years. The following discussion was a collaboration between my work and thought, in an iterative process with the writings of Dr. Todd Hoover, a colleague and one of my best friends. I am intertwining my lecture notes on the theory and model of provings and his historical writing throughout the remainder of this chapter.

Some Historical Problems with the *Materia Medica*

If we look back 200 years, what we find in the allopathic medical world is a *materia medica* that was riddled with what were called "specifics". Give *this* substance to treat *that* condition. And while many people did improve under such treatment, many did not. In fact many died not just from the disease but from the treatment administered. Even when the specific treatment makes sense from today's knowledge base, the overdosing was so severe that it hurt more than it helped. To put it simply, often the treatment back then was "kill or cure."

Let me give you an example from today's medical practice to give perspective. Think about radiation or chemotherapy. The idea behind both these therapies is to kill a part of the body without hurting the rest of it. It is a race between killing "bad parts" without negatively impacting the rest. Often the race is all too close. This is a good example of a current therapy. But think about it. With cancer, the medical world is dealing with an extreme situation. What if that was what *all* of our current therapies were like? What if treating an influenza or arthritis was the same thing?

Killing 'just enough,' so that the rest of the patient was left intact. Basically, that was the medical standard that existed during Hahnemann's time and is somewhat true today.

The other problem with the *materia medica* of that time had to do with inaccuracies. Although somewhat related to the first point above, it is a somewhat different issue. The exact question was this: which symptoms and diseases listed in the *materia medica* actually belonged to the medicinal substance in question and which symptoms did not? Which symptoms were to be truly listed for the drug and which belonged to a side effect, or another disease, or even another drug being used at the same time? In short, Hahnemann was attempting to achieve what we would now call pure science, where all the variables could be removed or at the very least, accounted for.

Approaching the Scientific Method

To find what symptoms should really be listed for any one drug, he fell upon a concept that all scientists use to this day. He reasoned that to attempt to understand any one drug we should try to *isolate* its effect. To do this, he would undergo a study, a test, of the drug in question, isolating everything else. If and when symptoms developed, they would be recorded as symptoms belonging to that particular drug. This 'test' or trial of the drug in German is called, "*Pruefung*." This word, and the process it represents, was anglicized to be called "proving." One proves, or tests a remedy, to tell which symptoms belong to the drug in question.

Hahnemann's goal was to create a better science, a better knowledge of the drugs. To that end he reasoned that we needed to know what each drug would do. Essentially, he reasoned that to test the pure effect, we need to create as clean a record as possible. He emphatically stated in his *Organon of Medicine*, Aphorism 108, "There is no other possible way of correctly ascertaining the characteristic action of medicines on human health—no single, surer, more natural way—than administering individual medicines experimentally to *healthy* people in moderate doses in order to ascertain what changes, symptoms, and effects each in particular brings about in the body and the psyche…" To this end, he created a framework for the methodology of investigating the nature of medicines–the provings. He developed the technique of provings as the most effective and precise method to define the exact nature of a medicinal substance. Hahnemann's early provings form the foundation of much of our *materia medica* to this day.

Most of Hahnemann's guidelines for provings boil down to the primary point which is to administer the test to someone who is not taking other drugs, is relatively healthy and is eating a simple diet. What was Hahnemann attempting to establish there? Remove all variables except one and then test that one variable. All changes will be attributed to that one intervention. Interestingly enough, his guidelines from 200 years ago still work well for a modern Phase 1 Drug Study. This is actually the most current version of pure science that we have now in medicine. Incredible foresight from someone living 200 years ago!

Instead of just accepting his words of how to conduct a proving and who to include in the proving, let's try something. Lets see if our models of *Stress* and *Strain*, and of *Cycles* and *Segments* are applicable to provings, as they are in case analysis.

Understanding *Stress* and *Strain*

We have in the last chapter very briefly defined *Stress* and *Strain*, as that has been described in the book *Stramonium*.

To review, any individual has a propensity or predisposition to experience a variety of interferences that in some way *Stresses* him. He or she responds to the interference in some way. The interference is the *Stress* and the response is the *Strain*. From this point of view, medicines create unique *Stresses* upon an organism. Additionally, *Stresses* created by medicinal substances generate very specific response patterns from an individual. And these specific responses are generated to better a person's health. This is why we give these medicines. The way that this was described before my model was that medicinal substances be defined as those substances that have a positive dynamic action upon the vitality of the organism—most especially the vital force.

From this new point of view, potentized substances can now be understood as being a subset of all medicines that provide a rather unique and highly specific *Stress* to the individual. If the potentized substance is 'homeopathically similar' to a sick person, then the *Straining* of the patient, responding to the *Stress* of the potentized substance is so specific as to ameliorate the person of their acute or chronic complaints. This is described more fully in my other books.

During a proving, when we give the medicine under experimental terms to a healthy person, the individual is impacted by this unique *Stress*, and will *Strain* in a manner consistent with their unique nature. As defined in my other books, the unique nature is the most energy efficient method that the individual has at its disposal to adapt/evolve due to the *Stress*.

During a proving one should therefore be able to observe both *Primary Symptoms* caused by the *Stress* of the drug upon the organism, and *Secondary Symptoms* produced as the individual *Strains* to adapt, evolve, or return to a more balanced state.

Primary and Secondary Symptoms

Primary symptoms in their grossest form can be thought of and seen in the toxicology of the drug. Kent states "When the patient is under the poisonous influence of a drug [what I call *Stress*-ph] it does not seem to flow in the direction of his life action, but when reaction comes [what I call *Strain*-ph] then the lingering effects of the drug seems to flow, as it were, in the stream of the vital action. The symptoms that arise are of the best order, and hence it is necessary in proving a drug to take such a portion of the drug only as will disturb and not suspend, as will flow in the stream of the vital order, in the order of the economy, establishing slightly perverted action, and causing symptoms, without suspending action, as we would, for example, with a large dose of *Opium*."

When the *Stress* of the drug is great, as in a toxic dose, only a fragment of the true picture of the remedy is seen. These are mostly the primary symptoms. Homeopaths throughout time have suggested that this type of information is incorrect and not to be relied upon.

Secondary effects are here described as those that are the result of the *Straining* back of the individual toward the healthy state. We, along with Kent, find that these symptoms reflecting this response are of greatest importance in defining the precise nature of a medicine.

However, one of the benefits of my model is that it finally gets rid of the rift of which symptoms to use. The topic of primary versus secondary symptoms is one that has dogged homeopathy for 200 years. In many cases we only paid attention to the secondary symptoms. Yet in other situations we paid attention to the primary symptoms. There was no clear answer until now. Truly, it comes down to a philosophical discussion akin to how many angels can stand on the head of a pin.

Using the model that incorporates *Stress* and *Strain*, and *Cycles* and *Segments*, we can see that the primary *and* secondary symptoms are both actions that occur to and with the individual and that they both can count. As such I have to respectfully correct the misconception that the primary action is to be discounted. It can not be discounted. It reflects symptoms that are occurring to and with the individual. At the very least, the primary action of the *Stress* is showing us the *predisposition* of the patient to that type of *Stress* and so is showing us qualities of the individual's state. Rather than saying that the primary effects are incorrect, I think a better way to look at them is that they form an *incomplete picture of the whole*. Similarly, the secondary symptoms are somewhat incomplete as well. They both reflect one part of the *Stress* and *Strain*, the dance of life, our cycle of existence.

As an aside, I want to highlight the fact that a good model should answer many more questions that were difficult before. As you go through these chapters and books, I think you have seen how the problems seem to fall away. Here we will show that the infighting and difficulty of understanding provings can be avoided. The answers lie in the simple model that we have developed.

Stress and *Strain* in Practice and in Provings

In my model, when treating a patient we have emphasized the importance of understanding this process of untuning and retuning. We seek to understand the *Stresses* that have pushed the individual out of the balance of health, and how the individual *Strains* to recover. We see how the individual constantly strives, more or less ineffectively, to throw off the *Stress*. The exact dimensions of how this individual *Strains* defines the clinical state of his pathology. By clearly perceiving the totality of the effort of the individual to return to natural health, to adapt more perfectly to his environment, we will understand the patient better, especially what symptoms need to be matched homeopathically.

It is the same in a proving. By perceiving the totality of symptoms produced solely by the potentized substance during a proving, we will understand the precise nature of that substance. By carefully documenting the symptoms that arise when a healthy patient takes a substance, what is it that we are doing? We are recording the *Stress* of the substance upon the individual (the primary effect) and even more importantly, recording the symptoms that the individual produces in response to that *Stress*, the *Strain* (the secondary effect). This is the short answer to what a proving is.

Stresses Effect Different Individuals Differently

Hahnemann wrote of this in the *Organon of Medicine*, aphorism #134. "All external forces, and especially medicines, have the propensity to produce specific changes in the health of the living organism in their own characteristic way. But the symptoms proper to a medicine do not all come out in one subject…"

We have defined medicines as substances that create or bring about *unique Strains* from *unique Stresses* upon the individual. Additionally, it is apparent from our practice and experience that human beings respond to similar *Stresses* in patterns consistent with their unique constitutional nature. Basically, while the *Stress* is the same, the responses are uniquely the individual's. We could therefore predict that a variety of individuals should produce a variety of responses to the *Stress* of the medicine being proven. *Susceptibility* or predisposition has a part in it, though. When the substance to be tested or proven is tested in a more toxic dose, it will *Stress* the largest number of individuals. The theory behind this has to do with the fact that *at a toxic dose, more individuals within a species share the same predisposition.* But as the substance is increasingly potentized, it is experienced as a *Stress* to an increasingly smaller number of individuals, just the ones that share the individual predisposition to be affected by a small amount of that substance.

Hahnemann similarly concludes in Aphorism 135, "The total picture of disease symptoms that a medicine can produce approaches completion only after multiple observations have been made on many suitable persons of both sexes, with various constitutions." And in Aphorism 136, "As we have said, in provings on healthy people, the changes in health which a medicine can produce cannot all be brought out in any one person, but only in many different people of various physical and psychic constitutions…"

What Really Happens as Seen From our Model

A medicine will theoretically tend to produce all symptoms in all provers, but in reality, when a proving is conducted *properly*, this does not happen. What we find is that some people develop many symptoms, some develop some symptoms, while others do not develop any symptoms to speak of. More often, some of the symptoms that are developed are common to many of the provers, while others are unique to certain individuals. Using our model, we finally have a way to understand this reality.

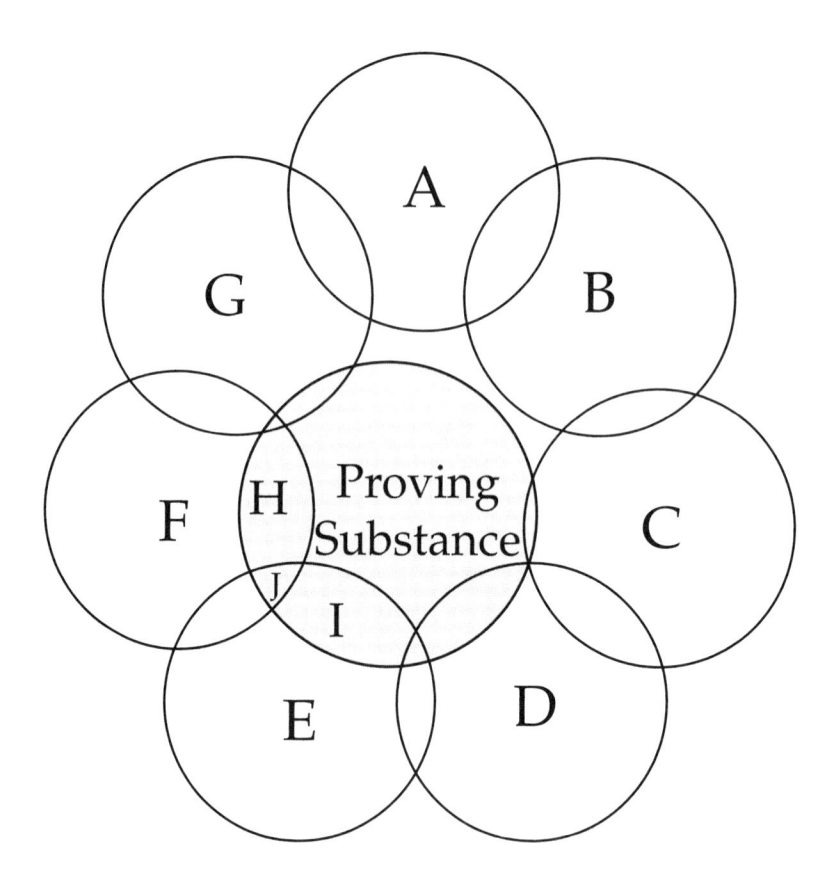

Figure 1

In Figure 1, we have constructed a simplified model of a proving. The central circle represents the symptom picture of the medicine being proved. This circle is either of the known symptoms of a proven substance or you can think of it as a *'potential'* circle, not yet filled with the symptoms because the proving has not yet taken place. In either case, think of that inner circle as the sum of the full potential of symptoms that that substance can produce in individuals.

Peripheral circles **A–G** represent provers with distinct constitutional predisposition and potential symptoms. Again think of these provers as either having symptoms or not, but that the circles represent the full total potential of all the symptoms that can be produced in these individuals. As can be seen, not all individuals and their constitutions share the same predisposition. Look at the Figure. Some provers, such as **E** and **F**, have a constitutional predisposition that substantially intersects with the medicine. What this means is that the constitutions of provers **E** and **F** both share a fair amount of potential symptoms with the substance **H & I**.

I have always called such symptoms *bridges* between remedies. For example, in practice we sometimes see a patient's remedy state change from one to another; perhaps from a constitutional state to an acute state. But if you were to look at the new condition and the old condition, you would find that the two states, and likewise, the two remedies, share a significant *bridge* between them. Another way of saying this is that any one state predisposes you to enter into another state, but only the ones that share some similar predisposition. (*This is not to say that patients being treated constitutionally need an acute remedy each time they develop an acute illness; sometimes they do, sometimes they need a repetition of their constitutional remedy and sometimes the best thing to do is to wait. Look for more on follow-up and the practical elements of practice in a different volume on that topic!*)

Both constitutions **E** and **F** share some similar predisposition with that of the substance to be tested. What we tend to find then is that people of these 2 constitutions are more greatly affected by the substance than other people who do not share these bridges. I have previously written the logic behind predisposition and why we are affected. This simply carries the same argument when comparing how a substance influences one type of individual as compared to another. In fact, if the constitution has a lot of similarity to the proving substance, then the proving will actually 'look' like an acute illness. For example, constitution **F** may be so similar to the proving substance, that they will develop a great deal of new symptoms, just as if they were going through an acute illness.

If you look again at Figure 1 you can see other persons represented. **A** and **B**, for example, have little or no intersection, little or no *bridge* with the substance tested. As such, it means that the overall predisposition, the overall sensitivities of individuals in group **A** and group **B** are substantially different from the substance being proven. As such, this means that we should notice little or no effects when these individuals try to test the substance in the proving, assuming that the *Stress* is not given at a toxic dose.

Some provers may actually have a constitution that needs the proving substance, a remedy that is identical to the circle represented by the proving substance. These individuals have a curative response from the substance, and contribute the most valuable information to the proving.

Figure 1 also illustrates an observation that was previously unexplainably found in provings. We sometimes find subsets of provers who develop the same symptoms, while others develop completely other symptoms. This model and Figure 1 conceptualize our findings. Some provers are of the same constitution and therefore develop more similar symptoms. For example, 2 different provers may be in constitution **E**. As such they share a good deal of predisposition and they respond to *Stress* similarly. When they prove the substance, they develop similar symptoms.

It follows that provers with different constitutions who have intersections with other provers may very well share similar symptoms of the remedy, while others may not. For example, in Figure 1, a prover in group **F** may develop similar symptoms to a prover in group **E** because groups **E** and **F** and the substance have a small space where they intersect. In the figure, it is represented by the intersecting circles of **E**, **F**, and the proving inner circle, **J**. However, other provers in group **F**, may still produce symptoms but not be similar to group **E**. In the figure that group is represented by the intersecting circles of group **F**, and in the inner circle but not the part that also intersects with group **E**, listed as **H**.

Still others may develop completely different symptoms. These individuals have a *bridge* of symptom potential with the inner circle, the substance to be proven, but do not share symptom *bridges* or potentials with other remedies mentioned thus far. In the diagram, group **C** is such a group. An individual in group **C** will produce symptoms. Those symptoms may very well be completely different from the symptoms produced by Group **E** and **F** as they do not share any symptom *bridges*. This is why Hahnemann mentions that we should prove a remedy on many individuals. He does not fully explain his reasoning, as I do, but this is clearly the intent.

Conceptually, this part of the discussion means that we are trying to find all the people who have a significant symptom *bridge*, i.e., have a sensitivity to the substance. Once we find these people, we should notice how the substance effects them in different ways. The sum total of that experience is what we will call the full potential of the *materia medica* of the proven substance. Once you removed all other variables, the effect is the effect. Brilliantly thought out by Hahnemann, given the fact that it predated modern science! It is all there in the *Organon of Medicine*, if you look for it.

It is a shame that older provings did not contain the constitutional makeup of the provers, as that information would be most valuable. Again, the fact that a model was missing meant that we did not fully appreciate why this would be important. With this model in hand, it becomes painfully obvious that we have to note the constitutions of the provers. With this model in place we say, "Of course, we have to note the constitution of the provers." But if you look back at all the previous provings, new and old, you find this information missing. A good model informs and heightens perceptions.

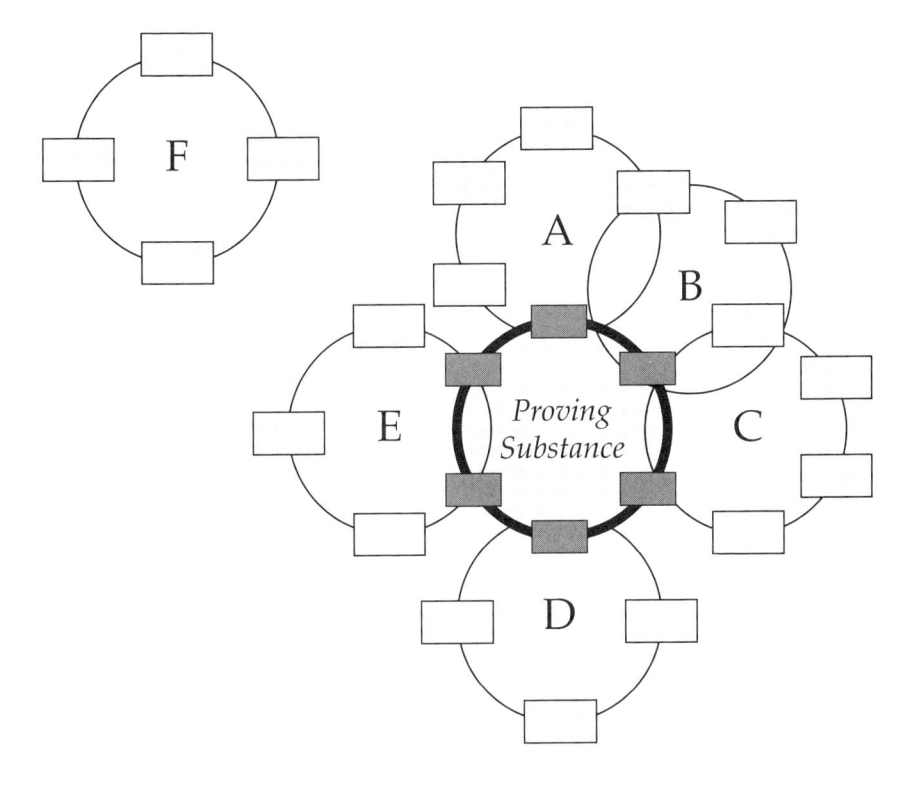

Figure 2

A more accurate model of a proving is shown in Figure 2. Here we see the *Cycle* of adaptation for each prover **A – F**, as well as the *Cycle* of the substance being proved. The *Cycle* is represented by a number of *Segments*. The *Segments* of these *Cycles* are represented by the boxes. Here we illustrate the relationship of different *Segments* of different remedy states to one another, as well as their relationship to the tested substance. We can illustrate that different provers may share *Segments* of the substance they are proving. These shared *Segments* will be seen in the reported symptoms of the provers that are directly related to the medicine. For example, all provers in group **A** will develop symptoms that fit within the *Segment* that is shared with the proving substance. In group **A** there is only one such *Segment*. Likewise, group **B** will develop Symptoms that fit into 2 *Segments*, as these are the ones shared with the substance. Group **C** will likewise develop symptoms that fit into 2 *Segments*.

Provers of similar constitutions may share common symptoms/*Segments* during the proving. For example, provers of Group **A** will share symptoms with provers in Group **B**, as these two states share one *Segment*. Likewise, Group **C** will share symptoms with Group **B** for the same reason. Note, however, that Group **A** and Group **C** do not share *Segments*.

Other symptoms of the medicine may only be experienced or proved by a single prover (i.e., subjects **D** and **E**). And some provers will experience no significant resonance with the medicine (i.e., subject **F**). Well constructed provings must be conducted with multiple subjects to clearly define the totality of the medicine under study. Incomplete data in our *materia medica* only serves to complicate our daily clinical practice.

Application

Provings should be both consistent with case taking as well as give us insight into our clinical philosophy. We have stated that provers will bring out only certain symptoms of the medicine. The symptoms being manifested are those in common between the nature of the medicine and the nature of that prover's constitutional state. At times, these symptoms become aggravated, and at other times they may even dissipate or resolve, resulting in an overall healthier state for the prover. Hahnemann and others even suggested that because of this observation, properly conducted provings actually strengthen the individual.

Even the best homeopaths will, at times, incorrectly prescribe. When a wrong remedy is given, the patient is unwittingly entering a proving. How could one distinguish between the two situations? We have shown in our proving model that if the medicine is similar to the constitution of the individual, or if the patient has a high degree of sensitivity, symptoms will be produced. Some symptoms will be the result of the *Stress* of the drug (primary symptoms). "Distinguishing symptoms produced by a simple medicine from those of the disease that it was taken to cure demands the highest discernment… Symptoms that were never before noticed, or what were perhaps noticed much earlier in the diseases, are new ones belonging to the medicine." — Hahnemann, aphorism 142.

Chapter 3 - Cycles & Segments and Stress & Strain

Some symptoms produced by the patient after an incorrect prescription, are actually the result of the patient *Straining* back against the *Stress* of the medicine (secondary symptoms). When medicines are prescribed in potentized form, primary toxic effects are for the most part minimized, while the majority of new symptoms produced will be solely due to the reactive *Straining* response of the patient. These secondary symptoms are common to the given drug *and* the *simillimum* of the patient (Figure 3). Those symptoms may resolve, increase in intensity, or lead to temporary or incomplete improvement of the patient.

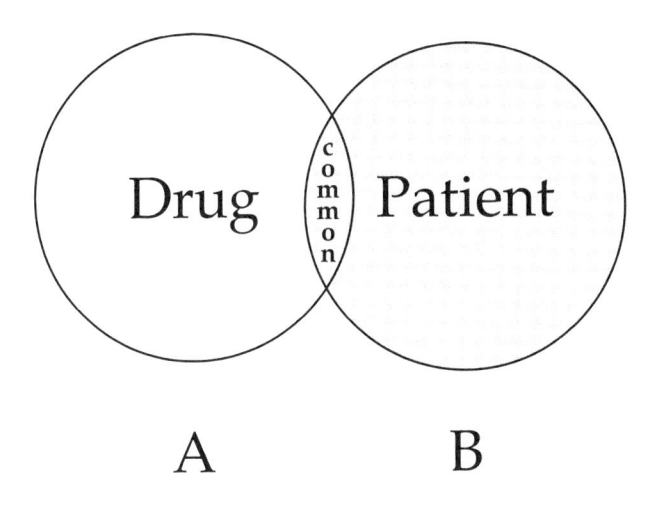

```
    Drug  [common]  Patient

     A              B
```

Figure 3

Most times, shared symptoms represent one or two shared *Segments* between the medicine given and the correct prescription for the patient. Figure 4, below, expands Figure 3 to show the segments. In Figure 4, Remedy **A** is given to the patient. The simillimum for the patient is actually described by the *Cycle* of Remedy **B**. The shared symptom *Segments* would be expected to show some change as a result of the patient coming under the influence of Remedy **A**. After the "proving" of Remedy **A** by the patient, two *Segments* of the true Simillimum **B** have been revealed. Special attention should therefore be awarded these clues to the true analysis of the patient's total pathology. Medicines that are similar or have been noted to follow well should be strongly considered as the next prescription. More on this topic can be found in the volume on patient management.

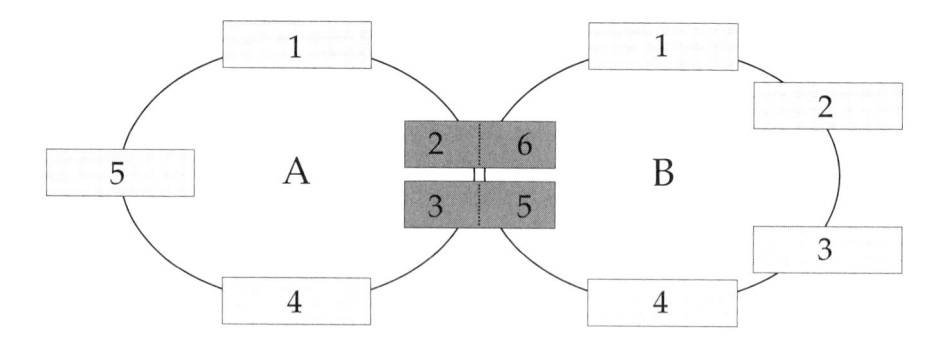

Figure 4

When a medicine is prescribed that has no apparent effect on the patient, it can generally be assumed that the prescription has little or nothing in common with the necessary remedy, as in Figure 5. (A similar case is described by prover **B** of Figure 1 and prover **F** of Figure 2.) A thorough review of the case and analysis is in order.

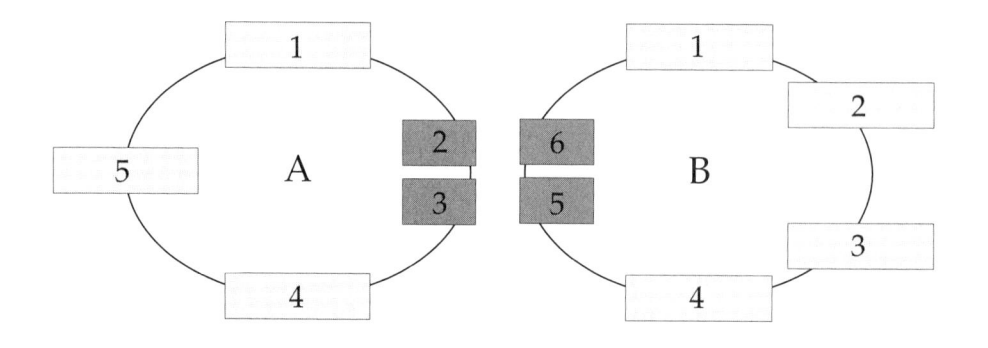

Figure 5

All Possible Reactions to the Proving Substance

A. Cure of patient. *As Hahnemann mentioned in aphorism 136 of the Organon, "... when the medicine is administered to a person who is sick with similar symptoms, it will exert all its powers, even those that it has seldom revealed in the healthy."* How does this occur? If an individual's constitution coincides fairly exactly with the nature of the medicine being proven, that person will have a dramatic and fairly complete picture of the medicine produced. This can often result in curative action of the medicine as well, based on our concept of homeopathy, of *Stress* and *Strain* as well as *Cycles* and *Segments*. In this situation, the medicine being proven is considered the simillimum, or at least very similar, to the constitution of the prover, and cure ensues. Many times *Strange, Rare,* or *Peculiar* symptoms will be noted in these people, as they are the most sensitive to the substance proven. These symptoms are quite unique to the medicine and have proven quite valuable to the clinical practice of homeopathy. The likelihood of this occurring is very slight. It depends mostly on how likely it is that the substance has interacted with our species.

B. Cure of some symptoms. In some provers, while the person is clearly not cured, they do lose *some* of their chronic symptoms. How can this occur? As demonstrated above, due to certain *Segments* being shared between the substance being tested and the true simillimum of the prover, when the substance *Stresses* the prover, the prover *Strains* back, and *Strains* efficiently enough to cure a symptom. This is explained in the above Figures.

C. New symptoms develop. Again, when a substance is taken by a person who shares some of the sensitivities, then the substance *Stresses* the individual. When the substance is in a toxic/strong dose, then most of the provers will develop symptoms, as they are all sensitive, due to our species sensitivity. When the substance is in a minute amount, potentized, then only the extremely sensitive people will develop symptoms. From our model we can say several things about these new symptoms. The people who develop them are people who either need this remedy or a remedy similar to it. We know this to be true because they share *bridge* symptoms. As such, if the substance is *not* the simillimum, at least it shares *Segments* with the simillimum.

Another point is that we do not know necessarily if the symptoms are due to the primary or secondary effects of the substance. But nevertheless, from our model, we can say they both count for us. We can use the symptoms regardless of how we view that particular point.

D. Altered symptoms. Again we may notice that at times a prover's constitutional symptoms are altered in some way. This shows that the prover has a sensitivity to the remedy and that the altered symptoms belong to the new remedy and, in some respect, to the old.

E. Past symptoms return. Here, symptoms that a person had not experienced in a long time return. The question has been to which remedy should these count? Actually to both remedies, the one he or she needs *and* the one being proven. Why? The person is sensitive enough to the substance to experience the *Stress* and to *Strain* in response. That *Straining* in response produces the symptom. The symptom belongs to both remedies, as illustrated in Figure 4, by the middle *Segments*.

F. No new symptoms. Here the symptoms that the person usually has have remained unchanged. In other words, the person did not have any sensitivity to the substance being proven. The symptoms did not change or go away, and the prover did not develop any new symptoms.

To sum up, a proving is therefore a basic scientific experiment of administering minute doses of substances to relatively healthy individuals and recording the changes that result. Medicines can be defined as substances that, in their gross form, have some physiologic, mental, or emotional effect on the organism. Our job in conducting the proving is to accurately record only the effects of this medicine on a variety of individuals. In so doing, a reliable symptom picture of the medicine will be produced. Reliable symptom pictures are essential to effective and reproducible results in prescribing.

Readings for this Chapter

Hahnemann's *Organon of Medicine* is divided into several large sections. For further understanding of this chapter as well as the next, please read his section on provings, which are Aphorisms 105 up to and including 145.

— Chapter 4 —
What Provings Add to the Medical Community

I would like to be clear about my intent with this chapter. While it is certainly educational, in that it corrects historical misconceptions that are prevalent in our community, my main attention is on political points. For many years we have been bombarded with criticism by our colleagues on the 'other side of the aisle.' The most frequent complaint is that our science is not tested, that there is not enough *science* in our science. For the most part we have had to defend ourselves, answering to questions and accusations that were levied against us by others, having to fight on their terms. Our defense tends to be both mediocre and incomplete, and in fact rarely changes any opinions.

What am I attempting to change in this chapter? Several things, all radical! First you, the homeopath. I would like to bring out in the open the fact that as a community we feel under-classed. No, I do not mean all of us. And no, I do not mean that we do not get brilliant results with some of our patients. What I mean is something much more insidious. What I mean is when in a debate with a physician on the other side, or a politician or a governing body, we fall flat. As a community there is a feeling that we are not as good, that we are second class citizens. I feel a great urgency to acknowledge this. For if not, we can never evolve from this place. We need to turn the tables and show what we are made of.

Let me make one point clear here. There is every reason for our community to feel inferior and even persecuted. As a community we have been under attack for 200 years. For two centuries, we have had to contend with political and strong financial opponents. Our adversaries have often set our agenda. For the most part we have had to *react* rather then *act*. This is a losing proposition from the start. Enough is enough!!!

To do this completely, this chapter will be a bit longer than previous ones. I include here an article to show colleagues, which adds to the pages.

In addition to changing our own self-definition, I also want to change the perception of our profession in the outside world: both in the medical community and the general public. The general community, for the most part, wants several things from us. They want to know that we can add something to the treatment of illness. They want to know that we adhere to certain standards and they want to know that we can work with other allied health professionals. In short, what do they get for supporting us? What benefit comes from seeing a homeopath?

While this point has been tackled on and on in different legislative bodies, we tend to have a tough fight for two reasons. First we have opponents that are powerful. Second, and more importantly, we do not know enough about our own history to defend ourselves properly. Of course the powerful have dictated our history for so long that it is natural to not know our full heritage but then it is *we* that are the losers. By knowing all that we have historically contributed to the field of science, perhaps we may have the opportunity to have them listen to our current work, both in the laboratory and in the field.

Many of our medical colleagues do not know us or understand what it is we do. It is an unfortunate truth that by suppressing parts of truths, you limit yourself. The medical profession has several problems with us. First, is what we call the 'tomato effect.' This term has its roots in history. Since tomatoes are in the nightshade family, for many years Americans did not eat them, in fact not eating them until the 1820's, because they were obviously poisonous and why would you want to eat something that is obviously going to kill you. It took time for the 'obvious' to be found to not be true, that tomatoes were indeed not poisonous. What is interesting is that it did not matter that their European counterparts were already eating tomatoes, the Americans were stubborn in their beliefs. Since that time we have used this term to express beliefs that are untested but strongly held to be true. The reception we receive is something like, "Since homeopathy is practiced with such dilute substances, it obviously can not work, so we will not listen to what you say are your clinical results." The tomato effect! Also, "Since you have no reliable, experimental evidence, we will not listen to you. The problem with natural medicine is that it is unproven, unlike our current practice of allopathic medicine."

I would like to change these opinions. I would like to share some tools to allow you to be able to answer these charges. Not just answer these charges but to do much, much more. I would like to show that homeopathy and homeopaths were in the forefront of medical thought. Yes, we fell back somewhat when we fell out of favor, but that does not mean we were not there.

Many of the homeopathic books written in the past decade focus on why these points are not important. They deflect, as a way to try to get around these issues. I wholeheartedly disagree with this approach for two reasons. First it does not work, it has not worked and it will most likely continue not to work. Second, this approach comes from not knowing our heritage and, as a result, blinds us even further. The truth of homeopathy's real contribution to history will hopefully win in the end and benefit all. I make the following points not to win a debate solely. I hope to show that by our medical colleagues knowing more fully our complete history and the *reasons* for our philosophy, that their craft will vastly improve. You see, I do not believe that we have been locked in a win/lose scenario, but instead in a lose/lose situation. I want to change that to a win/win and I think it can be done.

Provings and the History of Medicine

I think one of the best places to begin this climb back is to discuss the history of the provings in homeopathy As you know, Hahnemann began the process of testing individual drugs, as discussed in the last chapters. For a fuller description of his thoughts, see the *Organon* Aphorisms 105-145.

Let's think about what he was doing. He was attempting to find out what effect one drug had on an individual, at a time when polypharmacy was the norm and at a time when true effects were only conjectured at. In the aphorisms cited above, he pleads for honesty in testing and for a true accounting of medicine, to develop a true, pure *materia medica*.

By today's language we could say that it is hard to isolate effects from each other. It seems as though everything is related to something. However, the nature of any scientific endeavor is to try to understand the effect of one variable. To do that, therefore, you have to remove all the other variables, to try to design a test where everything is accounted for and only one variable is left, the one you are testing. What we try to do is remove what is called the 'noise' all around an event, to see what the pure event is. The best experiments do this well. The nature of all poor experimental design is that the experiment does not successfully isolate only one variable and test that variable. A poor experiment does not remove the 'noise.'

Hahnemann picked as healthy a prover as possible, so that he would not have to contend with the prover's 'noise.' He asked each subject not to take drugs, and to moderate foods and lifestyles, again to eliminate 'noise.'

He even suggested that if some strong influence occurred to the prover that he eliminate those symptoms, as being too much affected by the outside noise. As such, he was revolutionary in his time. His work flew in the face of what was current, but his work is the standard that the modern scientific world holds to now. He began the process of drug testing!

Currently, there is a very well-defined process of bringing a drug to market, developed about 40 years ago, comprised of different phases. Phase 1 comes very close to what we term a proving. The principal investigator tests a substance on a small number of people looking to see what sorts of effects the substance produces. How is the substance tolerated, how is it absorbed and metabolized by the body? This takes place with people who do not need the substance as a drug, i.e. they are not sick. Researchers are looking for physiologic tolerance without too many side effects; essentially, a proving.

Homeopaths pay attention to the opposite side of the coin. We push this process to the murky realm; that land that lies between health and illness, but we push it to see what symptoms, what 'side effects' we *can* find. It is those side effects that we will use to prescribe upon. Aside from the difference in what we are paying attention to and how we will use it, a Phase 1 trial is essentially a proving. I want to be clear here. Homeopaths began this process. We brought Phase 1 to the medical community, we began the trials. This is not a field that we have no experience in, or are late to adopt; we started it. Our colleagues on the other side of the aisle are the late ones. I have actually been in conversations where the physician tells me that we do not have enough proof for what we do. That is when I say, you mean like drug trials, like the phase 1, 2, 3 kinds of trials? When they say, "Yes, that is what I mean," I set the historical record straight right there. Let's go further.

Current homeopathic thinking and writing discusses how we do not need to mask the proving; how we do not need to have placebo trials. The discussion goes something like this. Hahnemann knew what he was proving. For goodness sake, most of the original provings were conducted by provers who made the medicines themselves. These were learned homeopaths who knew that they were proving a metal or herb, knew what the herb or metal was, potentized it themselves, knew the toxicology and poisoning effects of it and then set about proving it. Talk about poor technique, it may be hard to imagine anything sloppier. And yet the information we received from those provings is still the most important in our practice.

As the argument goes, it worked then, it has always worked for us, and we should not change it, just to fit in with what the scientific community wants from us.

I disagree with this posture mostly because it is factually incorrect, and what's more, flies against the spirit of how and why the provings came to be in the first place. It is a dangerous posture. It limits us on the one hand, and makes it possible to introduce mistakes into our work on the other.

Going back in history, recall what Hahnemann attempted. He pushed the boundaries forward many times in developing the proving process. His attempt was to clean up, as best he could, mistakes that were inherent in the testing process of that time, i.e. to push the science forward. There is no record of him ever stopping or slowing down in this desire. In the thirst for truth, he implored the testers to be honest, to love truth above all else; and he set about trying to regulate a fair amount of their lives so that only the substance being proven would be isolated in its effect. As rough as that may seem to us now, it was revolutionary thought back then.

Moving forward to our day, we hold as a standard tests that have multiple arms; arms with placebo versus active verum. And of course the test is masked, to the point that none of the participants know what it is that they are testing. "If only homeopathy could hold to that standard," says the outside world. We mostly argue back that that is not relevant for homeopathy, that we have different rules that we function under and that we should not be judged by others' rules. Let's take a moment to look at the reality of history.

Masked studies in medicine, where people did not know what was being tested, as well as placebo controls where blank pellets or sham surgeries were performed, were introduced to medicine in the 1920's. There is a sporadic mention of it before that time, but it was the 1920's that saw the benefits and merits of masking the study and having a placebo control arm. Essentially what they were looking for was nothing more than what Hahnemann began 100 years previously. How do we remove preconceptions to get at a more perfect truth. Hahnemann had his answers at his time. I conjecture that he would have kept on pushing with new innovations and would have adopted these thoughts in his method. There is anecdotal evidence from the 1840's that Hahnemann conducted a proving of *Aconite*, where he did not tell the provers what the substance was. This may have been one of the first masked studies in medicine. While that is conjecture the following is not!

What you are about to read is the earliest record of masking and placebo in medicine. It comes from page 147-154 of the *Transactions of the Thirty-Eighth Session of the American Institute of Homeopathy*, held at St. Louis, June 2-5, 1885, published in 1885. Notice the date 1885. This paper, discussing and adopting for our profession masked studies (point #1) as well as placebo (point #2), predates the beginning usage and adoption of these tools in the orthodox medical world by 45 years. I repeat, 45 years! This shows that homeopaths indeed followed in Hahnemann's footsteps and kept pushing the boundaries of research to help get at a more perfect truth. We began this. We began the use of masking, as well as the use of placebo in medical studies. We brought the rest of the medical profession with us. It did not happen the other way around. They have been hammering at us for so long, that they now believe their own rhetoric. And since we do not have institutional memory in our profession, as they have forgotten our history, so too have we.

REPORT OF THE DIRECTORS OF PROVINGS

By D.J. Mcguire, M.D. Detroit, Mich.

The Board of Directors of Provings begs hereby to make its first annual report.

This committee was appointed, as you remember, for the following definite purposes: To formulate and publish rules for the conduct of drug-experimentation and to review and pass judgment upon such unpublished provings as may be submitted to them with regard to their reliability and fitness for publication.

The slightest consideration will make it apparent to any one familiar with the history of the Hahnemannian materia medica, that the committee in accepting this work has undertaken a Herculean task. The undertaking is great, not only in the importance of the end to be accomplished, but in the multitude and intricacy of the means required and in the variety of the conflicting views to be met.

Immediately after receiving our commission we met at Deer Park, passed in review the work to be done, and organized by the selection of chairman and secretary. The secretary of the committee was requested to prepare a set of rules for proving, and to present them at a subsequent meeting for comment and criticism. From this time on our work has proceeded uninterruptedly till the present day.

In the month of September the committee held several meetings in Chicago, reviewing the work thus far done, and adopting resolutions embodying our more matured notions of the best methods of work. After long consultation and conference, there was reached at length an agreement on certain working rules.

PRINTED CIRCULAR

Chief among these rules are the following:

1st. In all experiments with drugs of various degrees of attenuation, the prover is to be kept in ignorance of the name and the nature of the medicine he is taking. This is believed to be an important safeguard against the admission of false symptoms.

2d. That blanks consisting of the medicine-vehicle only should be freely interspersed. This is believed to be another important and hitherto neglected safeguard against the admission of symptoms due to idiosyncrasy or imagination.

3d. That the consecutive order of the development of drug effects should not be interrupted by repetition of the dose. This rule is believed to be important in that it gives in the provings a more complete, more life-like and more useful picture of drug action than can be obtained from the confused, jumble of early and late, primary and secondary, direct and reactionary drug effects.

4th. That there should be a free use during the proving of the modern means of diagnosis, such as the thermometer, the opthalmoscope, chemical analysis, etc.

In the practical results of this year's work, we are pleased to be able to call your attention to the advantages to be derived from each of the foregoing improvements in method.

5th. For the sake of uniformity, the new provings have been carried on as far as practicable with drugs issued by the committee.

6th. In the dispensing of drugs for provings, the work has been divided so that the director who issued the drugs immediately to the prover was himself deprived of all bias in regard to attenuation and dose. The report of the pharmacist making known the attenuation and the dose was not given to the board until after the presentation of the provings. Thus, incidentally we reach valuable results in the settlement of the question of potentization and dose.

7th. The provings are to be performed by at least five persons for each drug, selecting for the purpose persons of different sex, age, temperament and residence, and there are to be a sufficient number of repetitions in each prover to produce convincing confirmatory results.

A circular letter was issued, setting forth the advantages to be derived from drug-experimentation under these improved methods. This was published in several of our medical journals. In addition to this the members of the board have used their personal influence to secure volunteer provers. Still further, the committee offered three prizes to meritorious provers—one of $100, one of $50 and one of $25. Here it is proper to mention the fact that Drs. T.F. Allen, F.H. Orme, J.P. Drake, A.I. Sawyer, A.R. Wright and I.T. Talbot have generously contributed to a fund for this purpose. The cost of drugs and the expense of travel, borne by individual members of the board at no inconsiderable personal sacrifice, have been freely given in the cause of science.

The prizes were made conditional upon the prover's conducting experiments in all three of the methods we recommend, including experiments on animals. The board regrets to report that not one of the numerous volunteers has conformed to this requirement, and that it is compelled to suffer another twelve months from pecuniary plethora.

Upwards of eighty persons volunteered to make provings. Of these twenty were physicians, and the remainder medical students. The great majority of these provers offered their services after personal solicitation by members of the board. Two of the board members have made provings in their own persons.

The accepted results of this work are not voluminous. We desire it to be borne in mind that this is but the inchoate beginning of our work, and that our striving is for quality rather than quantity.

Of these eighty provers many have made no report to the committee. Some have taken the parcels of the first or of the second series only, and reported that they got no symptoms worthy of record. Others have sent in reports which are gratifying to the board, not only on account of the external and internal evidence of the genuineness of the drug effects, but on account of the superiority of the style and character of the work accomplished.

Of these provings the following are deemed worthy of publication: Three series of experiments with *Aconitum*, showing in addition to the well-known prominent effects of this poison, the successive variations of bodily temperature produced in the healthy subject. The temperature curve of *Aconitum*, determined by actual thermic measurement, is not to be found as far as we know in any extant treatise on *materia medica* except one, which appeared immediately after these experiments of ours. I refer to that invaluable publication, the Cyclopedia of Drug Pathogenesy, published jointly by this Institute and the British Homeopathic Society.

Three partial provings of *Aletris farinosa*, one of *Convallaria majalis*, and two of *Lilium tigrinum*.

We have also a proving of *Arsenicum* by J.S. Robinson, which the committee think worthy of mention on account of its merits, but which brings out nothing with regard to the action of this drug not already published.

Several incomplete partial provings are in the hands of the board, which will be held for corroboration.

A running glance at these provings will illustrate the practical advantage of the methods we have adopted.

1. There is a notable absence of the irrelevant symptoms which most of us believe to be produced by causes other than drug action, namely, idiosyncrasies of provers, the influence of the imagination, antidotal interference and unassignable extraneous influences.

2. The clear distinction which we are able to make between the real and the imaginary. This is beautifully illustrated in one of the provings of *Stannum metallicum*.

3. The living, organized, unmangled, undissected character of the provings in the single-dose series contrasts favorably with the broken up and dismembered presentation of drug effects which is furnished by some of our earlier provings.

4. The close resemblance of the better provings one to another, extends not only to the individual symptoms, but to the chronological order in which they appear. To illustrate, we will call attention to two provings of *Lilium*, those of Dr. W. and Miss N. With Miss N. the first symptom was

a neuralgic pain in the right ovary. With Dr. W. the first symptom was a neuralgic pain in the left testicle. With Miss N. the second symptom was a neuralgic pain in the temple. With Dr. W. the second symptom was a neuralgic pain in the temple. With Miss N. the third symptom was lassitude and languor. With Dr. W. the third symptom was neuralgic pains in the extremities. (Both are spinal in origin). With Miss N. the fourth symptom was coated tongue. With Dr. W. the fourth symptom was offensive taste and salivation, followed by griping in the bowels and chilliness.

These remarks are offered merely for the purpose of calling attention to the prominent features of these provings. If your time and patience would permit, we should be pleased to read one of them as a sample.

In conclusion, your committee begs your kind indulgence as regards its shortcomings, and earnestly asks the cooperation of every member of this Institute in this work of experimentation. Without this cooperation our work must be a failure, with it the possibilities of success are boundless.

A NEW STANDARD OF CRITICISM FOR DRUG PROVINGS

By A.W. Woodward, M.D., Chicago, IL

As a member of the Committee on Drug Provings, I desire to state one difficulty with which we have had to contend. It is concerning the standard that shall govern the acceptance of drug provings. This, I believe, is a question that has never been settled authoritatively by the Institute, and is of great importance to the progress of our cause.

The practical nature of this question is seen at once, when we state that a large majority of those who have received medicines for proving, have either made no report, or have said "No results worthy of record." This brings prominently into view the prevailing sentiment of the profession, viz., that drug provings to be of any value must exhibit decided symptoms of a morbid character, and the greater the variety of these symptoms the better will the proving be considered.

This doubtless is a correct basis of judgement, if our object is to learn the pathogenetic effects of drugs; but in view of the assumed fact (as is claimed), that there is something else of equal if not greater importance than the pathogenesis itself that may be learned by new experiments, it would seem wise that a new standard of judgment should be adopted that shall vary according to the work intended.

Your committee has instituted three series of experiments; one by repeated doses, to elicit the full pathogenetic effects of the drug chosen, as has been the custom heretofore. A second is by a single dose less than toxic, to obtain such effects as it is capable of producing, each effect recorded in the order of their occurrence. A third experiment (but the first to be undertaken) is calculated to determine whether there is or is not a succession of organic derangements characteristic of each remedy, the same obtainable from many provers. This is a matter of the greatest importance to us as therapists, for, if it be true this succession of effects will furnish an unfailing guide to the one remedy. Under the law similia, we may expect not only that the local symptom of the disease and of the pathogenesis shall correspond, but they must coincide also in time of occurrence; and more than this, they must be attended by similar concomitant disorders in other parts of the body.

It may be well to say that the advocate of this doctrine was, for a number of years, baffled in his search for a uniform series of effects of one drug upon many provers. It was not difficult to obtain a sequence of effects; they may be seen in every proving ever made. The Cyclopedia of Drug Pathogenesy is full of them, but the sequence varies with every prover. This is the difficulty that must be overcome if the sequence of symptoms is to become of any value as a guide in therapeutics.

After many fruitless efforts it has been deemed impossible of attainment by the customary methods of dosage and observation. Hence we ask this society to adopt provisionally a new basis of judgment. We ask that you will admit as provings of the first series records that would be considered almost worthless by the old standard. The record of symptoms must begin in that border land that lies between health and disease, and it must include in the beginning every observable phenomena whether normal or abnormal, trivial or important. Gradually pathognomonic symptoms will appear, increasing in frequency toward the end, yet in many provings such symptoms may be few and unimportant in themselves.

That this method of observation will yield good results was indicated by our chairman in his report on *Lillium*. Two provers, male and female, experienced their first symptom in the sexual organs, soon followed by cerebral and later by spinal phenomena.

In the third proving of this drug by Dr. S., which is full of true symptoms from beginning to end, it will be observed his record begins with symptoms of the respiratory tract, similar to those experienced by the first prover toward the last of her record. Thus the third prover, whose proving is pathogenetically vastly superior, unequivocally contradicts and invalidates the two former provings that agree with each other in every important respect, and are more reliable as pathological guides, if not symptomatic, judging by our experience with this drug.

Again our difficulty in passing judgment on this new method of proving is illustrated by two provings of *Arsenicum* that were presented. They also presented a uniformity of organic effects, but the committee was not at liberty to accept, and recommend them for publication because they showed but few recognizable pathogenetic effects.

This indicates very briefly our desire that the Institute will recognize the necessity of receiving from us in this section of our work a class of provings that otherwise would not be received. We do not ask that every symptom the imagination can conceive shall be accepted. No provings will be submitted for our approval that does not exhibit indubitable evidences of its genuineness. Its individual value must be determined by the number of verifications it shall receive from other provers.

Not only should we be permitted to present provings of little pathogenetic value, but the necessity of such experiments should be made apparent to our provers, who, apprehensive lest their records appear imaginary and of no importance, will record only the serious symptoms observable in the later stages of a proving, thus failing to exhibit the true primary effects of the drug.

Thus is explained the poverty of our report that otherwise might have proved more interesting.

By the time Kent wrote his book on philosophy, he extolled the virtues of this method. It was already a given, not new to our profession at all. The date of the book is 1900, though the articles were written before that time.

Lectures on Homeopathic Philosophy
James Tyler Kent
Published in book form in 1900

Lecture XXVIII - THE STUDY OF PROVINGS

Aphorisms 105, et seq.

It may be well for you now to review thoroughly the first portion of the study of the *Organon*, containing the doctrines in general that may be hereafter found to be useful in the application of Homeopathy, including the oldest established rules and principles. The first step may be called theoretical Homeopathy, or the principles of Homeopathy after which we take up the homeopathic method of studying sicknesses. In this we have found that the study of sickness in our school is entirely different from the study of sickness under the old school. But up to this time the doctrines have not exhibited their purpose; we only get their purpose when we come to the third step, which deals with the use of the *Materia Medica*. We have seen that we must study sickness by gathering the symptoms of sick patients, relying upon the symptoms as the language of nature, and that the totality of the symptoms constitutes the nature and quality and all there is that is to be known of the disease.

The subject we will now take up and consider is, how to acquire a knowledge of the instruments that we shall make use of in combating human sicknesses. We know very well that in the old school there is no plan laid down for acquiring a knowledge of medicines except by experimenting with them upon the sick. This Hahnemann condemns as dangerous, because it subjects human sufferers to hardship and because of its uncertainty. Though this system has existed for many hundreds of years, it has never revealed a principle or method that one can take hold of the help in curing the sicknesses of the human family. His experiments in drug proving were made before he studied diseases. In other words, Hahnemann built the *Materia Medica* and then took up the plan of examining the patient to see what remedy the sickness looked like. Whereas now, after Homeopathy has been established, and the *Materia Medica* has been established, the examination of the patient precedes, in a particular case, the examination of the *Materia Medica*. But for the purpose of study they go hand in hand.

Before Hahnemann could examine the *Materia Medica* you may say he had to make one, for there was none to examine, there were no provings as yet; we now have the instruments before us to examine, we have the proved remedies. When the fallacy of old school medicine fully entered Hahnemann's mind; when he became disgusted with its method at the time his children were sick; when he placed himself in the stream of Providence and affirmed his trust that the Lord had not made these little ones to suffer, and then to be made worse from violent medicines; then his mind was in an attitude for discovery. It was a discountenancing of and disgust for the things that were useless, and this brought him to the state of acknowledgment of not knowing and that everything of man's own opinion must be thrown away. It brought him to a state of humility and the acknowledgment of Divine Providence.

That state of humility opens man's mind. You will find so long as man is in a position to trust himself he makes himself a god; he makes himself the infallible; he looks to himself and does not see beyond himself; his mind is then closed. When a man finds out that in himself he is a failure, that is the beginning of knowledge in any circumstance; the very opposite of this closes the mind and turns man away from knowledge.

I have been teaching long enough to observe, and I will tell you some things I have observed. I have observed quite a number of young people turn away from Homeopathy after once confessing it, and professing to practice it, and after seeming able in a certain degree to practice it. I often wondered why it was that after they had made public profession of it they turned away from it, and I found in every instance that it was due to a lack of humility. The great mistake comes from turning one's attention into self and relying upon self, with an attention that closes the mind and deprives one of knowledge and prevents clear perception. Man takes himself out of the stream of Providence when he becomes satisfied with himself and thinks "now that I have done so many things I have nothing more to study". This is a wrong attitude; for anything like self-conceit will blind man's eyes, will make him unable to use the means of cure and will prevent his becoming acquainted with the *Materia Medica*. The homeopathic physician, as much as the clergyman, ought to keep himself in a state of purity, a state of humility, a state of innocence. So sure as he does not that he will fall by the wayside. There is nothing that destroys a man so fast in the scientific world as conceit. We see in old-fashioned science men who are puffed up and corpulent with conceit. The scientific men who are in the greatest degree of simplicity are the most wise and the most worthy, and you need not tell me that those who are innocent and simple have not had a tremendous struggle, in order to keep self under control and to reach this state of simplicity.

Extensive knowledge makes man simple, makes him gentle. Extensive knowledge makes a man realize how little he knows, and what a small concern he is. A little knowledge makes a fool of a man, and makes him think he knows it all, and the more he forgets of what he has known the bigger man he feels he is. The smaller he feels he is the more he knows, you may rest assured. In order to do this, he must study and keep himself in a state of gravity and in a state of innocence.

In the scientific world we have all those horrible jealousies and feelings of hatred to those who know more than we do. A man who cannot control that and keep that down is not fit to enter the science of Homeopathy. He must be innocent of these things; he must put that aside and be willing to learn of all sources, providing the truth flows from these sources. In this frame of mind, and this frame of mind only, can the physician proceed to examine the *Materia Medica*.

We have already said that Hahnemann had no *Materia Medica* to start with. He could not go to books, and read, and meditate, and find remedies in the image of human sickness. He had so many remedies to study, and hence it was necessary to build up the *Materia Medica*. We can imagine that Hahnemann must have been almost in a state of despair, and inclined to say there is no knowledge upon the earth. He felt in his own mind that we should never know anything about the *Materia Medica* so long as we perceived its effects only in human sickness, but that a true and pure *Materia Medica* must be formed by observing the action of medicines upon the healthy human race. Hahnemann did not commence to feed these medicines to others; he took the Peruvian Bark himself, and felt its effects upon himself. He allowed it to manifest its symptoms, and when he had thus proved Peruvian Bark (which we call *China*) it might be then said that the first remedy known to man was discovered, and that the first drug effect was known and that *China* was born! Hahnemann searched the literature of the day to find out what other effects of *China* had been discovered accidentally, and accepted such as were in harmony with what he had discovered. We have already referred to the fact that Hahnemann was able, after proving

China, to see that in its action it closely resembled the intermittent fevers that had existed through all time; that there was the most abundant relation of similitude between *China* and intermittent fever. Do we wonder, then, that Hahnemann said to himself, can it be possible that the law of cure is the law of similars? Can it be possible that similars are cured by drugs that produce symptoms like unto the sickness? Every drug that he proved thereafter established the law more and more, made it appear more certain, and every drug that he proved added one more remedy to the instrument we call the *Materia Medica*, until it came to be what we now recognize as *Hahnemann's Materia Medica Pura* and the *Materia Medica of the Chronic Diseases*. This work was simply enormous and very thorough, but many additions have been made to it since the time of its publication, and these form the instruments that we have to examine.

The best way to study a remedy is to make a proving of it. Suppose we were about to do that; suppose this class were entering upon a proving. Each member of the class would devote, say, a week, in examining carefully all the symptoms that he or she is the victim of, or believes himself or herself to be the victim of, at the present time, and for many months back. Each student then proceeds to write down carefully all these symptoms and places them by themselves. This group of symptoms is recognized as the diseased state of that individual.

A master-prover is decided upon, who will prepare for the proving a substance unknown to the class and to all the provers, known only to himself. He will begin with the first or earliest form of the drug, it may be the tincture, and potentize it to the 30th potency, putting a portion of that potency into a separate vial for each member of the class. The provers do not know what they are taking, and they are requested not to make known to each other their symptoms. When their own original symptoms appear in the proving the effect of the remedy upon any one of these chronic symptoms is simply noted, whether cured or exaggerated, or whether not interfered with; but when the symptom occurs in its own natural way, without being increased or diminished, it may be looked upon as one of the natural things of that particular prover, and hence all the natural things of the prover are eliminated. Generally if a remedy takes marked hold of a prover all the chronic symptoms will subside, but when a proving only takes a partial hold it may only create of few symptoms. These few symptoms, when added to the symptoms that the other provers have felt, will go to make up the chronic effect of the remedy, which may be said to be the effect of the remedy upon the human race. Now as to the method.

After the master prover deals out these vials, each prover takes a single dose of the medicine and waits to see if the single dose takes effect. If he is sensitive to that medicine a single dose will produce symptoms, and then those symptoms must not be interfered with; they should be allowed to go their own way. In the proving of an acute remedy, like *Aconite*, the instructor, who knows something about the effect of the medicine, may be able to say to the class: "If you are going to get effects from this remedy you will get those effects in the next three to four days. "It will not be necessary to wait longer than that for *Aconite*, *Nux vomica*, or *Ignatia*, but longer for *Sulphur* or some of the antipsorics. If we were attempting to prove a remedy like *Silicate of Alumina*, the master prover would advise the class not to interfere with the medicine for at least thirty days, because its prodrome may be thirty days.

It is highly important to wait until the possible prodrome of a given remedy is surely passed. If it is a short-acting remedy, the action will come speedily. We must bear in mind the prodrome, the period of progress and the period of decline when studying the *Materia Medica* as well as when studying miasms. The master-prover will usually be able to indicate to the class whether they should wait a short time or a long time before taking another dose, and from this the class will only know whether the drug to be proved is acute or chronic.

If the first dose of medicine produces no effect, and enough time has been allowed to be sure that the prover is not sensitive to it, the next best thing to do is to create a sensitiveness to it. If we examine into the effects of poisons, we find those who have once been poisoned by *Rhus* are a dozen times more sensitive than before. Those who have been poisoned by *Arsenic* are extremely sensitive to *Arsenic* after they allow the first effects to pass off. If they continue, however, to keep on with the first effects they become less sensitive to it, so that they require larger and larger doses to take effect. This is a rule with all poisonous substances that are capable of affecting the human system markedly. Now, when the time has passed by which the prover knows he is not sensitive to that remedy, that he has not received an action from the single dose (and perhaps in the class of forty you will not get more than one or two that will make a proving from the 30th potency) to make the proving and to intensify the effect, dissolve the medicine in water and have him take it every two hours for 24 or 48 hours, unless symptoms arise sooner. By this means the prodromal period is shortened. The medicine seems to be intensified by the repetition, and the patient is brought under the influence, dynamically, of that remedy. As soon as the symptoms begin to show, it is time to cease taking the remedy.

No danger comes from giving the remedy in this way; danger comes from taking it for a few days and then stopping it, and then taking it again. For instance, say you are proving *Arsenicum*; you find that you are not at all sensitive to it, and after waiting thirty days you start out again and take it in water, for three to four days, and the symptoms arise; now wait. So long as you discontinue it, it will not do any damage. Now, the symptoms begin to arise; wait, and let the image-producing effect of *Arsenicum* wear off; let it come and spread and go away of itself; do not interfere with it; if you do interfere with it, the interference should be only by a true antidote; you should never interfere with it by a repetition of dose. That is one of the most dangerous things. If the *Arsenic* symptoms are coming and showing clearly, and at the end of a week or ten days you say: "Let us brighten this up a little, and do this thing more thoroughly," and to accomplish this you take a great deal more, you will engraft upon your constitution in that way the *Arsenicum* diathesis, from which you will never be cured. You are breaking right into the cycles of that remedy and it is a dangerous thing to do. At times that has been done and the provers have carried the effects of their proving to the end of their days. If you leave this *Arsenical* state alone it will pass off entirely, and the prover is very often left much better for it. A proving properly conducted will improve the health of anybody; it will help to turn things into order. It was Hahnemann's advice to young men to make provings.

Another portion of the class will not get symptoms, no matter how they abuse the remedy, and if it be *Arsenicum* they will have to take a crude dose of it to get any effect, and then the symptoms given forth are only the toxic effects, from which little can be gained. The toxicological results of poisons are provings of the grossest character; they do not give the finer details. For instance, you give *Opium* in such large doses that it immediately poisons; you see nothing but the grosser, overwhelming symptoms; the irregular, stertorous breathing, the unconsciousness, the contracted pupil and the mottled face and the irregular heart. The details are not there, you only have a view of the most common things.

The reproving of remedies is of great value. The Vienna Society did not fully endorse Hahnemann's provings. This society thought it impossible that such wonderful things could be brought out upon the sensations of people. The society did not endorse the 30th potency that was recommended by Hahnemann for proving. So this society gathered itself together and resolved to prove remedies, and to test the 30th potency, and it so happened that the society was honest. *Natrum mur.*, *Thuja* and other remedies were proved, and W____ was honest enough to say that although his convictions were decidedly against the provings he had to admit that the symptoms gathered from the 30th potency were very strong. The Vienna Society demonstrated by these reprovings that the polychrests of Hahnemann had been fully proved. Their provings of the 30th of *Natrum mur.* was a wonderful revelation to them; but W___, in spite of this result, held on to his prejudices. He acknowledged that he was wrong; but he continued to use potencies lower than the 15th. He could not get his mind elevated to the 30th; his prejudice was too strong. Dunham says of some of these, that in spite of the fact that they had seen better results from the 30th and higher potencies even, they were so prejudiced they could not bring themselves to a state of yielding. As Dunham humorously expressed it, "they are ossified in their cerebral convolutions as well as in their bony structure". That is to say, their minds were inelastic, they could not expand. We talk from appearance when we say the eyes are closed; it is the mind that is closed, the understanding that is closed.

Read Aphorisms 107-112. When the patient is under the poisonous influence of a drug it does not seem to flow in the direction of his life action, but when reaction comes then the lingering effects of the drug seems to flow, as it were, in the stream of the vital action. Then the symptoms that arise are of the best order, and hence it is necessary in proving a drug to take such a portion of the drug only as will disturb and not suspend, as will flow in the stream of the vital order, in the order of the economy, establishing slightly perverted action, and causing symptoms, without suspending action, as we would, for example, with a large dose of *Opium*. When a state of suspension exists in the dynamic economy, then we have a beclouding of all the activities of the economy; so giving a large dose of medicine to palliate pains and sufferings is dangerous. We have a suspension of the vital order when we give a medicine that does not flow in the stream of the vital influx. Homeopathy looks towards the administration of medicines that are given for the purpose of either creating order, and then always in the higher potencies, or for the purpose of disturbing, and then in the lower potencies. We should never resort to crude drugs for provings, unless for a momentary or temporary experiment. It should not be followed up, and no great weight should be put upon the provings that are made from the crude medicines. They only at best give a fragmentary idea. Unless the proving that has been made with strong doses becomes enlarged with the symptoms from small doses the information remains fragmentary and useless. If we had only the poisonous effects of *Opium*, we would be able only to use it in those conditions that simulate the poisonous effects of *Opium*, like apoplexy.

There are some prescribers who teach that for the primary effect one potency must be used and for the secondary effect another must be used. No such distinction need be made. I have many times been at the bedside of apoplectic patients when death would have followed had not the homeopathic remedy been administered. I have been at the bedside of some when the pulse was flickering, when the eye was glazed, when the countenance was besotted, stertorous breathing coming on, frothing at the mouth, and in a few minutes after the administration of *Opium* cm. I have seen the patient go into a sound sleep, remain quiet and rest, wake up to consciousness, and go on to recovery. *Alumina* has a similar state of stupor resembling apoplexy, and hence it is that *Alumina* and *Opium* are antidotes to each other. I remember a case of apoplexy once that puzzled many physicians for some days, and I was puzzled, too. The patient was in a profound stupor. *Opium* was administered by the physician in charge before I arrived, and it stopped the stertorous breathing, but the patient remained unconscious. Finally it was observed that one side was moving, whilst the other side had not moved for many days, and that on the paralyzed side there was fever, while on the well side there was no fever. That was observed after careful examination for many days. I asked the doctor if he did not consider that the natural state of a paralyzed side would be coldness; he thought so too. The whole paralyzed side of this patient had a feverish feeling to the hand, the other side was normal. That seemed to be the only strange thing in the case; no speech, no effort to do anything, no action of the bowels; a do nothing case. Upon a careful study of the *Materia Medica*, I came to the conclusion that *Alumina* was suited to the case, and in twelve hours after taking a dose of *Alumina* in a high potency that fever subsided on the paralyzed side and the patient returned to consciousness.

Thus ends our lengthy discourse by Kent. What is the bottom line here? The next time someone takes you to task about our profession and the scientific method and current study design, set the record straight. We developed it. Period! These points are the hallmark of a science. Now that we show that we have not only been there, but placed our flag there first, what excuse can they come up with next? You disarm them: you educate them.

The real difficulty this century has been *within* our own profession. Since we are ignorant of our past, we have had no recourse but to react and to react badly at that. Instead of following on with Hahnemann's love of truth, that which permeated many homeopaths including the two authors quoted in this chapter, many in our community have argued against these methods. Many have argued that these rules of research are incorrect. So while Hahnemann and those that followed him were attempting to get rid of the background noise, the current homeopathic community argues that there is no such thing as noise. A ridiculous proposition in any scientist's mind. I hope to see that end.

To summarize, since the conception of homeopathy, beginning with Hahnemann, one of the primary issues has been to find what the true effect of one drug is on a human being. We began single drug prescriptions. We began single drug testing to find the physiologic responses on healthy people. In other words we began Phase 1 drug trials. We began masked studies. We began placebo trials. And this was not by a year or two. This was ahead by 80 years in some instances and by 40 years in others. We were well ahead of the rest. We set the standard. The driving force has always been that we want to help our patients. The way to do that had always been to find the purer truth. Anything short of that has always been not up to the standard to our forebears.

Currently, since we do not have institutional memory, we are arguing from a ridiculous vantage point. Whether we are put in this vantage point or put ourselves here matters not at this point. It is we who keep ourselves here with ignorance. Hopefully this will change now. It is really up to each one of us to educate and help guide our community through this period, back to a unified approach based on the scientific method that we in part developed.

How Else Can the Medical Community Benefit From Us - The Point of This Chapter

The following three points grew out of a collaboration between my work and thoughts, in an iterative process with Dr. Christopher Ryan, a colleague and a best friend. The world of homeopathy suffered one of its greatest losses with his passing away in early 2000 and I personally will miss him dearly as a friend, colleague, poker buddy and man of tremendous talents and intellect.

Point One. One of the great liabilities of current medical science is the tremendous inefficiency inherent in selecting medicinal substances to investigate in the first place. There are trillions of natural and synthetic compounds which may be ingested, injected, or applied in some way to the human body. To randomly apply each, in varying doses and via different routes to even a population of laboratory animals *with disease states mimicking those we are interested in,* is still a vast and ultimately impossible proposition.

In fact, one of the great ironies or bizarre quirks of current medicine is that we have long become dependent on the natural. Pharmaceutical companies often begin new classes of drugs by observing traditional uses of natural substances. I say ironic because, on the one hand they can discount systems of natural medicine which use these substances, yet on the other embrace the substances to test and study. They use those systems that they discounted to at least narrow the field of potential substances and potential uses. Only later do they derive synthetics from active compounds discovered in this way, and then construct families of potential compounds based on chemical similarities to compounds with known activity. The whole process is at best hit-or-miss, with the discovery of entirely new classes of biologically active compounds dependent it seems entirely on chance!

Point two. Compare and contrast the current medical model with the process of administering a dose, small enough not to be toxic, but not necessarily "potentized." Take a substance to a group of *randomly selected healthy volunteers,* observe the effects over time, and use those effects to guide further investigations into particular classes of clinical problems.

How much more efficient is this path, compared with randomly testing compounds against diseases? How many fewer stones are left unturned, when in a proving, *every* action of a substance is discovered. It is the difference between asking an open-ended (proving) question—"what hurts?"—versus a closed-ended one (current testing)—"does this hurt your right wrist?" The use of clinical provings to define areas worthy of further investigation is not limited to homeopathy, but is an advance over current methodology, and that by itself merits further investigation!

In essence, what this does is change the current drug pipeline, changing the Preclinical and Phase 1 trials, making them more efficient and useful. **Currently, we test a drug to a disease. What we suggest is adding a step. This would be the open-ended step, where we test a substance on healthy volunteers, testing the substance at sub-toxic doses, but pushing the test to developing symptoms.** The symptoms would then show locations where the substance may have efficacy. Then testing the substance on diseases in that location would be the next step. Without this step we test a substance/drug against a myriad of diseases, sometimes visiting the drug again 30 years later to see if it has benefits in the treatment of a different disease in a different part of the body. This new step streamlines this process, removing quite a bit of guesswork. This new step is the process of provings begun 200 years ago by Hahnemann!

Point three. This is the one that matters to the practicing physician. Another potential use of provings as an adjunct to existing methods of investigation, is as an answer to the problem of "sub-group selection." That is, all forms of current clinical investigation as randomized clinical trials, case-control studies, retrospective studies, result, if properly done, in statements about the qualities of a *population* of people, of a group.

Applying that information to the *individual*, to the patient in front of you, who we may sometimes forget, is the only member of the group that matters at the moment, is, again, a proposition fraught with a high degree of chance. Will the person behave like the 70% who responded to the therapy, or the 30% who did not? Or will he respond like the 50% (including members from both of the previous groups) who suffered some form of undesirable "side effect". Or will he respond like the 2% who suffered a potentially fatal or catastrophic reaction?

Medical science recognizes the need for a way to distinguish between individuals in a group before giving the drug to the patient. To which group does my patient belong? But the question has always been how to tell.

Provings provide a possible way to address this vital issue by more finely characterizing the individual. Instead of making decisions that apply to groups of people sharing only 6 or 10 characteristics, the number of characteristics increases towards infinity.

Provings could in this way allow an interface that has never existed in medicine. There will finally exist an interface between clinical trials and clinical practice, undergoing a quantum leap in medicine equivalent to the leap from algebra to calculus.

Homeopaths already have this interface by use of the repertory. As a symptom is discovered in a proving it may enter the repertory as a plain type. But as we clinically use it successfully to treat that symptom, we change the type to italics and as the substance is used even more it becomes a bold type. So our interface is easy to see. We naturally drift from Phase 1 to Phase 2, 3 and 4 but the current medical model lacks this tool. As such, until they adopt such a method, they will never be able to tell which subgroup any particular patient will belong to. At times not knowing is a nuisance or bothersome, but at times this lack of knowledge is lethal.

It was Dr. Ryan's greatest hope that these thoughts provoke interdisciplinary discussion between the homeopathic community and the current medical community. He envisioned that his medical world colleagues might see the utility of even this one part of homeopathic theory and practice in their own world, and in this way move closer to bridge over the chasm of belief that currently we share.

While I share these hopes, I have more concrete hopes based on the spirit of Hahnemann and those that came after him. The search for the truth has been currently dampened in our camp, by the belief that we do not need to adhere to strict guidelines. As such, we are currently drowning our databases with what I call "noise." *This is why many provings have all the provers developing symptoms, even the ones taking placebo.* Our community is not sophisticated enough to understand that point. A great shame on us.

In our medical colleagues' camp, the truth is hampered by not including a method that could streamline their inquiry and by publicly acknowledging that their research of new drugs is often based on natural medicine systems of healing.

What is the outcome that I seek? That we take all of this together and capture the historical, moral and scientific higher ground. That is where we were last century and where we need to be again. It is ours to take and ours to lose. Not the outside world, but ours. We held the higher ground pushing the boundaries forward. There is no reason why that can not happen again.

I am proposing a change in the drug-testing pipeline. For those not familiar with the process of bringing a new drug to market, this is radical, since the pipeline had not changed in many years. Nevertheless, it is a logical step forward for the drug companies. I am placing this proposal here to mark once more in the homeopathic camp a first proposal, one that will come to pass in the future. This is the ground we own. This is the standard we should uphold.

What is the outcome that I seek? Truth. Should both camps come closer to this vision that Christopher and I share, then homeopathy will become less of an outside force, less unknown and closer to being part of the mainstream.

In the next chapter we focus on some current misconceptions in our community of what a proving is and what a proving is not; the roots of those misconceptions being exactly what we discussed in this chapter.

— Chapter 5 —
What Provings Are Not

In the last chapter I mentioned the fact that we do not know enough about our own past. I reproduced documents which illustrated that point. I also talked about truth and how truth is hampered and limited when we function in ignorance. In this chapter, I want to discuss specifically how this has negatively impacted our profession and its very self-definition.

I apologize for the fact that I will not be writing here about many specific remedies that were proven. Rather, I am attempting to correct misconceptions and mistaken ideas. *Unfortunately, we do not yet have a forum for debate.* As such, I would like to discuss these problems in a general way. *That way, we can discuss the concepts and not the prover; the idea, not the personalities involved.* This is a discussion of science and fact. I know all the people involved are doing their best, trying to help this profession as they see fit. As such, we can have a healthy, respectful discussion of the ideas purported, leaving out the homeopaths themselves.

I would like to begin with an interesting observation. In this current resurgence of homeopathy, no other country has spent as much time and energy contending with the issues of provings as has England. Here is the interesting point. We can neatly categorize English homeopaths who are studying provings into two very different groups. The first group is the one that finds many, many symptoms in all of their provings. No matter what the substance being proven, it seems as though there are more symptoms elicited than can conveniently fit into a book. Interestingly, most of the current provings that fit in this category have more symptoms elicited than Hahnemann ever managed.

In the other category, we have homeopaths who have spent a good deal of their professional lives studying provings. They can not find many and at times *any* symptoms that would be attributed to the substance, when compared to the always occurring background noise. In the 1940-70's most of the provings that found some symptoms to isolate had either a scant handful to a dozen or two symptoms at most, these symptoms rarely helped us in the clinical setting.

So my question is an obvious one. How can these two groups both be describing the same process that we call provings, yet have such different findings?

A Quick Review

Again, in this current climate of our profession, current homeopathic thinking and writing discusses how we do not need to adhere to the standards that have developed in testing. Through various arguments made, the discussion is that we do not need to and are not able to mask a proving, nor can we have placebo trials. The arguments are made, as illustrated in the last chapter, that we never needed it before and that we do not need it now.

As I stated in the last chapter, I wholeheartedly *disagree* with this posture because it is factually inaccurate, flies against the spirit of *how*, and most importantly, *why* provings came to be in the first place. I warned that it is, in fact, a dangerous opinion. It limits us on the one hand and makes it possible to introduce mistakes into our work on the other. In this chapter I want to discuss some of the errors and inaccuracies that are occurring in our profession at this time, based on the way many provings are being conducted.

To review, one concept of scientific study—all scientific study—is that it attempts to understand the effect of *one* variable. To do that, you have to factor out all the other variables, to try to design a test where everything is accounted for and only one variable is left, the one you are testing. What we try to do is remove what is called the 'noise' all around an event, to see what the pure event is. The best experiments do this well.

Hahnemann was confronted with a science of his time that was based on suppositions and concepts that *seemed* as though they might be true, but were not tested, such as the doctrine of signatures and the use of polypharmacy. There was literally no way to discern what effect any one drug had on the individual or on a disease. When he shifted polypharmacy to individual drugs, he was attempting to clarify this issue.

The next step was to test each of the drugs, to see what effect they had on the disease and on the person. And so the poisoning of individual substances eventually led to the process of provings. In effect what Hahnemann was attempting to accomplish in medicine was the same as what other great minds were attempting at the same time in biology, botany, chemistry, and astronomy. By the description in the *Organon of Medicine* about the do's and don'ts, and by the moderation required in the proving process, we know he was developing the testing that has come to be the gold standard in medicine. He worked on the ever-increasing precision of filtering out background noise to see the *pure effect*. He was one of the leaders in a new vision of science. But where are we now?

Let me give you some examples of current provings. The following examples are not bizarre and on the fringe of our profession. Many students are currently being taught these proving techniques by some of the most vocal teachers today. What is more, a casual reader can not tell from the symptom list that the proving was conducted in one fashion or another. More than that, and most alarming to me, is that the repertory is beginning to reflect the "information" from these provings, with additions made into specific rubrics. This is not a trivial matter. Our very practices are dictated by these provings and this technique. Here are five examples.

Proving a Remedy in Meditation

Much criticized by those who do not understand this process, this method is enjoying popularity in England. The method here is to prove a substance either by taking it or not, either by ingesting it or by simply being in its proximity. Once this part is done, the participants all meditate on the substance and on their internal processes. The concept here is to establish a group that meditates together perhaps weekly or monthly. By developing this core group, the concept is that the individuals somehow come together as a whole, and can come to understand the substance being proven better. Also, from entering into a meditative state, the concept is that one is more attuned to the self and the changes that occur and that should make it easier to find the symptoms produced by the substance.

Proving a Song/Word/Movie

Also criticized by some, this method is enjoying popularity in conferences in Europe. The method here is that you have several people all exposed to the same song, the same word, the same movie, etc. During and after the exposure, you write down your impressions, your ideas and concepts, your feelings, and perhaps your physical symptoms. The concept is an easy one. You are all experiencing the same stimuli, your response to it is a reflection of your susceptibility and should reflect the symptoms of the proving.

Provings That Occur in a Seminar

The proving is conducted by giving a known or unknown substance to participants in a homeopathic seminar. This is becoming more popular in Europe and the United States. The methodology differs here from one teacher to another. Some give the substance to a few, while others give it to many participants. The concept is that they are at the seminar to learn homeopathy and doing a proving is part of the work of homeopathy. The concept is also that you have willing participants. Also this may be considered an example of a 'Homeopathic Phase 1 Trial' where we develop some general indications of the substance. The two examples listed above may be *specific* examples of seminar provings.

Dream Provings

The method is simple and has become somewhat popular in Europe and is gaining interest in the United States. As the name suggests, this method involves proving a substance and focusing on the symptoms which it elicits in the unconscious play of dreams. Dream work is long established in many cultures and in some fields of study in psychology. The method is: either to take the remedy and record the dreams or sleep with the remedy under your pillow and record your dreams, or think about a remedy and record your dreams. The concept is that the dream-state in some way is influenced by the proving and that the changes mirror the mental/emotional state of the prover. This is sometimes done during a conference so is also an example of seminar provings.

N=Infinity

Here the concept of a proving is stretched to the ultimate. The method is to test a substance, whether it is in a seminar or not does not matter. The methodology allows you to include anything that happens in the outside world that somehow relates to the substance you are proving. It does not matter if everyone took the substance or not, the fact that the test is underway is enough to allow the inclusion of anyone's symptoms. The concept here is beyond Carl Jung's concept of collective unconscious and synchronicity. Since the test is underway, if anything happens involving the substance it fits within the remedy somehow. Here the great works of Jung and Sheldrake, among others are used to justify the approach.

There are several other forms of non-traditional provings. Actually it seems as though they develop daily, but I think the ones described above are enough to help me discuss the problems we now face. By illustrating the inherent difficulties in some of these methodologies; and by showing their inherent flaws, I hope to show that all these difficulties and many more occur because we, as a profession, have incorporated grave misconceptions and inaccuracies into the very nature of homeopathy in general and provings in particular. So let's go through these one by one.

I know many of the people who began these concepts. Many of them I count as friends. So it is not their character or their motives that I question. They are all honorable people. It is their methodology and thinking process that I find questionable. As such, this discussion should allow the originators of these systems to answer, defend, expand, refine, redefine, abandon, change any or all of their work. We all benefit from discussion of our basic assumptions.

Misconception #1 - We Don't Need Masking and Blinding

I addressed this in the last chapter. Not only is this historically incorrect but it flies in the face of the purpose of a proving. The reason we go through the trouble in the first place is to try to isolate the effect of this one substance from all other effects. By masking and placebo we diminish the preconceptions of the prover. This has been demonstrated in countless experiments in the world of science and has been demonstrated in our community, as can be read in Volume Two of this work.

Several times through the years, we have had people tell their provers that the remedy they are going to prove is one remedy, when in reality they either only gave placebo or gave a different remedy. In either instance, provers developed symptoms of the remedy they *thought* they were given. The point is clear. If all you have to do is mention a word and you develop the same symptoms as someone who takes a remedy, then there is no way to separate the effect of the substance from any background noise. This is one of the reasons why some homeopaths think that provings are meaningless, as there is no way to separate symptoms of the substance from background noise.

Misconception #2 - Dreams

Here, I feel I must take a bit of the blame. When I was working on my first book, the pediatric *materia medica*, I found myself going through a very methodical process. I looked at cured cases, and separated all the cured symptoms and indications found in the cases. I noted that in many cases the dreams and their interpretations fit nicely with their general overall mental/emotional state. I began to teach that and to write my *materia medica*, accordingly. I clearly recognized the relevance of dreams to our work. I was the first one in homeopathy to break with a long tradition of locating sleep symptoms toward the end of a *materia medica*; rather, when I wrote the *materia medica*, I placed sleep symptoms right after the mental/emotional symptoms, to reflect their significance and connectedness to the mental/emotional symptoms. This began in the mid 1980's.

A few years after that, different homeopaths took on the concept full-force. No one was sure who began what, but within a few years many teachers were teaching about the importance of sleep and most especially, dreams. Many began to prescribe solely basing their prescription on dreams reported. It was not a far stretch to learn that after a few more years, the dream provings began. After all, we can recall that the practice of homeopathy and the proving process are mirror images of themselves. If you introduce a concept into one side of that equilibrium, you will eventually see it in the other side.

It was never my intention for things to get to this point. I never conceived that some homeopaths would take the simple concept so out of context. My point was very simple. The *interpretation* of the dream by the patient may give us a hint, a reflection of the way they look at the rest of the world, especially the images and emotions that resonate with the rest of the case.

So dreaming of a snake or a dog or the rain did not matter as much as how the patient *related* to the dream. The prescribing of remedies based on dreams is wrong, pure and simple. I would say that about any part of the case; mental or emotional or physical. You have to pay attention to where the energy is. Sometimes the dreams are intense and relevant, sometimes the arthritis is. A homeopath must be adept enough to understand each symptom in context, not to merely grasp at particular symptoms or unique dreams. One must look to where the complaint is, not to just a part of the case. Looking at only a part will always lead to inaccuracies, especially when the most severe symptoms do not reside in the part examined.

While this type of proving may seem strange and bizarre to many of you, look at other provings that have hundreds and hundreds or thousands of symptoms. You will find many dreams listed there. Part of this dream proving concept has trickled into many provings. At the rate we are going, the dream section will likely become one of the largest sections of the repertory. What makes this work dangerous and full of inaccuracies is the following point.

Misconception #3 - Hawthorne Effect

In the 1920's, Western Electric experimented with some people in Hawthorne, Illinois. They varied the experiment by giving subjects various amounts of illumination—the variable tested, with some receiving a lot more than usual, some less than usual and some the same. It turned out they were all effected. This has been reported many times in many experiments. The concept here is that when you begin to pay attention to someone and ask them to become more introspective, to report about themselves, everyone (a person taking a substance or not) reports more symptoms. **By you showing interest, you are intruding in the experiment. Individual behavior is changed by the person knowing that he is the subject of a study.** This is not a placebo effect. Rather, think of it this way. If I ask you to tell me all the symptoms you felt in the last week, you could draw up a list. If I then ask you to write down for me all the symptoms as you are experiencing them for the upcoming week, you will come close to what this effect is. Almost all people will have a much longer list on the second week. This may be to please the tester, but mostly it is because we are asking the participant to pay extra attention. As you become more introspective, the threshold of becoming conscious of your internal state drops. Now you sense much more, now you are aware of much more.

Now, if you look at the different types of provings mentioned above, one thing is not only common but striking. All of them are *accentuating* the Hawthorne Effect. All of the above methodologies make the person increasingly introspective about his or her state and therefore make him more aware of the minute by minute experience of life. **In effect, we have dropped the threshold bar** *so* **low that we are now able to find many, many symptoms.**

The dream provings are a great example of this effect. Many people report an increased ability to recall dreams, and the dreams are more remarkable once they begin a proving. Of course this is also true for anyone doing dream work. A significant proportion of people doing any dream work will begin to recall their dreams better. Now it turns out a significant number of people doing dream work report dreams of snakes, of being chased, of their teeth falling out, etc. These have been entering the proving documents in an increasing way. In other words, the very process of recalling dreams for everyone, produces more dreams in the proving document. Provings ask us to pay more attention and therefore we now have many more dreams. *So we have two variables at work in these provings, the substance being proven and the Hawthorne Effect.*

I believe this is why some investigators can find many hundreds of symptoms and even thousands of symptoms, while others only find a handful. In the former, the bar is so low that many people will attribute many or all of their experiences to the proving. **Herein lies the mistake. We have not filtered out background noise well enough in the experimental design. We actually have 2 interventions. One is taking the substance and seeing what effect that substance has upon the individual. The second intervention is the proving test itself.** By asking a person to become more introspective–something inherent in the process of a proving–you are also testing what becoming introspective can do to a symptom list. As you can guess, it makes the symptom list grow by leaps and bounds, as is evident in many of the current provings.

Misconception #4 - What Are We Testing?

Here we find yet another problem with many of the designs above. This may in fact be the biggest problem of all. When we all meditate together, or are all in the same seminar or class, we have coalesced into a tighter experimental group. Now we have many things in common, so what is it that we are testing? Are we testing the substance? Are we testing the air? Are we testing the seminar? Are we testing the sound system? Are we testing the fact that we are away from home? Are we testing the new foods? What is it that we are testing?

Hahnemann tried to filter all these out. His design had us all stay individually as we were and test us as we were. He did not look for us to coalesce, as it becomes impossible to tell what it is that we are testing. Was his methodology perfect? Of course not. But it is important to recall what he was attempting. Hahnemann was traveling on a journey of discovery, marking steps towards where we are now. Knowledge is cumulative, he would have progressed, not gone backwards.

And here is the proof. Many who have been to a seminar such as this have told of how incredible the process was because the people who did not take the remedy developed the same symptoms as the people who did take it. Actually, in one trial, the best symptoms were all gotten from people who did not take the remedy, the placebo group in fact. The participants and teachers argue that this is possible because of the interconnectedness of all of us. That is why one person can take a remedy and twenty other people in the room can prove it.

As I wrote this I was looking at the last proving book I received in the mail from a colleague and friend. As I was looking at the book, I noticed that the placebo group symptoms were not only included, but they were listed as valid symptoms. The placebo group, mind you. I then turned to the new repertories and found that the symptoms were, and are, listed in the rubrics. The transfer from the placebo group to the proving group to the proving list to the repertory happened. This is not a future fear of mine, this is the reality of the situation at this time.

While I do not want to argue against interconnectedness, I would like to put forth a different possibility; one that fits all of the observations and our current experience of practice, as well as science. The threshold has dropped so low that a great deal of background noise is no longer being filtered out. As such, we are no longer filtering for only one substance but we are now including a great deal of our environment. Think about the last time you went to a conference; a great deal of your life changed during those days. With the bar lower, not only do you have the chance to give all of your new found symptoms but also the many new symptoms that are due to being in a new environment, eating away from home, being away from family, and so on. One can list dozens of factors that are altered by being at a conference and not at home.

Likewise, some of the factors are the same for all participants at a conference. There will be many symptoms that are similar among participants, because the stresses around them are similar. Yes, the symptoms of the proving substance will be present, but in an artificial environment with the threshold lowered and multiple common new stresses on the same group of people, you will develop new symptoms and there may be a similarity among the participants because they are in a similar environment. *Therefore the true symptom of the substance is buried within the multitude of symptoms from the lowered threshold.*

This is another reason, another explanation, besides the interconnectedness issue, that gives us these symptoms across people who take the remedy and people who do not. To be clear about this, having numerous people who did not take a substance or who took a placebo develop the same symptoms as the ones who *took* the substance is not a demonstration of our interconnectedness; rather it shows that the filters are so porous, and the threshold is so low that the experiment is faulty. Period!!!

I know this is going against the grain at the moment, but perhaps I write mostly for future generations! Let's go through this from the other side now. How is it possible that provers in general, up until some of this current crop, would develop many fewer symptoms but that now in many provings we see extreme sensitivity to substances that *many* people—those who took it and even those that did not—develop a myriad of symptoms?

Misconception #5 - Where is the Edge of a Proving? Where is the Boundary? Whose Proving is this Anyway?

You prove gasoline and OPEC raised the gas prices. You prove a particular flower and when you go to the movies, you see it in the film. You prove a substance from an animal that lives in a region of the world and while driving to work, while you are listening to the news on the radio, you hear news from that region of the world. Now, while this may sound odd to some of you, at this time entering this new millennium, many people conducting provings feel that there is absolutely a relationship in these types of occurrences. A colleague of mine is positive that by conducting a proving on a certain substance he managed to bring down the government of the country where that substance originates. To his humility, he does not say that *he* brought it down, nor that the conditions in that country made him prove that substance. To his credit he does not say any of this in public. But the belief is implicit and comes across in his teaching and writing. Proving done, government gone; you do the math! While I enjoy my colleague and his belief and this is left for a harmless philosophical discussion over a beer, it does reflect a certain belief system in some current proving circles.

In this new belief the proving really has no boundary, has no edge, has no limitation, other than the one you place on it. I would like to give you several examples. While proving a remedy, someone loses their vial, so they never take the remedy to prove. I know provings where the symptom of losing things was taken because of that. Not only that, but since the person was considered part of the proving then they continued to use any symptoms that they developed.

Because of these beliefs which are circulating, I know of provings that are currently published, where the symptoms were incorporated in the repertory, where the symptoms developed before the proving even began, sometimes before the person took the remedy by a day or by weeks and sometimes it is before the person turned out to take a placebo. It did not matter. The symptoms were included.

Another person proved a remedy of a tree and then heard about that type of tree falling on a road and causing an accident. So accidents, trauma, lying down, all become symptoms of the new remedy.

Another person proved a remedy made from a bird. He later heard that that bird is not nearing extinction as previously thought. Probably from the remedy proving.

Another prover had car troubles. His car was Japanese, and at the same time the Japanese economy was breaking down as well. Money troubles were then considered an important symptom in the proving. These examples are all about the prover and the world at large.

What about their interactions with the world and the people around them? Since there is no edge, no limit in a proving, *as demonstrated by the fact that the placebo group gets the same symptoms as the other provers and at times even better symptoms*, it becomes fair game to take the experiences of loved ones *around* the provers. So a prover takes the substance, and then his or her wife or husband develops symptoms; those symptoms now enter into our proving list. So if a prover comes home and her husband is unusually irritable, that makes it into the proving. If you take the proving substance and then your wife is in an accident, maybe the accident is part of the proving. I can give many examples here. This sort of thinking may seem humorous to some, but it is not; especially when these symptoms then make it into our materia medica and our repertories, making the tools of our trade full of misleading information, ultimately making the practice of homeopathy, already challenging, that much more difficult.

Misconception #6 - Can you Prove an Experience?

Can you prove an experience? It's a good question. Some people say you can. And as a result they prove music. People sit around listening to music and writing their impressions down. Other people have actually potentized music and then proved it. Some have potentized movies or books. For the people who believe this is possible, then how is it possible to prove a remedy in a seminar? Clearly the seminar *is an experience* that everyone is 'proving' at the same time that you are trying to 'conduct' a proving. How do you separate the experience of the joke, a minor proving, from the traffic jam to get there, 'proving' a frustrating experience. What about the fact that you are still 'proving' the movie from last night, while you are attempting to conduct a proving? In short, if you can prove an experience, then provings can never be conducted in the first place, because we are never devoid of experience. We are filled with many experiences every day, every moment. If experiences are proven, then we undergo thousands of provings daily, with every interaction we have. It would not be possible to isolate one variable, as Hahnemann was attempting to do and therefore this whole exercise would be meaningless.

Misconception #7 - Meditation Works

I have only good things to say about meditation. I think every person should begin his or her day by meditating. However, the process is wholly opposite to what we are trying to achieve in a proving. A proving has us being *Stressed* by a substance and the symptoms elicited are the ones of our individual *Straining* in response. A meditation first has us change our threshold, actually dropping it to as low as it can go, and then we basically reach out to the substance and developing impressions. This is taking a great idea, meditation, and misusing it, based on a lack of understanding of what the actual process of a proving is. It needs to reach us, so that our predisposition may feel that *Stress* and therefore *Strain* because of it, not the other way around.

Misconception #8 - Do Objects Have Attributes Outside of Their Constituent Parts?

Would potentizing a brick from a monastery be equivalent to potentizing a similar brick from a regular house? Would potentizing a glass that was used in sacred rituals be equivalent to potentizing a glass that came from the same period but was used in everyday affairs? Or what about a glass that was used for a particular function, but has sat in a museum for the past 100 years?

While these questions may seem odd or strange, we have a new remedy in our materia medica. It is called the *Berlin Wall*. The original proving, I believe, was a meditative proving, but the point for me here is something else. Can objects that are used in certain types of situations, or experiences, inherit some of those qualities? According to people who have used this remedy, it is used for power and for oppressing others. Now, while not arguing the *Berlin Wall* itself, my question comes to the attribute or the rocks themselves. Did the rocks themselves inherit in some way the attributes of what that wall was used for? Proponents argue the answer is yes. But to me the answer can not be yes.

Let me give you a short parody: I may have discovered something! I think the metal that makes a refrigerator may be a good substitute for Lycopodium when Lycopodium does not work. You know, all it is concerned with is getting filled up; constantly concerned with food. And you know, there is all the gas stuff in the back of the refrigerator. As an aside, maybe people are not milk intolerant. Maybe the milk being in the refrigerator somehow takes some of the attributes of the metal, and then we get Lycopodium-like symptoms when we drink the milk. And of course, that metal would be more psoric, as opposed to the same metal in a vacuum cleaner, which, being so thin, and constantly sucking up hungrily, would be more syphilitic, as opposed to the airplane metal which is all over the map, i.e., tubercular, except when they try to turn it more sycotic by painting the back all those interesting bright colors!!

Okay, so I am being a bit lighthearted here. But truth be told, I am not taking this whole approach to provings in jest. It is extremely serious—actually essential—for me. But it is my hope that comic relief, (or its attempt!) can help the discussion flow more easily!

So the basic idea is: can a substance, an object, take on qualities that we attribute to it through belief and use, and can those qualities pass on to the proving? Of course, objects take on significance. Think of all the bloodshed lost over arguing who owns a building, a castle, a ring. Think about the shroud of Turin, the scrolls in a synagogue, even the idea of facing to the East in prayer. How about finding an old photograph of a friend or your child. I think we all agree that objects take on incredible importance. The question is, does that quality get impregnated into the actual proving substance?

For me the answer is no. Where the quality is inherent in the substance, I believe that what is being overlooked is the concept of emergence. An emergent quality is one that is unpredicted from its parts. I write about this at length elsewhere. For example, the properties of hydrogen and oxygen are well known, but there is no way to conceptualize the properties of water from these two ingredients. The properties of water are emergent and part of the whole.

Once you reduce the picture to ashes, the building to rubble, the glass to shards, I do not think it would be possible to tell which parts came from where. The qualities that are missing were emergent ones and no longer apply.

Likewise, I do not think that the Berlin wall 'remembered' its use. If it had, then it should have recalled it all. How it suffocated in the ground. How people exploded it out of the ground, took hammers to it and chopped it into bits to be used in the wall. How it was drowned in water. How it spun and spun in a truck. How it stood silently as it had bloodshed poured on it, along with beer bottles, and bullets. How it got famous and was in so many movies. How it made a president come to talk to it. How it was rained on with water and pollution. How it was stepped on. How it was celebrated on, chipped away at, broken, and finally bottled and sold at a dear price. You see my point is, if you are going to anthropomorphize an object, how can you pick your particular quality? There are multitudinous images, experiences and time factors to choose from. Which one is right?

Another example. Take any plant we use. Was it stepped on, urinated upon, chewed at, flown over, finally picked, killed in its youth, and drowned in alcohol? I do not believe that those aspects should or do come out in the provings.

Lastly, did we prove *Pulsatilla*, or did we prove a specific plant that lived through several events that other *Pulsatilla* plants did not go through? If this is the case then not only do we need a specific remedy as a simillimum but also we need the specific plant from that species, the single one on that particular hill growing at this particular time in history. This is not what is found in practice, thank God. If not in practice then I think not in the proving as well. As I keep reiterating, they, by definition, mirror each other.

Misconception #9 - Doctrine of Signatures

My first interest in medicine, before homeopathy, was the *Doctrine of Signatures.* In fact, I believe I got into medical school from my writing on the subject. Not that I practiced it, I was pretty young. I mostly covered the whole history of it. I rejected it, for the same reason that it gets rejected each time it arises again. The main problem with it is that there is no real way to predict, other than from guesswork. For every example given to support its truth there are numerous examples against.

The main detriment to the theory is that it is a *lagging indicator* not a *predicting indicator*. In other words, only after we use substances in nature do we see the qualities that we attribute to it and pick those qualities to highlight. This flower is yellow and therefore is used for the liver complaints, but there are many other plants that are yellow and would make you sick if you used them for a liver complaint. Again for every example, there are countless others that prove it wrong. After you use a substance successfully you may say, "gosh, it looks like the brain and helps memory!" That is a *lagging indicator* and is misleading.

What many people do not know is that Hahnemann knew the concept and the practice of the *Doctrine of Signatures* very well. You see, it was a dominant player in the medical treatment of his time. He wrote pages and pages about why the practice of medicine by this doctrine was a great mistake. What some current homeopaths fail to appreciate is that he came up with the concept of provings as a way to test a substance and not have a predetermined assumption on how it may affect the person. *Provings arose in part, from attempting to eliminate the Doctrine of Signatures!! It is ironic, at best, though sad to me personally, that I see the homeopathic profession bring this back. Homeopathy was created as a science to draw us out of the darkness. I can not believe there are those that want to go backwards. It is a refutation and a rejection of the spirit of homeopathy. It breaks the direct line to Hahnemann.*

Misconception #10 - Is it a Proving or an Etiology?

This goes back to the point that you prove substances not experiences. Most etiologies, though not all, are experiences. We use them as clues to the remedies. In fact we use them as chief examples, as rubrics exemplifying and forming a *Segment*. Herein lies the difference between isopathy and homeopathy. In isopathy, you would take the substance that caused the problem. In contrast, in homeopathy we use a substance that produces the similar symptoms. If we were to see a frightening movie, the isopath would potentize the celluloid and give it to the patient, whereas the homeopath would give a substance, mineral, animal or plant, which produces similar symptoms. *Isopathy sometimes works, but when it does, it will be found that the substance is also homeopathic to the case.*

Let me give you an example of what I mean. Instead of giving a sad patient story, I will tell you a funny thing that happened to me as an example. I was sitting in a theater discussing a play with a gentleman who was becoming a friend. During a pause in the discussion, he asked me if we could talk about homeopathy for a few minutes. I was wanting to watch my daughter on the stage rehearsing but said sure. He asked me how long it takes for a remedy to begin to work. He was not a patient of mine, so I asked him how long he had been taking the remedy. He said several months, but he did not see any difference in his complaints. I asked him what remedy he was taking, I was getting curious. He said, "NYC." I said, "What? Can you say that again?" He said he was taking *"New York City."* He said that some of his complaints began during the busy life he had when living there, so that is what the homeopath gave him. I was dumfounded. In the awkwardness of the moment, I could not think of what to say, so I asked him what potency he took. He replied that it was a 30c. So there it was, After hearing about people potentizing dollar bills because of poverty issues, potentizing all sorts of things, it has finally come to potentizing New York City.

Misconception #11 - It's a Great Big Interconnected World Impacting You

So what we are left with is the belief from those conducting such provings that the world is totally interconnected and that when we prove a remedy, we are changing the fabric of life on this planet. I actually believe in an interconnectedness of all life. However, the point of a study is to design the experiment so that we isolate one variable and learn qualities about that variable. That essentially is the only difficult part of a study. If you do not do that well, the study becomes meaningless. If this whole view, reflected in the way some of these provings are conducted, is correct, then the concept of proving becomes null and void. *Since the process is designed to try to find the symptoms this one substance will elicit, this very definition and belief of the total seamless interconnectedness of everything can never allow a proving to exist.* It becomes null and void by its own definition. The result is just what would be expected. All the provers develop symptoms and all provers develop many symptoms but this is because the threshold is so low because there are no barriers between the proving and the rest of existence.

Misconception #12 - What We Find in Practice

One of the most troubling aspects of this new work has been the complete divorcing of the proving experience from actual practice; from our clinical experience. I give here two different examples. Very often when we give a remedy that is incorrect, symptoms arise in the person. But often it is our experience that nothing seems to happen. Some people are not sensitive to the wrong remedies that they take. Much of my practice is treating patients sent to me by other homeopaths. By careful history taking, I can see the remedies that impacted the person and the ones that did not. So from both situations, I understand that many times, we give a remedy and nothing happens. Likewise, I have been at seminars given by other homeopaths where, there too, nothing seemed to happen with the wrong remedy given.

This of course makes sense from our concept of individual predisposition. Not everyone is sensitive to substances equally. This forms the very foundation of homeopathy. What then can I make of the fact that most, if not all people in some of these provings develop all the same symptoms? If we say that they are all indeed proving the remedy, then we are negating our experience in practice that often nothing happens when giving the incorrect remedy. *More than that, we get rid of the concept of individuality and susceptibility, the definition and uniqueness of provings and case taking and, most importantly, the hallmark and promise of homeopathy. We do not have to find a special remedy that is similar. There are no special remedies. There are no similar remedies. Everything is connected. That is the natural extension of this idea.*

I believe that the mass of symptoms included in provings is the mirroring of our experience in case taking. When we elicit the history, we find many, many symptoms. It is up to us to make coherent sense from the mass of information elicited. We use the symptoms that will lead to the remedy. Yes we find many, many symptoms, but we say that they are common to the human experience. Some of the current provings do not do that well enough. It is this lowering of the bar that lets so many symptoms into the books now.

Misconception #13 - It Will Not Impact Your Practice

This is probably the worst implication of this faulty belief system. The proving model and procedure and concept of symptom selection is the mirror image of the case taking and selection of the remedy. So what is the implication of this system in practice? When you take a case history where does the history end? For example if your patient's husband fell, should your patient take *Arnica*? If on the way to work you heard that the Japanese economy is recovering should you give your first patient *Aurum*? If you look out the window and see a certain bird fly by, should you give that remedy?

One mirrors the other. If your borders are not tighter, if your threshold is not high enough, then your analysis of patients will eventually follow suit. One will mirror the other. I have seen my colleagues go through this for many years. It winds up being a painful process to all involved, at the end. The effect is frightening for me to see. The problems are so numerous that it will take a long time to correct.

I think one of the biggest problems is the repertory. The repertory does not necessarily tell us how the proving was conducted. It gives us the name of the prover only. Many of the newer repertories have raced to include all the new information. This means that we are including a great deal of 'noise' because the threshold is so low. One of two things is going to happen to that remedy in that rubric. Because the repertory is being bombarded with new remedies that are listed in thousands of rubrics, it means that the remedy will repertorize out often. This means that many people will prescribe it. Due to the high frequency of use, we will eventually get to understand the real image of the remedy. Most of the prescriptions will not be curative. However, some will. The high volume of prescriptions will allow that *some* people will benefit from its use. The information garnered from *those* patients will develop the real use of the remedy.

But this method is messy, imprecise, and ultimately dangerous to some of the people who do not receive a remedy in a timely fashion that could help them. The problem with the repertory is as follows. Once the 'noise' is included in the repertory, there is no easy way to extricate it.

One of the oddest concepts to come out of this currently popular view is that there is no such thing as polychrest remedies. This is obviously a forgone conclusion once you take this view into account. Most of our remedies, ones we have used for a hundred years do not have as many symptoms as some of these new proving remedies. So from this point of view there are no polychrests, or rather all remedies are polychrests. Right or wrong, I talk about this more in other places, but I mention it here because it is an implicit outcome of this belief system.

Let me end with this thought. I have my own concepts of how to conduct a proving and have conducted them accordingly. I do not believe there is a perfect way. I do believe that perfection should be sought, though. I mentioned several types of provings and some of the rationales used in conducting them. While I am not necessarily arguing against innovation,

I am arguing against sloppy process. I have my own concepts of why I like or do not like any of these methodologies. However, from the point of view of those conducting such provings, if you consider it as a whole, their very own theory argues against their very own methodology.

I once sat next to the editor of one of these books. The homeopath in charge of the proving was describing a case and wanted us to *"guess"* the remedy. The homeopathic editor whispered to me a new remedy, then a different or maybe a third new one that it could be; really so many common symptoms and nothing really to prescribe upon! This editor began to laugh, because it was all so funny! Not to me. We have included so many symptoms that all the remedies begin to look alike.

As I began to describe above, the question comes down to how low or how high to put the threshold bar. Too low and every symptom enters into the *materia medica.* Too high, and we find no symptoms at all. In the next chapter I would like to describe a process that I have developed to place the bar sufficiently high to eliminate much of the 'noise' but which still allows symptoms to be developed and counted.

— Chapter 6 —
What Provings Are or Great Exaptations

In the last chapter I discussed several methodologies for conducting provings that are gaining popularity at this time. While I applaud the desire and the urge to add to our knowledge base, I pointed out the shortcomings of those methods. Mostly, the problem has been the inclusion of too many symptoms that do not belong to the proven substance. As such, this means that the symptoms that *do* belong to the proving are buried in and amongst the symptoms that do not. Time will fix this problem. As homeopaths over-prescribe the remedy, they will eventually confirm the symptoms that indicate the remedy and let go of the other symptoms. This 'messiness' takes time, takes many incorrect prescriptions and places people in danger from *not* receiving the correct remedy.

A Possible History

We do not clearly have Hahnemann's history to find out how it was that he came up with the concept of provings, but there is enough that we do know about his history to put together a rough 'guess' of what it was, at least from the rational, scientific point of view. What I want to describe now is how a scientist works. You see, models and concepts not only must seem to work, they must have a certain elegance to them, they must be 'pretty' for lack of another term. Scientists know what I mean. All great scientific theory is pretty to look at. It is when it is not understood that it becomes 'bulky' with added concepts and added points. When Newton described the physical world or Einstein described relativity, their models were short and elegant.

Once Hahnemann came up with the concept of treating with similars—an elegant concept—then many, many other concepts flowed from there. Many of those concepts were not new to him but surrounded him most of his adult life. This then is the concept of *exaptation*. It is a leap of evolution, a leap of ability or thought, but with objects that have existed long before. (One of the greatest examples of *exaptation* is the development and evolution of voice and speech, which "jumped" into existence, even though the vocal cords were present for many years before.) A leap, an evolutionary large step forward, *exaptation*, that is what happened once the concept of similars became firmly entranced in Hahnemann's mind.

We know that when he gave up practice and went into translating and working with medical texts in general, he became involved in trying to understand the poisoning effect of different drugs. At that time, as now, physicians had to learn what the toxic effects are of any substance they dispense to patients. At that time, a fair number of substances prescribed were plants or minerals. The trick was trying to understand the toxic effects of any *one* substance. The practice of the time was *polypharmacy*. One dispensed several substances at once. To which did the toxic effect belong? This may sound bizarre or unscientific to us at this point, but at that time there was clear rationale for that method of practice. For a modern example of this method, just to put it in context with today's practice, we would have to look to Chinese medicine. In today's world it is not just customary but expected to prescribe more than one herb at a time; there is a whole cosmology to explain why and how one compounds six, eight, ten, or a dozen plants into one formula. Now, I am not denigrating it or claiming that there is a problem there, I am just giving the example of how, given a certain time in history, any one form of practice not only makes sense but is to be expected.

That is how it was then. Several to many drugs were given at a time. But it seems that even then, there were reports that described the effect of individual toxic plants. We know that Hahnemann was keenly aware of these reports and was interested in them as he wrote about that topic. Once we are aware of this area of research in his life, the rest of his development into the world of provings can be seen as a simple evolution of an idea. It can be seen as a progression, rather than the divine intervention that is currently perceived by our profession, without rationale or reason.

He was the consummate scientist. All his work shows that. Once he settled on the concept of treating by matching the similar, the next step for this work was to develop a rational map of the drugs and their toxic effects. One would have to poison people with individual substances to see the single effect. By reducing the experiment to just one drug, you were more likely to find the symptoms of that one substance and thereby have the symptoms to match, i.e., the simillimum.

Of course by poisoning people, you risk losing friends and going to jail! So, the solution was, and is, to test substances that are already in use, already in the pharmacopoeia. Now, since the testers would not be sick and would not actually *need* the drug at that time, it seemed unnecessary to take them at the lethal or toxic dose. And so began the process of diminishing the amount of substance which a proving would test.

The next step was again a small one. Give minute amounts that would produce symptoms and use those symptoms to prescribe upon. Once the drug is diminished greatly, one finds an interesting point. Some people are more sensitive than others. Some develop a few symptoms while others develop many symptoms. Some develop minor symptoms while others develop intense, exaggerated symptoms. And you once again confirm the concept of individual predisposition.

While we do not have it all laid out like this in his words, all the pieces were there and in play during his life. We know that. As such, it seems extremely probable that his work synthesized his main interests of codifying medicines in some large scheme. The scheme he settled on was treating by the matching of symptoms, by the simillimum. Once that decision was made, then the next ones follow naturally: test individual substances to find their toxic effects, test them one at a time, test them in less than lethal doses, test them in not quite toxic doses, test them in minute doses having individuals who are sensitive to the substance develop the clearer symptoms; and, using healthy subjects for the same reason as using one drug, to limit the symptoms that may confound us. While all these may seem like major innovations in thinking, they are all minor modifications, minor refinements upon his original idea.

His process led us to the provings as we know them in the *Organon of Medicine*, as well as to Phase 1 Drug Trials. The process was to remove as much as you can of any kind of 'noise' that might hide what the real substance's symptomatology might be. Obviously, this would be the most important part of homeopathy. If you did not include the correct symptoms of the toxicology of the substance, how could you ever try to match them to a patient; homeopathy would fail before it began because the *homeo* part of homeopathy would be missing. Hahnemann's search was for the truth. Medical testing and experimentation has moved forward since Hahnemann's methodology, but still maintains the concept of testing to find more perfect truths.

With that in mind it seems backwards in thinking to include symptoms into provings that the method had aimed at removing in the first place. He worked on removing *Signatures* and folklore and replacing them with a perfect truth that he saw in the concept of the Simillimum. Many of today's provings actually do go backwards. It is for that very reason that they contain so many symptoms, as opposed to older provings. We are including things we should not be including. We are including symptoms that do not really belong to the substance being proven. As I mentioned before, this eventually will get worked out by time and by trial and error but in the meantime there will be many wrong prescriptions, and it will warp our *materia medica* and repertory.

Here is a sobering fact to illustrate my point. There are several remedies new to homeopathy which contain 1,000–2,000 symptoms. There will be more and more in the near future. It places these remedies in the top percents of the remedies that we have. Many of the remedies we use daily are listed in less rubrics than that. How is it possible that we proved and used these remedies for a hundred years and still have only hundreds of symptoms after thousands of cures. How is it possible that we have so many new remedies that have so many symptoms? Like it or not, we are experiencing a warping of our *materia medica*.

How is it possible that we have had so many provings in the past with so many fewer symptoms than many of the provings occurring today? One possible answer is that what we call provings today are in some way *different* from what we called provings in the past; they must differ in some essential ways.

This confusion around what to include and what to exclude—the most important first step in any scientific model—has led in many of the new provings to burying the symptoms that *should* be there within the mundane symptoms that should not really be there in the first place and that will not lead to the remedy selection.

I have focused most of the previous chapters on the problem of inclusion, that we are including much too many symptoms. This is because we do not have a clear model of what occurs in a proving. Also possible is the opposite phenomenon in the homeopathic world. There are some homeopaths who have researched provings and have come up with the conclusion that there are *no* reliable symptoms that occur in the proving that can not be attributed to the background noise. To them it all looks like random noise. Here it is the same exact problem. Without a clear model of a proving, not just of the methodology but of what actually occurs in a proving, it could easily all look random.

ANATOMY OF A PROVING

This time, I will describe one way to conduct a proving. How can we keep the bar high enough up and still find the symptoms that the substance really does cause? This is how I do it. This is my thinking process. It is what I consider as the best way to work the difficulties inherent in the process. Is it the best way? Probably not. But it is one way. Whether you adhere to these guidelines or others, or develop your own, one thing is clear. You have to have an epistemology, a guiding principle, a model that can at the same time explain the proving process and be coherent with other aspects of homeopathic theory and practice. It must come closer to reality.

Size of proving

The size of the proving should match the purpose of the proving. If the proving is conducted as a personal experience, just to see what it is like to prove a substance, or to try to understand a substance, then the size could just be one person. While this is a test of the remedy, it probably will not count as a full proving.

A full proving should have enough people participating so that a full picture is elicited. Here, I suggest between 15-40 people, hopefully closer to 30. This number allows for dropouts, as most experiments have them, as well as for placebo arms of the test. The number fits very well with the model that we devised for what actually happens in the proving. As you recall from previous chapters, the model for the proving is as follows:

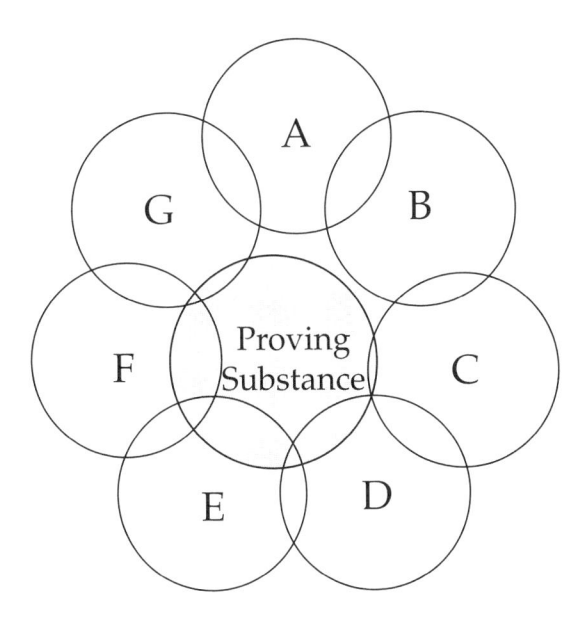

Figure 1

Figure 1 illustrates the model whereby different provers, having different constitutions will have a variety of sensitivities to the remedy. Some will be very sensitive, while others will have no appreciable sensitivity to the proving substance. *This model then insists or drives the design so that we have enough participants to make sure that we develop a full picture of the remedy.*

To illustrate the point, lets turn to Figure 1: If we had a small cohort of provers and they were in the constitution **A**, then few, if any, proving symptoms will develop. Likewise, if we had only provers who were in a constitutional state that needed **D** or **E**, then while we do develop proving symptoms, they are only of that part of the verum. In other words the full picture is not developed because we are not seeing what the **C**, **F**, and **G** provers of those constitutions will produce.

The more people one has involved in the proving, the more likely it is that we will have different constitutional sensitivities towards the verum and therefore be more likely to develop a fuller image of the remedy.

Size does become impractical and unwieldy, expensive and perhaps unnecessary. Keeping track of hundreds of participants over a long period of time becomes very difficult, though possible. The purpose for a large group, though, becomes questionable from the viewpoint of my model. (In my proving of *Alcoholus*, I actually had over 100 provers. Why? I conducted the proving as several separate provings. Each year a different group of 30-40 people would prove the same substance. While not necessary for the proving, I did that to test my model at the same time. So, my proving was conducted for the remedy but also for fine-tuning and checking on the methodology.)

Let's recall that the purpose of a proving is to give us some of the symptoms to prescribe upon. Once we have those symptoms and prescribe, we begin to find the symptoms that are useful for successful prescriptions and which ones are not. We shift from the testing/experimenting phase to the maturing phase of understanding a remedy. A mid-size group is large enough to show us the symptoms that we will prescribe upon. After that we have mostly duplication.

The only benefit of a larger group, after the original test, is if we can determine who was sensitive to the substance and who produced clear and important symptoms. We do not know that until a later date, until the first phase is over. Once we finish the proving and find the sensitive people, we can reprove the remedy using them or we can reprove the remedy with other people who are very similar constitutionally to the sensitive people from the first phase of the test. Simply duplicating information, using all people of constitutional states that are not sensitive to the remedy adds very little to the goal—finding symptoms to prescribe upon.

If one does wish to use a large cohort, then the purpose should be to use that first stage for the express purpose of finding the really sensitive people and excluding the rest. Here if you wish to start with 300, 400 or even 500 provers, that is fine, but then only use the provers showing a keen sensitivity to the substance.

A second reason for having a larger cohort is to have the study be multi-centered or even multi-cultural, to see if we find variations in the proving. For example, some people in some cultures may prove, or at the very least, may pay attention to different things. This has been confirmed already in older studies. While some studies have shown exactly the same symptoms even though they were conducted in different countries, others have shown different symptoms in different countries.

Aside from these two reasons, there is no purpose to having a larger cohort. The proving test is to get us to the clinical phase and 15-40 people will do that well.

The Constitution

There is one aspect to size that has not been discussed or thought of enough in conducting provings. **The thinking process about the predisposition of the prover has not been addressed in our profession, but clearly must be.** We know this for a fact, as the provers are rarely mentioned in terms of their constitutions. *The reason for this omission is obvious. Since there was no model of what was happening, there was no need to discuss the constitutional makeup of the provers, aside from occasional general descriptions.* I am afraid that this is an *un-homeopathic* view of people, as we are treating them all as equals. But clearly they are not.

From the homeopathic point of view, and according to this model, predispositions control so much of our interactions and responses to the outside world that they clearly also must control our responses to the substance being proven. *So the provers' predispositions are equal partners with the proving substance: one contributing the Stress and the other the predisposition to the Stress and then the response, the Strain.* Not thinking about the constitution of the prover is as negligent as not thinking about the proving substance. Just as we look at the substance in accidental poisonings to glean information about the substance, so too must we glean from the person's constitution and predispositions what kind of person may need a particular substance. In other words to what kind of person might the substance become homeopathic?

In many ways this should be considered some of the most important information that we discover. For example, in our proving of *Alcoholus*, we discovered that people who had a strong family history of alcoholism, as well as people who needed *Nux vomica* and *Lycopodium* constitutionally, were effected by the substance proven more than others. Now once you understand the remedy more fully and read about the liver symptoms of the remedy, then we can easily recognize some important points. For example the relationship between *Lycopodium* and *Alcoholus* makes sense when you think about the liver. That those needing *Nux vomica* would be sensitive to *Alcoholus* makes sense because of the desire for and aggravation from alcohol in many of those needing *Nux vomica*. Clearly, we begin to understand the substance being proven more if we know the type of constitutional makeup of people who are influenced by it. We also begin to see relationships between the new remedy and other existing remedies. This is a very important point that has been missed in all provings to date.

Therefore, much more important than the number of provers is the total number of different types of constitutional types. This adds a complication to the statistics, but think about it. Having 30 people of only 3 constitutions is definitely not as beneficial to us as having 10 people of varying constitutional types. Your likelihood of developing proving symptoms goes up from this diverse group. So when we talk about proving size, we need to think about two sizes: first the total number of provers and second the total number of constitutional predispositions involved. Both numbers need to be adequate for us to develop a fuller understanding of the proving substance.

Substance to be proven

Here is an interesting topic that is not often thought about. What should we prove? The answer to that question is slightly complicated and I have two different answers. First the simple one. The material to be proven should be one that the principle investigator is excited about, as conducting a proving is incredibly time-consuming. To all the people who have participated in provings of whatever method, I tip my hat. Your dedication is obvious to anyone who knows the process. As such, prove something you're excited about proving. Otherwise, the proving becomes a chore. After all, Hahnemann proved *Sepia*, after observing a painter who constantly dipped his brush in sepia ink and also licked it. So he proved a substance after observing a minor poisoning. You too can prove anything in the world. Any substance can be proven and so it is up to you.

I have another answer, closer to my reality, which is logical if you think of previous chapters and books and the concepts of *Stress* and *Strain*, evolution, and of predisposition. With that as the background, to choose a substance to prove becomes a much less daunting task. Those up for consideration fall into 3 categories. One group of substances to prove are all the substances that people have been interacting with for a long time, especially things that were used as medicines, or foods. Why? Both foods and medicines are in some way beneficial to us. They are not neutral to us, but have interacted with us, on the cellular level, for millennium. This should mean that they are an integral part of our constitutions.

If we look at Figure 1 once more, we would be able to substitute any food with any of the intersecting circles such as **E** or **F**. That is why we eat it in the first place, or have used it as medicine for hundreds of years. This means that if I, personally, had to pick a bird to prove, instead of proving a condor or vulture, I would prove a chicken or turkey instead. Why? We have personally interacted with these birds for years. We have lived with them, grown them, and eaten them. We should have more in common with them than with birds that we do not interact with. It may not be a 'sexy' substance to prove, but I think it will produce good symptoms, especially if you choose provers that are sensitive to the food. For example, to test *Lac defloratum,* pick people with milk allergies. Likewise, medicines that we have used over the millennium are medicines because they interact with us in some way already. We know we are sensitive to these substances already. It only becomes a matter of process to find the full picture. Hahnemann picked these readily.

The second group to prove would be any substance that living beings are made of; humans, in particular. Any substance that we are constituted of, that we have a lot of, should be useful, as it is integral to our makeup. This is especially so if used to maintain homeostasis. This is why remedies such as *Sulphur*, *Natrum muriaticum, Phosphorus,* and the *Calcareas* are such profound remedies.

I think one of the strangest aspects of homeopathy at this crossroads of our profession is the feeling that in some way the remedies that we have used for so long are just coincidentally polychrests. The idea being floated about now is that the polychrests are given so often only because they were proven first, and that over time, a more equal even playing field will emerge where all remedies are equal and given in roughly the same amount of time.

I think this is completely incorrect. For me, it shows two things. First, that there is a serious lack of understanding of why remedies act. The lack of a model for these colleagues of ours leads them to misunderstanding. More than that, it puts into question their results. The fact is that many homeopaths *do* good work with these polychrests, so how is it possible that the practitioners working with these old polychrests get good results if it is all one level playing field? Equality in all substances is not in our world-view of biochemical individuality. The possibility of all substances in the world being prescribed equally in frequency and effectiveness is ludicrous for me. Living beings, people, are not made up of all substances equally. We need different amounts of different things to function.

We need salt to function immediately. Likewise we need calcium and sulfur. Without these in proper amounts, we die! Too much or too little and we become very symptomatic. That is not the same with all elements. Therefore, even though we have a full periodic table, our bodies do not contain these in equal amounts. The elements that we use, that we have in important concentrations, controlled tightly, are the ones that will always be polychrests and will always be used much more frequently than other substances. Think about it.

The third group of substances are the ones that poison us. Any substance that easily poisons us is going to be a great remedy. Why? A poisoning means that we already know we are sensitive to a certain substance; we already know there is a predisposition, a relationship to the substance. We already know a fair amount of the symptoms from the poisoning effect. It is only a question of finding out in a proving the full symptom picture of the substance.

Part of the poisonings category are plants that are toxic in some respect and animals and insects that cause us harm. We know them and have a full description of the toxic effects already. As a result, part of our work is done already. It is only the subtle part of the proving that is left to discover.

So what do we prove? If we look at the first group of substances originally proven to make remedies to be used homeopathically, we find that they were often from one of these three categories and often a combination. For example, *Mercurius* was a drug used to treat disease for many years.

Humanity interacted with it for a long time, so much so, it was as if it was used as a food additive. In addition, we were so sensitive to it *and* many were poisoned by it. A natural choice. It was the same with many plants that people mistakenly ate and were poisoned or killed by, or plants that we used in medicine that caused strong side effects or poisonings.

Obviously, I am not suggesting that this be a strict guideline, though it is mine. Nature is bountiful and there are many things that can be proven. It is your work, if you are the one that is doing all of it; you should be excited by whatever the substance is you decide upon. Also, this is not the only way to find remedies that are going to be very useful. I am only suggesting this as a method to narrow down the choices, so that the remedy your work describes will be of great benefit to our profession and our patients.

Dose

The dose one proves is also something that has been questioned. Reviewing the literature, we find that the results of provings and information about substances was gathered from many different potencies. At first, the lowest potencies were used. We have many symptoms in our *materia medica* produced by the tincture or the 2, 3, 4, 5 centecimal potencies.

By the time Hahnemann wrote/lectured on potency for provings, he was suggesting the 30C dose. However, let us be clear. He was a constant experimenter. Given another few years he may have suggested yet a different potency. After Hahnemann, we found that many provings were conducted with potencies ranging from tincture to the 1M doses. While Hahnemann was trying to get the 30C to be the potency used, we kept on experimenting. So the question comes to us now. What potency should *I* use in *my* proving?

Using my model, a method of approaching this subject arises. If we think of the model of *Stress* and *Strain* and of the question of susceptibility, we come up with tools to understand how to answer this question. After all, what is it that we are attempting to accomplish? We are trying to find symptoms that are elicited by *Stressing* the individual with a certain substance. As such, we need to find the people who are susceptible to the substance. The best way to do that is to *'generalize the susceptibility.'* This is my term for trying to find the maximum number of people who will be sensitive to a substance. Here,

I am looking for as many people as possible to be sensitive to the substance. The way that is done is to use the lowest possible potencies that will elicit symptoms, as the cruder the dose, the more people will be effected.

The lowest dose producing symptoms are poisonings of that substance that we can find from the literature, if the crude substance is toxic. If the crude substance is not toxic, using low potencies will achieve the same goal of finding the most number of sensitive people. I personally believe that this is why the first set of provings had used toxic doses and 1C, 2C, 3C doses. They elicited many symptoms as the substances tested were very strong and at times toxic, and so most provers were sensitive to them.

Using that same formula, we can say that toxic substances at the material dose would create a wonderful proving with lots of symptoms, but with injured provers. So the tendency quickly changed to giving slightly higher potencies, ones that would not poison the prover.

Also, the proving of the toxic substance at the low potencies gives us the strong general features of the substance, but it may lack some of the best individual characteristics. For those symptoms, we need to go a further step. We need to find the individuals that have a particular affinity to the substance. These people are much more predisposed to be sensitive to the substance. As a result they produce more symptoms, stronger symptoms, as they experience the substance as a stronger *Stress*.

In a proving we are especially trying to find these people. These are the people who are more sensitive to the remedy. These are the people who find the substance most toxic. These are the people who produce the strongest symptoms. Homeopathy is attempting to replace the symptom group of the patient with the symptom group of the remedy, which should be similar. As a result of this, what we are trying to find in the proving is how the most sensitive provers respond to the substance. It is their characteristic responses that will lead to the remedy description and eventually to the remedy selection in practice.

*So what a typical proving result really is, from our model, is that some people who are not sensitive do not contribute to the proving symptoms. A lot of other people who have a low sensitivity to the substance in low potencies will contribute a great deal of the **general characteristics**. And a few provers who have a great sensitivity to the substance will contribute a great deal of not just general characteristics but also of some **specific characteristics** that will typify the substance once it is a remedy.*

If this is so, then logic would dictate that an ideal proving be conducted in three phases. Phase 1 is the symptoms elicited by the poisoning of the substance. This is essentially a data search, since many substances have a long record of their toxic effects. Phase 2 is the proving conducted on a mid sized group of provers to find the general characteristics. Phase 3 would be a repeat of the proving using any people who showed extreme sensitivity in Phase 2. In this Phase 3 group, we would use a higher potency, to stress the individuals even more and thereby elicit even clearer individual symptoms.

Practically speaking then, we can see why many provings used low potencies, as they gave us the sub-toxic symptomatology without injuring the provers. Over time, to diminish the toxic effect, we began to use more potentized substances. Eventually we settled on 30C potencies. Why? It seemed that enough people would still be sensitive to the substance but there would no longer be any danger of toxicity.

In fact it is the 30C that I use in provings for the Phase 2 portion. The potency is high enough so that the proving bar is lifted high. As such, there are definitely people who no longer show much sensitivity to the substance. There are also people who show great sensitivity to the substance. As you use too low a potency, you run the risk of toxicity. As you go up in potency, *your susceptibly* needs to be more precise, more specific to that substance. As such, we begin to lose too many people when we use 1M.

30C is a good dose but not the only one. For example, if the substance is not toxic, then surely a lower dose would be advisable. If a substance is toxic, then a lower dose would be questionable. There is also the middle ground as well. There are many plants that in tincture dose would cause agony but at a 6C or 12C produce only symptoms and yet are no longer lethal.

What I am attempting to give here is the rationale of what potencies to use. That rationale is fluid enough to explain why some potencies were used in the past, why to use differing potencies at different times, and with different substances. For example, for a non-toxic substance, a low potency, such as 3C, 6C, 12C would suffice for the Phase 2 part. Once identifying the sensitive people, then 30C, 200C, 1M, or 10M would work well. For toxic substances, I would use the poisoning record for Phase 1, 30C for Phase 2, and 200C or 1M for Phase 3.

Repetition

A question that is related to potency is how often to give the substance. Again, there is great debate here as well. The simple answer would be to give it until we elicit symptoms. But from this model, I would like to give a better framework. If Figure 1 is true, as it seems to be, since homeopathy is based on it, then we have some clues as to how often to repeat. Recall what it is that we are attempting to find. We are trying to find the sensitive people and especially the supersensitive people who would elicit symptoms because of their susceptibility to the substance. If this is so, then if you have to repeat a dose often until you elicit symptoms, then by virtue of this model, we can say that that person has very little sensitivity to the substance. If this is so, why use any of the symptoms elicited there?

The prover's regular symptoms and the ones he may develop from the proving would be indistinguishable, as the level of susceptibility to the substance is so low, just as it is to so many other substances. In other words, in those people, the likelihood of the symptoms being from the substance being proven is not sufficiently higher then other objects and events in the person's life. It is too buried within the background noise.

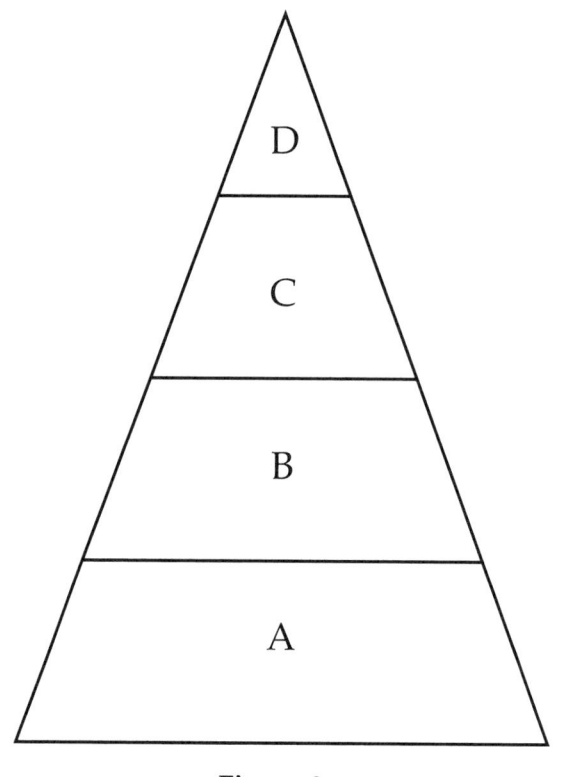

Figure 2

Figure 2 is a simple illustration to demonstrate what I mean. Take the triangle as representing a number of individuals. The people in Group **A** have little sensitivity to the substance. They live their life below the first bar, the first line. Remember they are living breathing human beings. They do have sensitivities and predispositions to many things in their environment. Being below this bar means that they are more sensitive to things in their environment than they are to the substance being proven. These people are poor provers in relation to the substance in question.

People in Group **B** are above the bar and show some symptoms from the substance. But their level of susceptibility is so low that it may be difficult to determine which symptoms belong and which do not. Those questionable provers should most likely not be included in the final list. This is not to say that they do not produce symptoms. Simply, they add confusion by the fact that they add too many symptoms that are not part of the proving. There is so much to sift through, that their value is lost and actually they turn into a detriment.

People in Group **C** definitely produce symptoms. If you take the first bar line as the one that represents all the sensitivities of an individual, Group **C** individuals are so many levels above those regular day to day sensitivities that it is easy to see which symptoms should be used. Group **D** is the most unique of all the groups and easiest to spot. When they take the substance being proven, their symptoms shift so dramatically, that it is as if they are under the influence of an acute illness. In other words, the proving for them acts as if they have a true acute ailment, with chronic symptoms disappearing as new ones appear. When the proving is over for them, their acute symptoms cease and their chronic symptoms return. Provings are conducted to find symptoms. But to do that we are trying to find Group **C** and Group **D** individuals, in regards to their response to the substance.

By this logic we are looking for people who can develop symptoms with only a few repetitions, ideally with only one administration of the substance. Those are the Group **C**, and **D** individuals. The other provers, though well-meaning, should not have any symptoms input into the record. Why? They are so close to their steady state bar line that the symptoms may or may not be due to the substance. But even if they are, they will not add any remarkable symptoms that are not found in the best Groups. They simply muddy the waters. As you read Volume Two, you will note that many studies that found no difference between placebo and verum took all the provers' results, regardless of susceptibility. Those tests were doomed to fail because they lacked the model that would have allowed them to select the provers that should be included, those in the Group **C** and Group **D**.

As a result of this model, I have several modes of application, of repetition. If the substance is toxic, I will give at most 3 doses of the substance in the 30 C, in the Phase 2. I repeat after a few hours if there has been no response. If there is no response, then it means that that prover should not be used. I give only one dose of 200C or 1M in the Phase 3. I do not go lower than the 30C in toxic substances.

In the non toxic substance I can repeat a 3C or 6C up to a dozen times, in the Phase 2 portion, also after a couple of hours of no symptoms, and can give 200C, 1M, 10M in the Phase 3 part. In either case, as soon as we find that the prover is influenced by the substance, no more of it should be given. Continuing to dispense the substance may place the prover in difficulty.

Let's face it, not only is this in keeping with my model, but it makes sense. It allows us to test substances without hurting people. But since we are no longer bombarding people with the toxic doses, we need to find the provers that are most sensitive to the substance so that we can elicit symptoms with a sub-toxic dose. This method accomplishes that. Obviously we are sacrificing or giving up many symptoms and provers' time in not using a more toxic level of the substance, but this does do the job, and since the drug trial standards have been set and agreed to by civilized society, this method adheres to it.

I have a final point to make here, in regards to potency and sensitivity and repetition. There are many provings conducted these days, where most provers develop many symptoms, with non toxic substances, with 30C potencies that are not repeated that often. I frankly cannot understand this, for two reasons. First, it does not match the practice. In practice, homeopaths often give remedies that seem not to work, to not impact the person. That is an all too painful part of the reality of practice. How is it possible that so many people in some of these provings have so many symptoms and all seem to be sensitive to the substance?

This finding also makes no sense from my model. And since my model really does encapsulate our current understanding of homeopathic philosophy, from the *Organon* onward, I cannot understand it. It is as if we are saying that all of a sudden every individual is sensitive to everything, and that is the reason why all substances are producing symptoms in everyone in some provings. From the homeopathic point of view, this cannot be. It gets rid of homeopathy and the concept of the simillimum. And how is it possible that some of these provings have more symptoms than any other proving conducted thus far, in two hundred years? I can only explain this dichotomy in one way. What some people are calling provings is not what others call provings. The bar is left too low such that there are too many symptoms from Group **A** and Group **B** people that are being included within the body of the text.

Masked Provings

The next four topics discuss the trial design. Here we examine briefly the masked design. In this design, only a few people know what the substance being tested is. No one taking the substance nor their homeopaths know. I have mentioned the benefits of this earlier, quoting sources showing that homeopaths were the first to adopt this method. This insures yet another safeguard in the testing method. The scientific testing method of our time adheres to this design. This is even more important when you consider that we are no longer giving very toxic doses but potentized substances to semi-sensitive provers. Keeping suggestions away becomes more important. In our provings, a maximum of three people know the substance to be tested: the primary investigator, the pharmacist who potentizes the substance, and at times a third person conducting the literature search on the toxicology. No one else knows the substance.

Placebo Provings

Here, likewise, I included the quotes from past sources showing that homeopaths were the first to use placebo in trial studies, seeing this as yet another way to keep the prover honest. I usually include about 5 placebo tubes in the 40 people receiving a vial in a proving. There are several reasons for this. First I tell them ahead of time that there are placebo vials included. I tell them this at the same time that I attempt to instill in them the reasons why. I tell them that I am trying to limit suggestion. I am trying to limit people thinking that they will absolutely develop symptoms. I cannot overemphasize this point. I want to say this loud and clear.

Here I reject the concept that the collective unconscious and/or group dynamics in some way influence the placebo arm of the trial and lead them to have the same symptoms. I reject it as it does not happen in practice. I reject it as it does not happen in other trials. I reject it as it does not happen in other provings. And most of all, I reject it because it completely nullifies homeopathy.

If you assume, as any reasonable person would, that the proving in some way mirrors practice, then what some are saying is that through the collective unconscious, we are affected in such a way by others as we need the same remedy they need. That means that if your husband falls, you the wife may need *Arnica*. Worse, if you need *Silica* or *Natrum muriaticum* or *Sulphur* as the homeopath, then everyone you see will need the same remedy, as they are effected by you in the way that makes them into those remedy types. Obviously, I can go on and on with this topic and lay down all the examples and reasons but I will not. Simply put, if you need a remedy, you need a remedy. The proving and the practice methodology must mirror each other.

Cross-over Trials

The next aspect of design I want to mention here involves cross-over trial. By cross-over we mean people at first take verum and later placebo, or placebo and later verum. For homeopathic purposes only one direction makes sense. Since the effect of potentized substances lasts for various amounts of time, one can not take the verum and later the placebo and attempt to judge differences. The substance may still be active. It does however make sense to give placebo and later switch to active verum. The reason for doing this is to take the person to the extreme of their symptomatology and see if they are so suggestible, or if by the Hawthorne effect we are producing more symptoms, or just becoming more aware of symptoms. Should this be done, then the most relevant way to conduct this is to give daily doses of placebo, but on a certain day of the trial, say day 10 or 12 or 14, you give the active verum. All that came before is considered below the bar line and will not be included.

The Pre-trial Phase

In some way we need to eliminate or at the very least diminish the Hawthorne effect. One of the best ways of doing this is to embrace it fully. Tell the provers about this and tell them that to diminish it we need to hyperfocus on *the prover* at this time. You are asking them to pay particular attention at this time in order to create an adequate base level for them.

This is currently being done by some provers. *However*, it is not done with the seriousness that it should be. I must tell you that this phase *is* the most important aspect of the whole trial. Currently it is at times being incorporated but done with too cavalier an attitude. It is sometimes considered a nuisance or busywork, but that is not so. We need the bar to be at the proper level for each and every prover. To do this, we ask people to spend an incredible amount of time analyzing their symptoms before the verum is given. We may lose some symptoms in this way by the bar being too high, but any symptom we have will at least be a good one.

When the pre-proving period is incorporated, because the full importance of why this is done is not fully appreciated, exactly the opposite outcome is now observed in some of the current provings. Some people include symptoms from prover's journals that occurred only prior to taking the remedy. I have an example of such a proving sitting on my shelf, where the symptom accepted was not only from before taking a remedy, it was taken from one of the people who received placebo.

The general concept with all four of the preceding sections is that we are attempting to filter out the people in Groups **A**, **B**, and some of **C**, in Figure 2 in exchange for a purer record of Group **D** and some of **C**. Further, we are attempting to clearly record the prover's steady state symptoms; how they respond to the world they find themselves in.

Who are the Provers

Who should be the provers? Hahnemann as well as some other authors have insisted that the provers be healthy. Others insist that there is no such thing as a 'healthy' person. So who should these provers be? First there is the legal requirements. The provers, taking part in a drug test, must be consenting adults, (at least 18 years old) and they should not be pregnant.

As it turns out, it is true that we cannot find too many people who do not have symptoms. And so to that extent there are no 'healthy' people. However, thinking back to our intent and our model, we begin to look at this differently. We are attempting to find the symptoms that the substance elicits in the patient. Period!!! As long as we have a very clear baseline, where we can differentiate all the symptoms of the patient from the symptoms of the substance we are all right. As such, 'healthy' does not mean *asymptomatic*. Rather it means a steady state that does not shift too easily, does not change constantly. This is a state that we can define and enumerate.

This definition does limit several groups, though. Any person on regular medications should be eliminated as the medication is complicating the symptom picture. Are the symptoms that the medication covers important? Are they not? Is there a drug effect from the medication? These people also represent polypharmacy, the taking of more than one substance at a time.

Also excluded are people who, for lack of a better term, are hysterical by nature. By this I mean people who seem to be effected by everything. There is no steady state for them that *is* measurable. Everything is not only possible for them but probable. For these people you may never be able to establish a reliable baseline.

Pregnant women go through changes constantly, inherent in growing the child, so the steady state may be elusive there.

Any person who has an illness that is progressive and very symptomatic should be excluded for similar reasons. People with chemical or environmental sensitivities should also be excluded. Their illness is so severe and with such a wide constellation of symptoms that are constantly changing that a steady state is difficult to find. The effect of the substance being proven will be only one among many substances that they react to strongly.

Lastly, people who are not aware sufficiently about themselves are excluded. If they are unable to verbalize their state to you, then the proving will not count for much with them.

I think that some of the provers being homeopaths is fine, but I also think it is important to have non-homeopaths as provers. They add a different language to the proving than do the homeopaths. With non-homeopathic provers, it is at times almost like a cross-cultural experience.

Lifestyle

The way one leads their life during a proving is also something that has been confusing. Historically, provings have been held in every conceivable situation. Some currently feel that the patient should be secluded, almost cloistered so that they may pay attention to their internal milieu. I reject this as well, much for the same reasons. What we are attempting to do is find the symptoms that are elicited from the *Stress* of the substance and only those symptoms. Changing locations, moving, cloistering one's self, all change one's lifestyle. That change always causes changes in how we experience ourselves. Some miss their loved ones, some feel serene, some get anxious and have loose stools, some become constipated, all from the move itself. Change brings change. That method I reject because we are testing several things at the same time: the substance, the change to a new location, the change from an old location, the lack of company, the new company, the lack of sex, the change in foods.

Much more logical is to find provers who are not going through any major upheaval. Provers who have a lifestyle that is not being traumatized, changed, or unduly stressed. That should help us develop a baseline for the steady state. I would like to give you two examples of what I mean. A wife acts a certain way towards her husband and children. By cloistering her, without husband or children, her feelings of aloneness, or loss, or peace and calm are all accounted for, having nothing to do with the proving.

A second example is the provings that are conducted in seminars. There are so many changes that occur to every single person there, and at the same time there are so many factors that are the same. Everyone's baseline is shifted differently, so there is no way to test any one substance. You might as well be proving the seminar, the air in the room, the hotel, or the food. Again, the experiment is not limited to one factor here.

In terms of diet, provers should keep on eating the foods they are accustomed to. If there is a recreational drug that they take, such as *Cannabis indica*, they should be disqualified from the proving, as the symptoms may be long-lasting. If they took a homeopathic remedy in the previous 3 months they should be disqualified, as new symptoms may still be due to that dose. If their symptoms are changing from a current acute or from the last remedy being given and there is no steady state they should be disqualified. If they proved a remedy in the previous 3 months and were sensitive to it, they should be disqualified. If the prover is going through a big change or *Stress*, they too should be disqualified. From the homeopathic point of view, these *Stresses* alone will elicit new symptoms. Without a steady state, it will not be possible to know which symptoms belong to the proving and which are there because of the other new *Stresses*.

To end, let me say that one of the most trying aspects of the proving discussion is that there are so many opinions based on many things. What I hoped to accomplish here was to give reasons, to show that there is an elegance to process once a model is in place. Should this be the only model? No. This writing serves as a template for others to develop their own models. The only criterion is that there is an internal coherence and that it mirrors practice.

Essentially, these are the elements that go into the proving design and execution. In the next chapter, I will discuss the actual proving design and provide some easy-to-use resources for those conducting provings.

— Chapter 7 —
Conducting a Proving
One Method, With Tools

In this chapter, I present the steps of a proving as the culminating end product of these past chapters. It is the *actions* or *application* part of the model I propose, in this case as related to provings. It is a type of coherent summary of the past chapters, and puts theory into practice.

The steps involved are similar to most scientific experiments. The ten steps described below are the steps involved to convert a substance into a remedy, to convert any 'thing' into a medicine that we can prescribe confidently. I begin by outlining the 10 steps and then going into each one in further depth.

1. **Step one is the design and interpersonal phase.** Here we decide on the substance to be proven, on the design, on how we will set the bar, and on who will be part of the proving.

2. **Step two is the beginning of the interactions.** Investigators meet homeopaths to give them guidelines and supplies; homeopaths meet provers and discuss guidelines.

3. **Step three is actually having the homeopath establish the steady state.** Homeopaths take the prover's case and follow the symptoms for some period of time, until both are satisfied that a steady state can and has been documented.

4. **Step four is giving the substance and writing down all elicited symptoms.** The homeopath discusses all symptoms with the prover.

5. **Step five is agreeing and clarifying which symptoms are above the bar** and may fit in the proving as symptoms elicited by the substance.

6. **Step six is developing the catalogue.** Here we combine all the agreed upon symptoms of all the provers into one big catalogue of symptoms.

7. **Step seven is the refinement.** Here we remove symptoms from the catalogue that do not seem to fit the general qualities of the majority of symptoms.

8. **Step eight is the re-testing of sensitive provers.**

9. Step nine is publishing the material.

10. **Step ten is the *materia medica*.** Here the remedy is finally described not just from the proving point of view but also from clinical experience. The *materia medica* does not just list the symptoms found in the proving but also the toxicology of the substance and descriptions of the curative effect of the substance used as a remedy.

1. Step One. Design and Interpersonal Phase.

A. Primary Investigator (PI). The first step is to decide upon a primary investigator (PI). This is the master prover as defined by the article from the 1880's. The primary investigator, with a cohort, helps to design and conduct the whole project. Ultimately the PI decides which substance to prove, as well as the people who will be involved in the proving.

B. The Substance. The PI must have the substance prepared for the study. This involves either preparing the substance or having a pharmacist prepare it. The PI needs to decide upon the proper method of preparation. If the substance is already a remedy, the preparation should conform to the pharmacopoeia description. If it is not a remedy yet, then the PI should consult the pharmacopoeia that exists in their country, for the needed information and method of acquiring the substance and its preparation. This is so that the work in preparing the substance, should it prove to be a worthwhile remedy, be easily reproducible in the future by other pharmacies.

The pharmacopoeia gives details of everything needed for the collecting, identifying, and producing a potentized medicine from any specific substance. It is incredibly important to do this part correctly. Pharmacists need to know how to prepare the remedy 100 years from now. Documenting everything properly allows this to happen. There is only one thing I would add to the description in the pharmacopoeia. With today's technology, I would also include digital photographs of the substance, if relevant or possible.

C. Literature Search. The PI should either attain or assign someone to conduct a literature search on the toxicology of the substance. Some of that information will enter the proving. The toxicological information found in databases around the world *informs us as to the effect of the substance on humankind, in general. This forms the general tendency of the remedy,* and absolutely fits within the concept of the proving. It is not specific enough but most definitely reflects the substance.

D. The Homeopaths. The PI should find homeopaths who will track the prover's symptomatology. It is essential that there be one homeopath per prover. The homeopaths are the ones who are going to track every symptom. They are the linchpins in this process. They must be well versed enough in homeopathic theory and technique to be able to take a case initially, and then to be able to see the changes as they occur. They are going to need to be able to assess and qualify all symptom changes so that a full description of each symptom is elicited. They must also be able to recognize changes as soon as they occur. When a prover takes a substance, if the homeopath does not recognize that the proving has begun, with new symptoms developing, then the prover may incorrectly take another dose and this may create difficulties for the prover.

E. The Provers. The provers are the individuals who actually take the substance. These people need to be able to identify clearly a steady state that does not vary wildly. The provers should be people who are not on medication and do not take recreational drugs. They should not have taken remedies for a few months, not been in a proving where the substance effected them for 3 months and not be pregnant. They should not be overly effected by their environment with an over-production of symptoms, and they should also not be people who are under an undue amount of *Stress* either new or prolonged. The prover needs to be able to be coherent, precise and correct in their self-descriptions; the more articulate the better. The people should be going through their regular lives as best they can.

F. The Design. The PI decides on the type of proving they want to conduct. Do they want it to be for themselves, an experience for others, or a proving that will enter the homeopathic records? For purposes of the rest of this chapter, I am assuming the latter.

The design needs to include mechanisms to ensure that we are able to easily differentiate the steady state of individuals from the symptoms elicited only from the *Stress* brought about by the taking of the proving substance. To do this, one has to diminish the Hawthorne Effect as well as any other suggestions to the prover. We have the proving masked, so that no one knows what the substance is and has no preconceptions as to the substance. We include placebo controls and tell them why we do that. We include about 1 placebo to every 8 provers, so about 5 in 40 provers. You may even decide to have a cross-over study, where you give everyone a dose a day. However, the actual provers who are taking the substance will have the verum given to them at a certain time within that sequence.

The design should also include a search of the pharmacopoeia for the details of how one brings the final information to the community. Decide how you will publish it, before you begin the study. If you plan on having the information included in the pharmacopoeia, then check it first. You will find that there are several requirements that you may not have considered before. Build them into your design. That way we will all benefit from your work.

2. Step two is the beginning of the interactions.

The PI and the initial cohort meet the homeopaths and educate them in the process of the proving, agreeing upon the guidelines of the philosophy and methodology. They also arrange for any supplies that need to be dispensed. The substance is given to the homeopaths. A notebook or access to computer is made available for the recording of symptoms. At this stage, the homeopaths need to have a clear concept of what the PI is looking for, that being the clear steady state in a reasonable prover, as well as the ability to perceive changes that may ensue after the substance is given.

While we can not teach them all of homeopathic theory and practice, we have to feel comfortable enough with the homeopaths' case taking and analysis skills that they will be able to differentiate symptoms that are elicited by the substance as opposed to all the other *Stresses* in their life. We also must make sure that their follow-up analysis is up to par, as trying to find the changes after a substance is given in a proving is the same process. If they can not do that well, then three problems may occur. They attribute symptoms to the substance that they should not, they do not attribute symptoms to the substance that they should, and perhaps most damaging, they do not see that the substance has impacted the prover and so they continue giving him the substance even though he or she is already producing symptoms. Because of this potential danger, we limit the repetition of the substance to a maximum of three times for any toxic substance.

Homeopaths also meet the provers and establish the same guidelines and inform the prover as to what the general process is going to be.

3. Step three is actually having the homeopath establish the steady state.

A homeopath takes the prover's case and follows the symptoms for some period of time, until both are satisfied that a steady state can and has been documented.

To diminish the Hawthorne Effect, the design sets about a period of evaluation of symptoms *before* the substance is given. Here the homeopath takes the case of the prover *in detail*. This helps to establish the mindset of the prover as they begin paying a great deal of attention to themselves *before* the substance is given. Once it is given, the Hawthorne Effect is diminished already, as they have been paying attention intensely already. This period of time may be 4 days, one week, or two weeks. That is up to the PI and the design of the study. The main point here is not the number of days. Rather it is to establish clearly the steady state. Once that is done, this phase of the proving is complete.

At this phase of the proving, if the homeopath finds that the prover is too unaware, or unable to talk to us to explain their symptoms clearly enough, they should be excluded and a new prover should take their place. This process repeats until there is a prover who is well versed in his or her own symptoms, and who can be clear enough in descriptions. The homeopath then follows the symptoms for a period of days, to make sure that there is a steady state delineated. If the symptoms shift frequently, then the prover should be excused, and a new prover found. We need to find people who have steady states that are somewhat predictable. Once we found these people we carefully ask them about their symptoms daily until the day the substance is given. This part is crucial as it carefully establishes this prover's steady state that we will use in the elimination of symptoms phase. All symptoms are carefully recorded. The homeopath must understand not just the symptoms intimately, but also what brings them on and what happens because of these symptoms.

The homeopath at this point should not only find out what symptoms the person has usually, but what remedies they respond to, if there is a remedy that effects them constitutionally, or what remedy they may need constitutionally.

Since the homeopath will not be with the prover every minute of the day, the prover needs to be educated about writing down the information about their symptoms as clearly and fully as possible.

For an exact copy of our handout to the homeopaths and the provers, see the handout at the end of this chapter.

4. Step four is giving the substance and writing down all elicited symptoms.

The substance is given. The homeopath is present at the time. The homeopath and prover record all symptoms that are experienced. If there are no symptoms after three hours, the prover takes a second dose. If the substance is toxic, then no more doses are given after a third dose, if no symptoms were elicited .

As soon as symptoms develop, no more of the substance is taken. Now the homeopath begins to focus in on the symptoms that may be above the bar, changes from the steady state. These symptoms fall into 5 general categories and are the same categories that we have when analyzing a follow-up. These are:

OLD symptoms. The prover's regular symptom remains unchanged.

ALTERED symptoms. The prover tends to have this symptom but it has altered in its location, sensation, intensity or modality.

CURED symptoms. The prover tends to have this symptom but not since taking the remedy.

PAST symptoms. These are symptoms from the distant past that have returned during the proving.

NEW symptoms. The prover had not had this symptom before or has not had it on a regular basis.

Again, to understand the full image of the elicited symptoms, to turn this substance into a remedy, I think it is also very important to understand the flow of the symptoms. This part, missing from previous provings has half-crippled our understanding of those provings. By delving into the sequences of symptoms, we can begin to see the larger patterns that they form, the *Cycle*, full of *Segments*.

The prover and homeopath meet daily at first, as most symptoms that occur in a proving occur in the first few days. As the symptoms become fewer and fewer, and as the prover becomes more aware of what is required, the debriefing interviews happen further and further apart. They finally cease when the steady state is overpowering any new symptoms. At this time it becomes difficult to tell if the *Stress* of the substance is eliciting symptoms versus other factors in the environment. Again to see what we tell the homeopaths and provers about this, please turn to our handout.

5. Step five is agreeing and clarifying which symptoms are above the bar.

All during the proving, as well as at the end of the proving, the homeopath and the prover meet and discuss symptoms experienced by the prover. The goal is twofold. First is to understand fully the symptom within the greater complex human being. Second, to document it as clearly as possible so that one does not depend on memory and so that it can be transmitted to the community correctly.

The homeopath and prover must not only understand a symptom fully, but must also gauge whether the symptom is being elicited by the substance or not. This is a sifting process that occurs at the end of the proving.

For a description of one such document, see my handout to provers and homeopaths.

6. Step six is developing the catalogue.

Once all the symptoms have been analyzed by the prover and homeopath, once they are all understood and once they are sifted through and distilled to the ones that are most likely to be elicited by the substance, then these are sent to the PI.

The PI catalogues all these proving symptoms into a major catalogue that combines all the provers. At this time a few interesting points will be found.

First the numbers game. From the list of provers, it will be found that a few will actually provide most of the symptoms that are of quality and quantity They were the most sensitive, the Group **C** and **D** from Figure 2 of the last chapter. This is to be expected. These people's symptoms should be particularly explored. From your group of 40, you may have 1-8 that may fit this description. In the proving of *Alcoholus*, out of 114 people, we found 25 that fit the criteria.

Another thing that becomes apparent is that there are several repetitive symptoms found within a prover, or within several provers. These symptoms will probably be common examples of *Segments* of the remedy. These should be explored in detail.

Another thing that is noted is that there are many unspecific, general symptoms that appear in many provers. These are common to provings and to many provers. Many will be happy or irritable, or have this or that pain developing. This was noted from the first provers onward. It is important here to note them but to make sure that they do not muddy the waters for us. These symptoms must be kept in proper proportion to the rest of the proving.

Another thing noticed will be that the *Cycle* should come together very easily. Why? Because by the inquiry of the provers and homeopaths, we found not just the symptoms but what came before and after. Looking at the symptom catalogue in this way, one will find that many of the symptoms begin to coalesce into major groupings and that these groupings flow from one to the other to form a circle. The groupings are the *Segments* that typify the *Cycle* of the remedy developed. If the *Cycle* does not come together easily then there is something wrong in the proving. At the very least the symptoms were not explored in detail or the proving is incomplete.

7. Step seven is the refinement.

Once the *Segments* and *Cycle* have been developed, there are still two pieces of work to do. Here, though, it becomes less of a science and more of an art. There are probably more definable rules, but at the moment they are in evolution in my mind and experience.

Looking at your symptom list and *Segments* and the *Cycle*, you must make sure that the unique features of the remedy outshine the non-unique features. Think about it. There are some symptoms that are produced by every substance proven. The more you stuff the record with those symptoms, the less unique your new remedy becomes. The greater the percentage of common non-unique symptoms, the less differentiated your remedy is and the less likely it is that it will be easily understood.

How do you do this? What the PI has to do at this point is to look at the *Segments* and pick the chief, unique, or strong symptoms that typify that *Segment*. Also possible is a common symptom that was listed, but only if it was experienced by several of the provers and intensely at that. In this way, even though you have 100 symptoms listed in one *Segment*, you may at first only list 5 or 10 of them. After all the *Segments* are sampled in this way, the *Cycle* becomes more crisp. Now you can go back and fill in each of the *Segments* with as many symptoms as you wish that were found, but keep the balance equal. Make sure that the symptoms that you deemed most important, stay most important, and are not buried by minutia. Aside from the problem of balance in the repertory, the remedy becomes too amorphous if every symptom is included. Balance is the key. You will see what I mean when you read part 2 of this book, on the proving of *Alcoholus*.

The second piece of work that needs to be done has to do with symptoms that do not seem to fit into any *Segment*. Some of these will turn out to not be symptoms of the remedy, but artifacts, mistakes that entered the proving. Others may be symptoms that fit the remedy nature, but the PI can not see their relationship to the overall pattern. My suggestion is that if the symptom really does not fit the overall pattern, unless it is striking in its qualities, I would leave it out of the catalogue. Why introduce uncertainties. For the other symptoms that may fit the overall pattern and are striking, include them, but with a qualifier stating that that particular symptom is questionable. Let history correct you there.

8. Retest the Sensitive Provers.

Here, the PI may contact the provers that were most remarkably sensitive to the remedy and repeat the proving with them, with the provers taking a higher potency. We do this to elicit even more remarkable, individualizing symptoms of the substance. When this step is done we repeat all the steps that precede here. When this step is done, it should be after a long break from the proving. We need time to pass, so that the effect of the first proving ceases. It is not fair or healthy to bombard a sensitive person with a strong *Stress* that causes them to *Strain* so vigorously.

9. Step nine is publishing the material.

The work can only become important to the community if it is published, read, and incorporated into the communal understanding of remedies. For a new remedy to be included in the pharmacopoeia of some countries it absolutely must be published. There are various ways that the work can be published. It can be published as a book, booklet, or monograph as is done currently. It can be published in journals, which is also being done now. It can also be broadcast electronically.

The choice is ultimately with the PI. I only have one clear suggestion. Check the pharmacopoeia of the country you work in. The pharmacopoeia often has the requirements of how the monograph should be detailed. There are provings conducted and published today that do not meet those requirements. It is a shame that the PI was not aware of the requirements ahead of time.

10. Step ten is the *materia medica*.

After the proving is published, the remedy is produced in pharmacies and the remedy is finally being prescribed by homeopaths in the treatment of disease. After successful and failed trials, after cases are discussed at conferences and published in the literature, we begin to understand the remedy in a fuller way. We begin to understand the remedy's uses better. The remedy is finally described in a *materia medica*. Here the proving symptoms and the clinical experiences are intermixed. Finally, a substance has been fully transformed into a homeopathic remedy!

Document #1

I would like to offer to the community the following document with a disclaimer form. Both forms are written for the specifications of the USA for the mid-1990's. They were drawn in part by a fine legal team and cost a total of approximately $4,300 in legal fees. They are meant to be an illustration of the type of document that needs to be created, explained to and then signed by every prover and homeopath. Every medical experiment must have some form of documentation. It is the legal requisite in our society for this form of disclosure. These documents were compiled from other such standard documents, used in research centers and hospitals in Boston, Massachusetts. I suggest when you decide to conduct a proving, you check with a local legal authority to have such documents drawn up to reflect the proper legal disclaimer for informed consent in your country.

TO THE PROVER AND SUPERVISING HOMEOPATH

Please read both sections

TO THE PROVER

Thank you for taking part in this proving!

The object of this experiment is to conduct a proving, that is, to find the changes which a substance is able to produce or elicit in the mental, emotional, and physical functioning of the healthy volunteer. This data is then collected into a proving record that will form the backbone of the homeopathic *materia medica* of that substance, from now on called a remedy. This information, together with toxicological data, as well as reported cured cases, will form the *materia medica* of the remedy. It is this *materia medica* image and data that homeopaths match to the sick patient to practice homeopathy and have a cure ensue.

The first part of this document is for the prover and the second part is for the supervising homeopath.

Please read both parts and sign one copy at the end of the document. This signifies that you understand your responsibility and agree to follow the protocol as stated. Please give the signed copy to the supervising homeopath, who will send the copy to us.

A proving is conducted to create a new remedy out of a substance. The remedy is created to help rid people's suffering. The ultimate goal of the process is health, and that includes you, the prover and supervising homeopath. Thus, if any reason arises—a health emergency or a possible health emergency or even if you are in need of some medical care—please stop the proving immediately and seek appropriate care. We will still be able to use your proving symptoms up to the time you needed to stop. Your health is the most important thing. **If at any time you wish to stop the experiment, do so**. If at any time you feel that some medical intervention is needed, please seek it out as quickly as possible. Be advised that you can stop being a part of the proving at any time. Your health, as any patient's health, is paramount. Your free willingness is the necessary ingredient to make your part of the study successful.

One of the aspects of this proving is that it is a 'blinded' study. This means that neither you nor your supervising homeopath knows what the remedy is. Why is this necessary? It is peculiar to the nature of homeopathy that we look for the *individual* response. Whereas current drug studies focus only on the large, common symptoms, we look at both common and uncommon symptoms, looking for how the substance effects any of the individuals. Thus, certain symptoms may not be included in the proving record of the substance solely by having several people show that symptom, because the symptoms are explainable. Alternately, we may still include a symptom into the proving record if only one prover shows a symptom, because it is unexplainable and is clearly produced as a response of the substance being proven.

In other words, provings have a tremendous amount of 'background noise'. These are symptoms that we all may experience. What we are trying to do in the study is find which symptoms are *not* part of the prover's regular 'steady state.' Everybody has different 'regular symptoms.' Since we are looking for the individual response to the substance, there is no way for us to separate symptoms by looking at any one symptom or group of symptoms. In this study, you are your own control of the experiment. The symptoms that you identify as part of *your* steady state form your background pattern that we will later match to the total pattern during the proving. By subtracting the former from the latter, we know which are the proving symptoms which may be included in the record. By not knowing what the substance is, you are less likely to have any preconceived impressions of that substance's influence on you.

Therefore, it is desirable that the prover and supervising homeopath not share their symptom experience with other provers or supervising homeopaths, besides the supervising homeopath you are working with. We do not wish to have you influence other provers' records. You can, however, feel free to discuss any part of this proving with anyone else, just not with other people involved in the proving—at least until it is 'unblinded'. As much as possible, it is also desirable to avoid any contact with these other participants. If you have to be with other provers or supervising homeopaths for extended periods of time, please consult with your supervising homeopath. This will ensure that your symptoms will be, as much as possible, only yours, unaffected (or affected as minimally as possible), by others taking part in the proving.

One other peculiar aspect of provings is that while we are trying to find symptoms, we certainly do not wish to cause disease. This is why we give only dilute amounts of the substance. We do expect to see symptoms arise in some of the provers, but not disease. Thus you may not exhibit strong symptoms but only subtle ones. *You may not even be aware of them. This is why you need to be in contact with your supervising homeopath.* His or her questioning will help you focus on whatever symptoms may be developing, or passing through, no matter how subtle.

To make the proving successful, we need to ask for your greatest assistance in the following ways. First, we would like you to stay away from any substance that may cause a strong sensation in itself. For example, coffee or alcohol or frequent hot-tubbing can all cause symptoms by themselves. If any of these are already a part of your regular routine, it may be best to continue them, but at a slightly reduced rate, so that the very act of eliminating them will not bring on symptoms. Please mark down when you do drink alcohol or use any substance that might produce a symptom of its own, an intervention, or a possible antidote.

Secondly, you need a crash course in paying attention to the symptoms you feel on a daily basis. We all become so used to our own symptoms that we mostly live without feeling them consciously. So we would like you to write down all your symptoms for 4 days before you take the substance. This has two benefits: (a) it trains you to describe your symptoms fully, and (b) it allows you to document your regular, steady state fully, paying close attention to it for the first time. These symptoms may then be eliminated at the end of the proving.

The greatest benefit of these 4 days is that as you review your record with the supervising homeopath twice during this time, it will allow you to refine your note taking so that you will learn to write down your symptoms, in a more complete, and therefore more useful, manner. It is important that you and your supervising homeopath can come up with a common language, as there cannot be any unexplained discrepancies between your two record books.

Please take the first dose with your supervising homeopath present, on the morning that you and your supervising homeopath agree upon. Take only one pellet, and let it melt on the tongue. Do not eat or drink anything for fifteen minutes before or after taking the pellet. Also have your notebook ready, to write down any symptoms you develop.

After three hours, if you feel that no proving symptoms have developed, take another dose, but only after your supervising homeopath meets with you again and concludes that no proving symptoms have developed. After a second three hours, if no proving symptoms have developed, and your supervising homeopath concurs, please take the third and final dose. Meet with your supervising homeopath again at the end of that evening, and again on the following day. You are to take no more than three doses.

Proving Symptoms

What are proving symptoms? They are any new symptoms or sensations, or any symptoms that tend to be changing in any way at all.

In a typical proving, some provers develop symptoms from the substance and some do not. If, as the month comes to an end, you have not developed symptoms of the substance, you may not be sensitive to this substance. Perhaps you will be sensitive to other substances in future provings. Thank you for your work and dedication.. Your lack of sensitivity to the substance fits nicely in homeopathic theory of sensitivity and will figure somehow in the final picture of the remedy. In other words, your lack of sensitivity to this substance is both informative and important to us!

If proving symptoms do develop in you, this means that you are sensitive to the substance being proved, and your symptoms may very well be the most important ones of the experiment. **As soon as you develop new symptoms you must not take any more doses of the remedy.**

Please note these symptoms carefully and write them down as completely as possibly. For completeness, we need the following for each symptom. Forget medical terminology for now. Give us the symptoms in the common everyday language used in your culture.

These are the essential things to look for and record in your notes:

1. SENSATION: What does it feel like. Please give us examples, for example, burning as in hot, or burning as in a chemical burn, or burning as in after touching fire.

2. LOCATION: Where is the symptom located. Draw a simple diagram if you need to but please be specific.

3. DIRECTION: Does the symptom move or shift from one location to another. For example, pain shifting from the left temple to the eye.

4. CONCOMITANT SYMPTOMS: What else is happening at the same time as the other symptom is occurring? What are your feelings at this time?

5. MODALITIES: This is one of the most important points that we look for. What can you do to make the sensation occur or become worse or better? Please try out as many possibilities as you can. If you have a pain, is it better from hot or cold or standing or lying? Try as many things as possible because the more modalities recorded, the better we understand the remedy.

6. INTENSITY: How severe is the symptom? This is compared to other symptoms you have had and as compared to what you are feeling now.

7. DURATION OF SYMPTOMS: Does the symptom last seconds or minutes or hours or days? Does it come and go every hour or day? Is it intermitting? All these are very important to the proving.

8. ONSET: The actual date and time, hours and minutes should be recorded. This will help us develop a pattern of unfolding for the remedy.

9. SEQUENCE OF EVENTS: Your circumstances before you developed the symptom should be recorded. This is one of the most important aspects of the proving. What were you doing or thinking? How did the symptom come on? It is also important to write down what the symptom made you do. That is, did you have to lie down, or pace, or talk to someone or what? This will help us develop a broader picture of the pattern of the remedy, the *Cycle* of the remedy.

Please use a new page at the beginning of each day. This will greatly simplify our record keeping.

Please note next to each symptom how it compares to your regular, natural pattern in the following way:

O - This stands for **OLD** symptoms. You regularly have this symptom and it is unchanged.

A - This stands for **ALTERED** symptoms. You tend to have this symptom but it has altered in its location, sensation, intensity or modality (that which makes it feel better or worse).

C - This stands for **CURED** symptoms. You tend to have this symptom but not since taking the remedy. For example, you tend to have menstrual cramps but did not have them this time, or you tend to have headaches in the rain but not since the remedy, or you have chronic sinusitis but it is gone now.

P - This stands for **PAST** symptoms. These are symptoms from the distant past that have returned during the proving.

N - This stands for **NEW** symptoms. You have not had this symptom before or have not had it regularly.

Coding the symptoms in this way will help us to tell which symptoms may represent the substance and which are incidental to the proving, the background noise mentioned before.

Also, please leave some blank space between each symptom you write down. This will give us room to record additional comments next to each symptom and discuss every symptom in context when the study draws to a conclusion.

Three times daily! Even if you do not feel any specific symptom, please review your overall condition three times daily. What is your mood in general? Also, has it altered in any way? Anything about your mental faculty, your ability to think clearly, finding the right word, your memory?

Please review your general physical state as well. Are you more or less fatigued? Are you chillier or warmer? How are you in general?

Please tell us about your sleep. Did anything change? Position, covers or none? Perspiration, grinding of teeth, spasms, drooling, jerking?

What are you dreaming about these days? Please be specific as to whether the dream is new, or if it is different from what you tend to dream about. Did the dream repeat, or have you had other dreams that shared the same feeling or motif? How did you feel during the dream? How did you feel when you woke up? Is there a reason for the dream? How intense was the dream? Most importantly, what do you make of that dream? How do you interpret the dream?

Please review your different body parts, pretty much going downward, from head to toe: Head, eyes, ears, nose, mouth, face, throat, esophagus, stomach, abdomen, rectum, urinary system, sexual sphere, lungs and bronchi, back, extremities, and skin.

As you can see there may be a great deal to think about during this time. Because of that, we would like you to pick a period of time to do this work when your life is more regular and more stress free. We ask this not because you will not get symptoms but because you may have so much on your mind that you do not write down the symptoms. It is important to write down the symptoms when you feel them. This is because it is at that time that you can check modalities and really go deeper into the symptom. It would be a wasted opportunity not to pay attention in that detail.

If you are planning to have an operation or to take new medications or to have dental work, please do not be a prover at this time. There needs to be only one major intervention at one time. Other interventions may bring about their own symptoms.

Pregnancy likewise brings about too many changes. As far as is known, provings do not harm the fetus. Be that as it may, pregnancy brings about so many changes that it would be very difficult to assess which symptoms should be considered in the proving. As such, pregnant women should not be included in the study.

If you are younger than 18, please do not be a prover.

If you are not reasonably healthy, please do not be a prover.

If you had taken a homeopathic remedy in the past three months that is working well, please do not be a prover.

If you have taken a homeopathic remedy in the last two months that is not working, please do not be a prover.

Please be in contact with your supervisor every day the first week and twice a week from then on. The proving is officially over for symptom collection when there are no new symptoms for one month. For women, the proving is over when there are no new symptoms for one month, but at least 2 menstrual cycles.

For those that are truly sensitive to the remedy, a future proving in one to two years in a 200C or 1M potency of the substance, should produce quite a few symptoms that will further refine and individualize the information regarding the substance in question. Those symptoms will probably be the best of the group, as they will truly and clearly define the remedy. However, just as we wait with a case until the remedy stops acting completely before repeating it, so too with a proving substance we must wait until it stops having an effect. And if the prover is sensitive to the substance, it may be cautious to wait for a year to pass before giving the higher potencies.

The substance is prepared in the 30C potency. This means that the substance was diluted 1 part in 99 parts, shaken vigorously. Then again, 1 part was diluted in 99 parts, and shaken. This process was repeated 30 times, to create the 30C potency. 10 % of the bottles contain placebo, looking and tasting identically to the other bottles.

One in ten of the provers will receive a placebo, a pellet that looks like the tested substance in all ways. Only the pharmacist knows which bottle is placebo; neither the supervising homeopath nor the principle investigator will know until the proving is 'unblinded.' The purpose of the placebo arm in the proving is to show a steady state for the population at large. For example, they will provide symptoms that may effect the whole testing population at large, as in an epidemic of influenza or gastroenteritis. This arm, though smaller than the traditional placebo arm, is invaluable to the experiment for this reason.

A NOTE TO THE SUPERVISING HOMEOPATH

Essentially your role in this proving is to act as the prescribing homeopath. You prescribe a remedy, and as soon as you see any reaction, you wait. Then as the patient reports to you, it is your job to question them to determine what really happened and what is really happening at this time.

You will need to take the case of the prover before the proving starts. Then you will meet with the prover a few days before the substance is given. The first step is to help you understand your patient and his symptoms as well as the way he articulates and lives with his symptoms. The second step is to make sure you can communicate effectively, via the notebook, and that the prover and you both understand what is meant by a complete symptom.

If the patient has many emotional or mental symptoms, please contact the principle investigator. It may be that the volunteer will have too many symptoms to make his work valid, i.e., his 'background noise' of symptoms is too loud.

Once the prover takes the remedy, your role is to again make sure whether or not symptoms of a proving have begun to develop. You may be the only one who can tell whether the proving has begun. The patient may not notice the new symptoms. Only your careful questioning and observation can determine whether to repeat the dose or not.

As the proving continues, your job will be to: help facilitate the uncovering of symptoms, fill them out carefully to help clarify their meaning and expression, find all the modalities and help the prover describe the symptom as clearly as possible to determine whether these symptoms are new or old. You should find out what happened before or after the symptom. Find the symptom and describe it just the same way you would like to see it in the *materia medica*, within context, not dangling alone in a meaningless, unconnected way. Finally, you will help separate the symptoms of the substance from the regular symptoms of the prover.

You will also be responsible for asking for clarifications when needed, and for giving the prover constant feedback regarding the symptoms in order to sharpen the prover's perception and understanding.

To summarize, you should meet daily at first, and then every two days and then twice a week until the proving is over.

Remember, keep your prover safe and the notes clear and pure. That is the bottom line for the supervising homeopath.

What follows are the legal implications of this work. For the material to be useful, it needs to be presented to the homeopathic community. As such we need to enter into a legal document that clarifies and transfers rights. Please read this part carefully, and if you agree to these stipulations, please sign the document and send it to the supervising homeopath who will likewise sign it and keep on file at NESH.

PROVING AND INTERVIEW CONSENT AND RELEASE

I may decline to write or answer any questions that I may be asked, but I will not be permitted to exercise any editorial control over the text, images and sounds that are the product of the experiment. The audio and visual recording of my participation may be edited as desired and used in whole or in part, or not at all, at the sole discretion of NESH and the producers of the proving.

I will advise you immediately if I should feel any discomfort in the course of conducting the proving. I understand that the proving will be terminated if I am pregnant, have a medical intervention, have a big stress. I have the right to end any interview at any time and to refuse further interviews.

I further understand and agree that all recorded products of my part of the proving may be duplicated by NESH or the FHE for publication. I also consent to your making available all or any portion of such products on the Internet in any manner that will permit the same to be viewed and extracted by anyone throughout the world.

To the extent that, during any of my interviews or texts, if I disclose information that would otherwise be covered by a doctor-patient privilege,

I agree to waive such privilege, but only to the extent of the statements that I voluntarily make during the course of any such interview. I understand that my name will not be used in conjunction with the text.

In addition to the foregoing, I hereby irrevocably grant NESH (i) the right to use, reproduce, prepare derivative works of, distribute copies to the public in any manner, publicly display, perform, sell and publish in any medium, in whole or in part, the recorded products of interviews with me for any purpose, including but not limited to educational, advertising, or promotional activities, and (ii) any copyright interest of any nature that I may have in photographs, videotapes, recordings and audio visual materials.

I hereby release and discharge NESH, FHE and the producers, their agents, assigns and designees, from any and all claims and demands arising out of or in connection with the use of my texts and interview(s), including but not limited to any claims for defamation, invasion of privacy or appropriation of rights of publicity.

I acknowledge that I am of legal age and of physical and mental capacity sufficient to enter into this Agreement. I understand that if I have any other questions about this project, I can contact Paul Herscu or Amy Rothenberg at the New England School of Homeopathy, (413) 256-5949.

DATE:_____

PROVER:_____

SUPERVISING HOMEOPATH:_____

Documents #2 and #3

I would like to also offer to the community a tool to allow provings to be conducted with less time being consumed in the documenting, extracting and collation, organization studying and printing of the data. The tool is used in the following way. The proving is conducted as usual. When the prover demonstrates a symptom that should be included in the proving, then the homeopath enters that information into a database. The PI is able to search through the symptoms and sort them in various ways. From the symptoms being entered in to the catalogue, to the refining and writing phases at least a year of work is simplified. I offer this tool to the community. Below is the explanation of how to use this important tool. It is written by Graham Hall, a tech wizard by day, and homeopathic student and practitioner by night. He was enrolled in the New England School of Homeopathy Three Year Professional Course (1997-2000), and has written the computer script to my specs. Graham has been a good friend and an important person in this process. For information on how to get on this site go to www.nesh.com.

Document #2

Instructions for Primary Investigators

This help file will describe the functionality available to you as a proving supervisor.

Overview

The Proving Web Site enables a homeopathic proving to be conducted 'online' with all of the provers (or rather their supervising homeopath) entering their proving symptoms into a database via a web browser. Once all the symptoms have been electronically entered, the proving supervisor can examine and analyze the proving with a web browser or download the proving's database to their workstation and manipulate the proving data using Microsoft Access 97 (or a modified version of the Archibel ProveIt program). Conducting a proving in this way expedites the process of collecting proving symptoms and allows flexible data analysis. For example, it is straightforward to select all the MIND symptoms with an intensity of greater or equal to 5 for a single prover or all provers.

Logging on to Your Proving

Before you can work with your proving online, the database for your proving and information about you has to be added to the system by the server administrator. After this has been completed you will be informed of the name of your proving and be given a URL and a password to login to the Proving Web Site.

After you have connected to the internet with your computer, start your web browser and enter the URL provided to you. You will then be shown a login screen that looks similar to this:

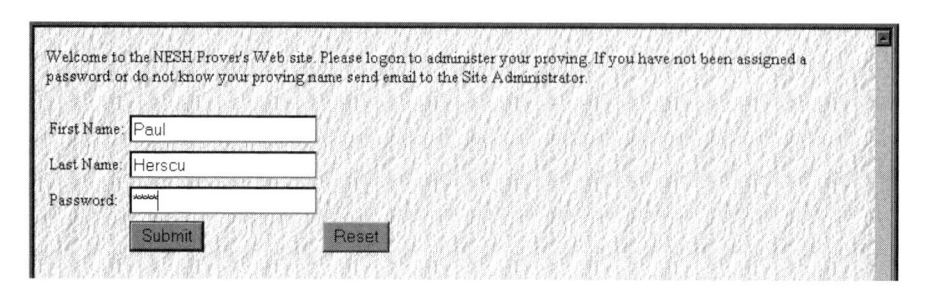

Enter your first name and last name and the password provided to you by the server administrator. Then click on the Submit button.

Once you have entered your information correctly you will see the following screen (with your name displayed instead of Paul Herscu):

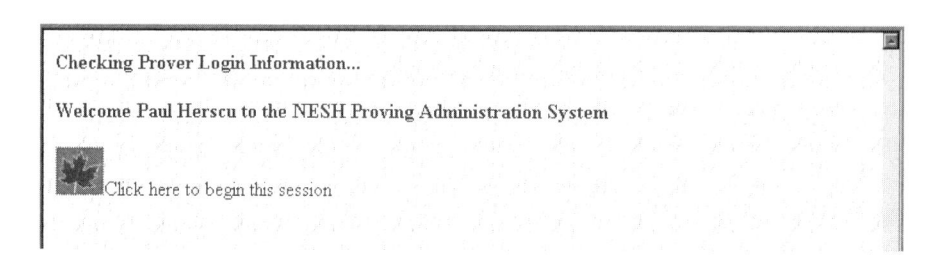

Click on the leaf icon to begin your session.

Adding Provers

Your first responsibility as a proving supervisor is to add the names and allocate passwords for all of your proving's provers.

To do this click on the radio button next to the menu option *"Add new prover to proving"* and click on the Submit button.

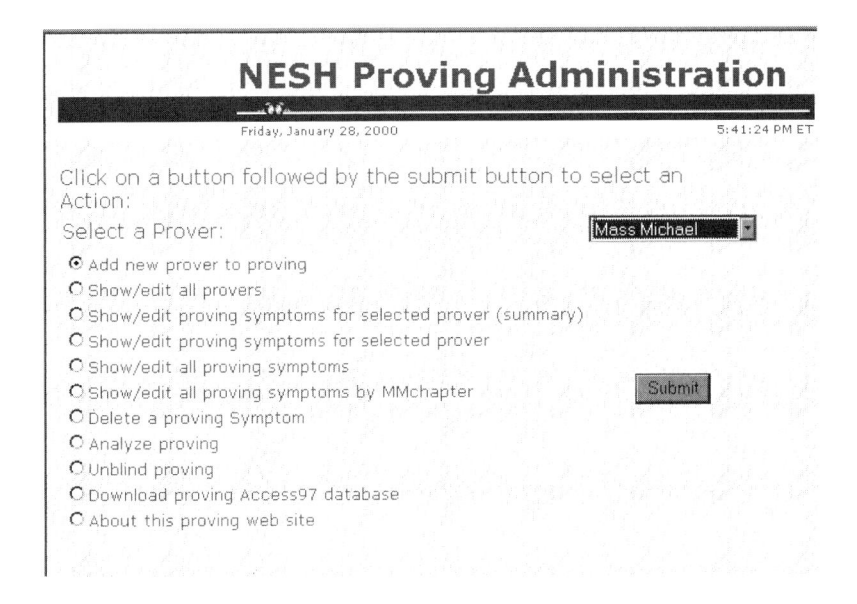

```
                        NESH Proving Administration

           Friday, January 28, 2000                              5:41:24 PM ET

    Click on a button followed by the submit button to select an
    Action:
    Select a Prover:                                     [Mass Michael  ▼]

    ⦿ Add new prover to proving
    ○ Show/edit all provers
    ○ Show/edit proving symptoms for selected prover (summary)
    ○ Show/edit proving symptoms for selected prover
    ○ Show/edit all proving symptoms
    ○ Show/edit all proving symptoms by MMchapter        [ Submit ]
    ○ Delete a proving Symptom
    ○ Analyze proving
    ○ Unblind proving
    ○ Download proving Access97 database
    ○ About this proving web site
```

A screen will be displayed for you to enter a single prover's first name, last name and password. IMPORTANT: The password must be exactly four characters in length.

After you have entered this information click on the submit button and then repeat these steps for each prover. You can display the prover information you have entered by clicking on the *Show/edit all provers* menu option followed by the Submit button.

Informing the Provers of How to Logon to the Proving Web Site

After you have entered all the provers into your proving's database you need to inform each of the prover's the URL to login to the proving site, the name of the proving and their unique password. You should also send them a copy of the help information for provers (which follows below). Each prover will then add their own demographic information and the date they started the proving. They can then add their proving symptoms to the proving database.

Viewing Your Proving's Symptoms

As the proving supervisor, only you can view all the proving symptoms entered by the provers. Individual provers can only view symptoms they have entered. There are several ways to view this information. These are described below.

Show/Edit Proving Symptoms for Selected Prover (Summary)

This option displays a summary of all the proving symptoms for a single prover at a time. First select the name of the prover from the pull down menu at the top right of the main menu screen. Then click on the radio button next to the *Show/edit proving symptoms for selected prover (summary)* menu option. Finally click on the Submit button. All of the symptoms for the selected prover will be listed in order of Materia Medica section name (ie. MIND symptoms first, followed by VERTIGO symptoms and finally GENERAL symptoms). The following symptom summary is listed: the *Materia Medica* Chapter, *Materia Medica* Sub Chapter, the symptom description, remarks concerning the symptom, the symptom intensity, and the date and time the prover first experienced the symptom. For a complete description of the symptom including symptom characteristics and the second and third times the symptom was experienced the menu option *Show/edit proving symptoms for selected prover* should be used. Alternatively, click on the symptom's ID number in the first column bring up an edit screen with all the symptoms fields filled in.

Show/Edit Proving Symptoms for Selected Prover

This option displays all of the proving symptoms for a single prover.

First select the name of the prover from the pull down menu at the top right of the main menu screen. Then click on the radio button next to the *Show/edit proving symptoms for selected prover* menu option. Finally click on the Submit button. All of the provers symptoms are listed in the order that the symptoms were entered by the prover. To edit any of the symptoms click on the symptom's ID number in the first column.

Show/Edit all Proving Symptoms

This option displays all of the proving symptoms listed in the order the provers entered them to the proving database. To select this option click on the radio button to the left of the *Show/edit all proving symptoms* button and then click the Submit button. (It is not necessary to select the name of the prover as in the two options above since the list of symptoms is for all provers). To edit any of the symptoms click on the symptom's Id number in the first column.

Show/Edit all Proving Symptoms by MMChapter

This option displays a summary of all the proving symptoms of all the provers organized by Materia Medica section name (ie. MIND symptoms first, followed by VERTIGO symptoms and finally GENERAL symptoms). The following symptom summary is listed: the Materia Medica Chapter, Materia Medica Sub Chapter, the symptom description, remarks concerning the symptom, the symptom intensity and the date and time the prover first experienced the symptom. To edit any of the symptoms click on the symptom's ID number in the first column.

Analyze Proving

This option allows specification of a selection criteria which the symptoms have to match to be displayed. You can select the prover name, the materia medica section, the intensity of the symptom, if the symptom characteristics are to be displayed and if symptoms entered by a prover who has taken placebo will be displayed (for this option to work the proving must be unblinded as described in the *Unblinding your proving* section). To see the full information about any of the symptoms that are displayed, click on the symptom's ID number in the first column.

Deleting a Proving Symptom

To delete any symptom from the proving, click on the radio button next to the *Delete a proving Symptom* menu option and then click on the Submit button. A list of all the proving symptoms will be displayed. Click on the symptom's ID number in the first column to select the symptom to delete. You will be prompted to confirm that you really want to delete the symptom before the symptom is permanently removed from the proving database. You should probably only use this option after all the prover's have completed entering and modifying their symptoms (since they could be confused if a symptom they entered is no longer available to edit).

Unblinding Your Proving

The proving web site is intended to be used for double-blind provings. Only after all the proving symptoms have been recorded will the proving supervisor get to know which of the provers took placebo and which took an active remedy (verum). To unblind all the proving symptoms click on the radio button next to the *Unblind proving* menu option and then click on the submit button. A list of all the provers names with a field to enter the potency of the remedy and radio buttons to specify whether they took placebo or verum is displayed. For each prover click on the appropriate radio button and, if they took an active remedy enter the potency. Then click on the Submit button. A program on the server will then set the placebo/verum field for each of the prover's symptoms to the appropriate value to indicate whether the symptom was from a prover that took an active remedy or placebo.

Downloading Your Proving Database

When all provers have finished entering and editing their symptoms you can download the Microsoft Access 97 database from the server to your computer (if you are using a Windows computer). After you have downloaded the database you can open it with Microsoft Access 97 and use Access' powerful query and reporting tools to work with your proving data.

It is also possible to open the proving database with a special version of the Archibel program ProveIT. Contact *<enter contact name here>* for more information. Note: not all of the attributes of the proving symptoms will be accessible from the ProveIT program.

Document #3

Instructions for Provers and Homeopaths Using the Internet Proving Site

Overview

The Proving Web Site enables a homeopathic proving to be conducted 'online' with all of the provers (or their supervising homeopath) entering their proving symptoms into a database via a web browser. Once all the symptoms have been electronically entered, the proving supervisor can examine and analyze the proving with a web browser or download the proving's database to their workstation and manipulate the proving data using Microsoft Access 97 (or a modified version of the Archibel ProveIt program). Conducting a proving in this way expedites the process of collecting proving symptoms and allows flexible data analysis.

This help file will describe the functionality available to provers.

Login on to Your Proving

Before you can enter your proving symptoms online your proving supervisor must add your first and last name and a password to the proving database. You will be sent the name of your proving and a URL and password to login to the proving web site.

After you have connected to the internet with your computer, start your web browser and enter the URL provided to you. You will then be shown a login screen that looks similar to this:

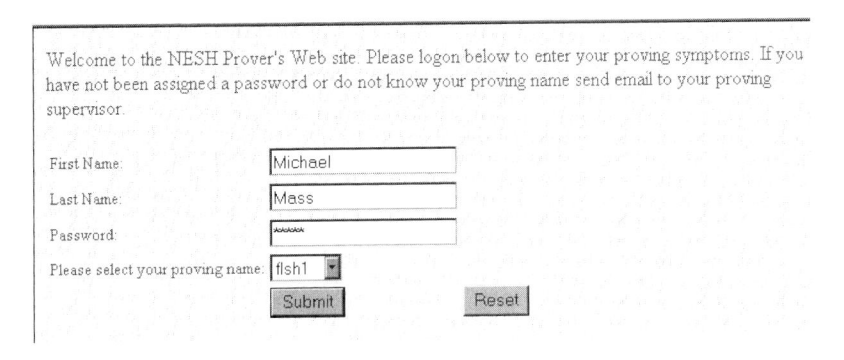

```
Welcome to the NESH Prover's Web site. Please logon below to enter your proving symptoms. If you
have not been assigned a password or do not know your proving name send email to your proving
supervisor.

First Name:                    Michael
Last Name:                     Mass
Password:                      ******
Please select your proving name: flsh1
                              Submit        Reset
```

Enter your first name and last name and the password provided to you by your proving administrator and click on the pull down list to select your proving name. Then click the Submit button.

Once you have entered your information correctly you will see the following screen (with your name displayed instead of Michael Mass):

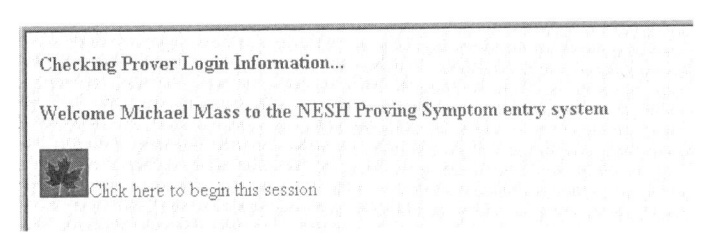

```
Checking Prover Login Information...

Welcome Michael Mass to the NESH Proving Symptom entry system

   Click here to begin this session
```

Click on the leaf icon to begin your session. If an error message is displayed make sure you have typed your name and password correctly and that you have selected the correct proving name from the pull down list.

Adding Information About Yourself

Before you enter your proving symptoms you need to enter your sex, email address (optional), your age, and the date you started to take the remedy. Click on the radio button to the left of the *Add my Prover information* menu option. After you have entered this information you are ready to enter your proving symptoms.

Adding Your Proving Symptoms

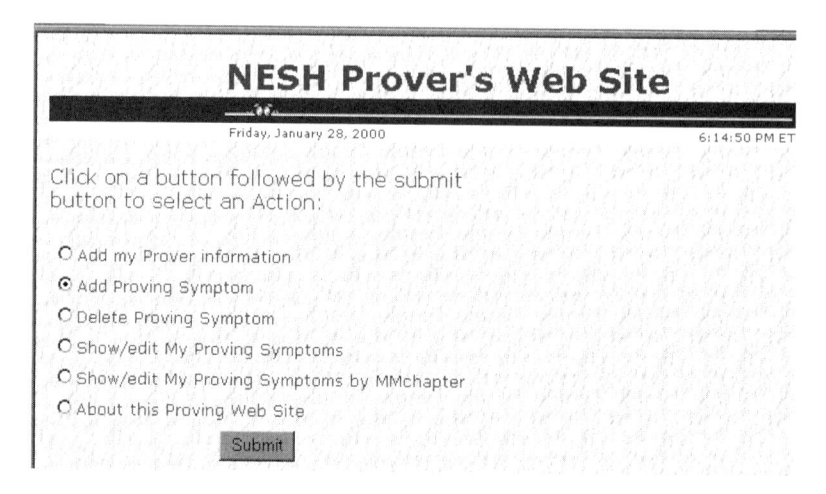

<screenshot of NESH Prover's Web Site showing radio button options: Add my Prover information, Add Proving Symptom (selected), Delete Proving Symptom, Show/edit My Proving Symptoms, Show/edit My Proving Symptoms by MMchapter, About this Proving Web Site, with a Submit button>

To add a proving symptom, ensure that the radio button to the left of the *Add Proving Symptom* is selected. Then click on the Submit button.

A web form will be displayed with fields to enter your symptom information. When you have finished entering your symptom information, click on the Submit button at the bottom of the form. If you have made a mistake typing in a date or time or have left a required field blank an error screen will be displayed. Click on your web browser's Back button to go back to the web form and make the necessary corrections. Then click on the Submit button again.

Viewing Your Symptoms

There are two ways to view the symptoms that you have entered. These are described below.

Show/Edit My Proving Symptoms

Click on the radio button next to the *Show/edit My Proving Symptoms* menu option. Then click on the Submit button. All of your symptoms are listed in the order that you entered them to the proving database. To edit any of the symptoms click on the symptom's ID number in the first column. The Add Symptom form will be displayed filled out with the information you previously entered. Make your changes and then click on the Submit button at the bottom of the form.

Show/Edit My Proving Symptoms by MM Chapter

This option displays a summary of all your proving symptoms organized by Materia Medica section name (ie. MIND symptoms first, followed by VERTIGO symptoms and finally GENERAL symptoms). The following symptom summary is listed: the Materia Medica Chapter, Materia Medica Sub Chapter, the symptom description, remarks concerning the symptom, the symptom intensity and the date and time the prover first experienced the symptom. To edit any of the symptoms, click on the symptom's ID number in the first column.

Deleting a Proving Symptom

To delete any of the symptoms you previously entered, click on the radio button next to the *Delete Proving Symptom* menu option and then click on the Submit button. A list of your proving symptoms will be displayed. Click on the symptom's ID number in the first column to select the symptom to delete. You will be prompted to confirm that you really want to delete the symptom before the symptom is permanently removed from the proving database.

— Chapter 8 —
Conclusion

The story of provings is the story of homeopathy. Our understanding of provings reflects our understanding of homeopathy. It is therefore not surprising to me to find that through our history we have had constant arguments about what provings are and how to conduct them. As with the questions, "What is a keynote?" and, "What are characteristic symptoms?" much was left unsaid and left unclear. As a result we have either clung superstitiously to methodologies we did not understand, or not paid attention to underlying issues at all. This lack of clarity has transferred directly into the practices of many homeopaths at one time or another.

Let me make the history of this short and clear. Think about my model of *Stress* and *Strain*. Provings began with very strong, near toxic doses. As such the *Stress* was so strong that it could elicit many symptoms from many people. We all were forced to *Strain* back. But as the dosage became increasingly less toxic, the balance had to shift. Now, only the predisposed people could react to the substance, the others would not be aware of it as a *Stress* in the first place; they were not predisposed to it. So now we need increasingly sensitive people to show us what symptoms the remedy can elicit. As the toxicity diminishes, we gain a benefit and we also run a danger.

The *benefit* we gain is that we find out who the most sensitive people are and we find out what symptoms they produce. What does this mean? By finding out what symptoms they produce we are finding out what a "sick" person who will need this remedy looks like. We are finding out in fact not just that this substance effects people in general, we are finding out exactly which people will experience a curative effect by taking this remedy. This is the zenith in the individualizing process we are looking for.

The *danger* is that as the dose becomes less and less toxic, we are no longer heavily *Stressed* by the substance. Instead of the 'heavy' shove we got before, we now only get a 'gentle' nudge. We no longer have a dramatic event occur. Rather, in many cases, we see a minor event. As such, it approaches our normal day-to-day *Straining* to the *Stresses* of life. *As the Strain elicited by the Stress of the potentized substance approaches in intensity, that of the day-to-day Strain, the difficulty arises in separating what is causing what?*

I argue that we are including too many symptoms. The danger has in fact become the reality. We are so close to the bar that we no longer know there is a difference and now lack the skill to differentiate. How does this play into practice? When a patient comes in with an infection, did the *Stress* of the bacteria cause a new remedy to arise? After we gave a remedy, and the patient returns for a follow-up, can we tell if the remedy effected them in this or that change? Can we attribute this or that to the action of the remedy? The fuzziness that is seen in our profession on these topics is the direct mirror image of the fuzziness we are seeing in provings.

It is because of this fuzziness that I add the following: Your homeopathic practice will benefit if you conduct or participate in a proving. Your understandings of the intricacies of case taking, follow-up and case analysis will all improve, if you participate in a properly conducted proving. Your appreciation for the balance of the *Repertory* deepens. *Aside from practice, there is no better teacher.*

Participating in provings should hone your skill in both developing a quick understanding of a steady state of your daily patient and being able to perceive what changes have occurred to that steady state from your giving the patient a remedy. Ultimately, you have to ask yourself the following question. "After conducting numerous provings, after participating in numerous provings, have your patients benefited? Has your skill level improved due to these experiments and have your patients become the beneficiaries of that skill?" If you can answer, "Yes," you are on your way. If not, you have to examine your proving design and your basic belief system about what provings are. The practice is there to keep you honest.

I would like to end with proposing an answer to a question I asked before. How is it possible that some provings have all or almost all provers describe symptoms, while other provings have few or none describe any symptoms? My question was, how can these two groups, both living in the same country, both be describing the same process that we call provings, yet have such different findings?

For me, I have come to realize that the answers lie in a few places. First, the *lack of definitions* in our profession has led or misled good people. The *lack of a model* has led and misled good people, and most of all the *lack of experimental design* that removes doubt has led and misled good people. I know these people. They are great people and friends. However, my conclusion is that, unknowingly, they moved the bar up and down not knowing there is a bar in the first place and included or excluded symptoms because there was no clearly agreed upon model. There was not even the awareness that a model was needed.

Again, let me state my disclaimer and hope. This is *my* model and these are *my* concepts. They incorporate a great deal of homeopathic history, philosophy, and experimental technique. I attempt to provide a forum for all to be able to discuss and understand their own findings as well as others' findings. Is this the best design? It is for me at this time. Hopefully it is for you for a while. And hopefully it will not be after a while. I hope you evolve it, change it, grow it, develop it to be a more perfect reflection of reality. The greatest possible outcome is that this design is studied, tested, and improved upon. In this way, the design evolves and at the same time our ability to prescribe correctly, evolves with it.

At this time, I see the application and design as I have outlined in this book as the best design possible. I cannot tell you a better way to do this now. I can, however, give you a big gauge to future methodologies and improvements upon this design. **The proving must always reflect the clinical practice**. If you meditate in the proving, you must meditate in the case taking. If you include experiences of people who did not take the substance in the proving, then you must include experiences of people who are not your patient in your clinical practice. In reality, the proving always reflects the practice. When they do not, when one diverges from the other, then you are running into a problem. The information included in the proving will be incorrect and many people will wind up receiving the wrong remedy as a result. Your practice will suffer.

The corollary is true as well. I hope that there are constant improvements to proving designs and understandings. If there are, then it means that those improvements will directly transfer into our clinical abilities and understanding. And most importantly, our patients will benefit.

Let's turn to part 2 of this book and see how all of this modeling came together into the application, the proving of *Alcoholus*.

Part Two
The Proving of *Alcoholus*

Introduction

The second part of this book is dedicated to the remedy *Alcoholus* and contains the following chapters:

Chapter 9 is devoted to the question, "Why choose this remedy to be proven?" It also contains information about the preparation of the remedy as well as a brief overview of the methodology of the proving. (For a more detailed description of the methodology, please refer back to Part One of this book.)

Chapter 10 describes the interaction between alcohol and humanity throughout time. This further underscores why it was necessary to conduct a modern proving of this remedy.

Chapter 11 focuses on the pathophysiology of alcohol ingestion, i.e., the effect upon human beings.

Chapter 12 puts forth the *materia medica* of *Alcoholus*. It is based on the information gleaned from the provings and those symptoms confirmed in the clinical setting with patients.

Chapter 13 describes a case of a child needing *Alcoholus*.

Chapter 14 lists the rubrics I have added *Alcoholus* to.

Chapter 15 is the copy from the actual journals of eighteen provers. In presenting the material of the proving, I was faced with the difficulty of how to actually present the symptoms in a more user-friendly manner.

Essentially, there are two different needs from the proving. The first is to elicit the actual symptoms. The second is to make it possible for the homeopath to find those symptoms. I settled on the following format. I would present one prover journal after the next, just as their journals went, rather then dividing them into different regions of the body. Lets face it, it is a lot easier to read about what actually happened, rather than having to read symptoms that are not related to the overall feel of what the prover was experiencing. In a sense, that is one of the complaints that people are discussing now. When we go back to some of our oldest provings, we only have symptoms without a sense of where they came from or what was going on with the person at the time. I have always held the essential notion that all symptoms are *context dependent* and this is also true for symptoms of a proving.

The second need is to make the material readily accessible to the practitioner. The *materia medica* takes care of that particular need. It also makes it easier to transfer the symptoms into the repertory.

There are some general comments I would like to make about this section. First, as I mentioned in the first chapter, I am a clinician; I treat people. That prejudice is seen through this description of *Alcoholus*. I do not delve into the mythology or poetry or anything else like that. I care about how the chemical impacts the individual. Period!

Second, the *materia medica* of *Alcoholus* is well described here. We did have a prior description in T.F. Allen's *Encyclopedia of Pure Materia Medica*, but the description was sketchy enough to make it almost worthless. This proving changes that. What I want to stress is that this is not a small remedy that might be used now and then for those difficult to help patients. This is a remedy that is closer to a nosode than anything else. Based on the history of alcohol and our species, I am quite certain that this remedy will be used at least as often as *Cannabis indica* or *Opium*.

I also want to say that this is not a new remedy to us. Homeopaths for the past 100 years have used this remedy but have prescribed on only the bare minimum of indications. The most common one was when a well indicated remedy failed and there was a strong history of alcoholism, either in the person or their family. Even with so little information, there *have* been brilliant cures based on a paucity of symptoms or perhaps based simply on conjecture. It is my hope and my belief that because of this proving, the frequency of prescribing this remedy correctly will go up, thereby enabling us to help more of our patients.

It was my intent to attain specific and accurate information about this remedy so that the proving would be reliable. As a consequence of these desires, many provers' symptoms were read and discarded. As I have posited in Part One of this book, a good proving cannot be based upon *all* of the symptoms that are experienced. Rather, a good proving is measured by the ability of the homeopath supervising the person who took the remedy, to screen out irrelevant symptoms. As an illustration, prover #7 had a lengthy journal of many pages, but less than one page could be included. The homeopath supervising prover #7 was an experienced homeopath. Moreover, she had participated in conducting provings before and was skilled in both case taking and eliciting symptoms from the prover. For her to come up with a whole volume of information but settle for only those few symptoms meant a great deal to me, as it helped insure that our information would remain both specific and accurate.

There are wrong reasons for having a newly proven remedy prescribed with more frequency and we have seen this in our times. Some provings are so voluminous that the remedy winds up being listed in many, if not most, of the important rubrics in the repertory. As a result, no matter what type of repertorization is performed, the new remedies appear. This is one of the inherent dangers in provings conducted without careful analysis as to which symptoms ought to be taken and which are superfluous. As I have argued in Part One of the book, a good proving should not be judged by *all* the symptoms that are included. Rather, a good proving is measured by the ability to screen out irrelevant symptoms.

There were many people in this proving, both provers and their supervisors, who greatly wanted to "have symptoms." Many supervisors were sorely disappointed that their prover did not produce symptoms that met the criteria of inclusion. While they were disheartened, I had to thank them, as they formed the most important part of the proving. They tested the method and found it working. It would have been so nice for them to include the myriad of symptoms that their prover described. However, their clear thinking, as well as a desire for true science, led them elsewhere. I deeply thank each prover and supervising homeopath for the time, effort and commitment it required to take part in this sometimes tedious process.

Lastly, I attempted to accomplish several goals with this proving. Besides understanding of a remedy which I wanted to know about, I was also testing out a model and a methodology. I needed to know what worked and what did not. As a result, instead of a regular proving which would contain only 15-40 people, I conducted the same regular proving of 15-40 people five times. But let me say here, each group confirmed and reinforced the other groups' findings. Though we had several proving times, at different times of the year, over a five year period, the symptoms garnered were essentially the same.

— Chapter 9 —
Why Me?
Why Prove the Substance Alcohol?
How do you prepare it?

This proving was not an easy task for me to undertake. No proving, if conducted correctly, is easy. From the choosing of the remedy to the collection and coordination of the data, from supervising the initial interviews to writing the *materia medica*, it is an exceedingly detail-oriented, time consuming, challenging, albeit rewarding, effort.

I am, foremost, a clinician; I treat patients and have had the enormous privilege to teach and write about that experience. Provings are on the other side of the equation for me, they are not where my primary interests lie. But to test my model of *Cycles* and *Segments*, my theories on *Stress* and *Strain*—to see how these ideas permeate throughout *all* of homeopathy, I needed to address the topic of provings in writing. In order to address this topic honestly and from a perspective of understanding, I needed to see first hand the process and outcome of a proving. This proving has enabled me to further understand how substances influence people and, to adjust, rework and improve my own understanding of this medical art. So whereas many students, colleagues and friends have wanted me to write more books on the *materia medica* of children, the body of work that interests me most, I found myself immersed in the world of provings. I suppose because all aspects of homeopathy stimulate my mind, I took this as both an exercise in learning something new as much as the opportunity to bring forth to our community an essential and deep acting remedy.

To embark on a project this massive and outside my main fields of interest, I needed to feel that there would be a very strong likelihood that whatever substance we proved would greatly benefit our patients. There are so many substances, thousands of minerals in various combinations, so many toxins in the world, so many medications and plants, so many compounds and chemicals, both new and old, how was I going to choose one I felt would be most useful in the clinic?

To guarantee the likelihood of a remedy that would be useful, I decided to follow the criteria that I laid out in the first part of this book. First, I wanted to choose a substance that a great number of people would be sensitive to. I wanted that because it increases the likelihood that more provers would be sensitive to it. It also increases the chance that it would be used as a remedy, as theoretically, many people would be sensitive to it.

I wanted to find a substance that people have interacted with for a long time. The more toxic a substance is that people have interacted with for generation upon generation, the more likely it would be that provers would develop symptoms and then the more likely patients would need it.

I wanted a substance that people still interact with on a daily or almost daily basis. Given the other points above, the likelihood of symptoms to develop in the proving would be very high.

Another point is a selfish one. If I had to test out a substance, I wanted to pick something that would be highly likely to help the patient population that I have the most expertise in. I wanted a remedy that would help children with genetic, chromosomal, neurologic, learning, and mental and emotional problems. I wanted a remedy that would help children that are failing in their school, social and family lives. If I had to test a new remedy, I wanted to develop a new tool for my own use.

Looking at the criterion that I laid out for myself, I looked for a toxic substance that people have interacted with for millennia, that people use regularly, and that causes either birth defects or impacts brain functioning. Looking at a potential remedy in this way, proving alcohol became an easy first choice. Alcohol is toxic, is addictive and is used by most populations the world over at one point or another. It has been used by our species for millennia and is not going away anytime soon.

Further and most interesting to me is the fact that alcohol is teratogenic, it causes birth defects. It is also the main and only cause of Fetal Alcohol Syndrome and Fetal Alcohol Effect, where hyperactivity, impulsivity, mood disorder, poor attention, and lower intelligence are keynotes. These traits are also commonly found in the patient population that I treat. I think it is safe to say that I have attended more of these children than most other homeopaths and from that vantage point there is one point that is very clear to me. We need more tools to be able to help them. We need more remedies than the ones we have. While the remedies we have help the majority of these children, there are still others that do not fit the known remedies. *Alcoholus* is one such remedy.

Alcoholus is a remedy that I and other homeopaths have used for years, though only on the barest of symptoms; we did not have a full symptom picture of the remedy. Many of us have used the remedy when other remedies have failed and at the same time found that there was a family history of alcoholism. If I had to conduct a proving, it would be on alcohol. I would help to define and clarify the symptoms of this remedy.

Alcohol and the Homeopath

There is an odd relationship between alcohol and homeopathy. Alcohol presents many problems for the homeopath:

A relationship to alcohol is mentioned in many remedies, for example, *Lachesis*, *Sulphur*, *Nux vomica* as well as scores of other remedies listed in the *materia medica*. Well, where do those symptoms belong? Do they belong in the remedy *Lachesis* or the remedy *Alcoholus*?

For example, when we discuss *Cannabis indica* or *Opium*, we discuss the effect, the symptoms produced and then list them under the remedy *Cannabis indica* or *Opium*. But it was a person who needs *Sulphur* or *Calcarea carbonica* who smoked those drugs. Sometimes we place those symptoms under the larger remedy, but sometimes under the drug. Why is it that we place the symptoms of *Opium* or *Cannabis indica* under the drug, but when it comes to alcohol we keep them all in the other remedies, not in the remedy *Alcoholus*?

Consider the following from T. F Allen, in his great magnum opus, the *Encyclopedia of Pure Materia Medica*. He begins the description of *Alcoholus* with the following most unlikely beginning to any remedy:

> "The following symptoms have been collected from various sources, and though incorporated with some hesitation, are believed to be reliable."

Can you imagine any other remedy being offered up with this sort of doubt?

To bring the point even clearer, consider this. Even though alcohol is the most common drug used by our species for millennia, even though it is so toxic, even though it causes so much agony and pain, it appears in a scant 200 rubrics in the repertory and is not mentioned in the majority of our *materia medica*. Just open up any *materia medica* that you have nearby. You will see what I mean. Even though, historically, it is *the* most toxic substance that we interact with daily, it is one of the most ignored remedies. So while the search is on for different new remedies that are exotic or unusual for one reason or another, I feel like I am addressing the story of the *Emperor with No Clothes*; homeopaths have avoided the subject of alcohol completely. If we leave out the obvious social, cultural reasons, there is a real and major reason why homeopaths have turned a blind eye to this substance.

To produce remedies we potentize substances. The process is to take one part of the substance and add it to 99 parts of *alcohol*. After that we take one part of that first mixture (being mostly alcohol) and add it to 99 parts of alcohol, and so the process goes, with succussing the mixture as you dilute it. As a result, what we can say is that *every* remedy has alcohol as one of the ingredients that has become potentized. I personally know pharmacists that say that *Alcoholus* can not be a remedy because it is present in *all* remedies. This is the *tomato effect* all over again. In other words, without a lack of understanding of the underlying processes, it is and has been easier to make believe the remedy did not exist, and when Allen put it into his *materia medica* he did it reluctantly, as he could not answer these pertinent questions. But there is an answer!

What was lacking for alcohol to become a remedy was a model to explain what happens during treatment, and the same model to explain what happens during a proving, and to explain what happens when you take a substance in the crude form. I believe my model provides such a framework.

As to the first problem, whose symptom is it? When a *Sulphur* patient drinks alcohol or takes *Alcoholus* 30c, the symptom that is elicited is definitely a symptom of the *Sulphur* patient. It may also be a symptom of the *Alcoholus*. In the same way as when a patient needing *Sulphur* smokes *Cannabis indica* or takes *Cannabis indica* 30c, the symptoms are definitely *Sulphur* and they may be *Cannabis indica* as well. The diagrams I drew in the first section of this book illustrate the point clearly:

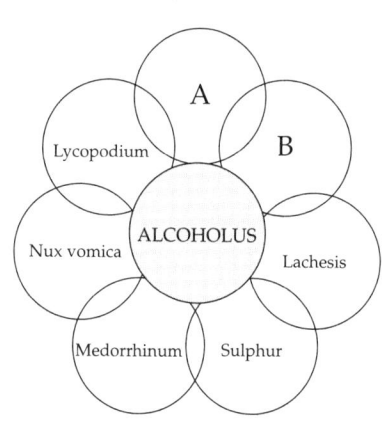

As you look at the proving records, you will see that the people that needed *Sulphur, Medorrhinum, Nux vomica, Lycopodium,* and *Lachesis* had a sensitivity to the remedy during the proving. They share symptomatology with the remedy. Interestingly, and I say not coincidentally, these are also the remedies that are listed in the rubric Alcoholism.

The second question is a little easier to contend with, though some may not like it. Every remedy that has been produced by using alcohol in the process, contains the potentized alcohol. As an example, the remedy *Pulsatilla* is actually a combination of the remedy *Pulsatilla* and the remedy *Alcoholus*. This is also true for the other remedies. To take this point a little further. Even though the person is taking a remedy that contains these two remedies in them, they will only be sensitive to the *Alcoholus* part if they share symptoms with that part of the remedy.

Now this is not really a problem for the homeopath. It does not matter what material you begin with, how many substances you begin the process with, as long as you list them. Once you begin the potentizing process, all those substances become *one* new remedy. So the fact that alcohol is in the remedies does not matter. **What matters is that the proven substance, the one that is written and recorded in our *materia medica* be the same substance that we use in practice. That is homeopathy.**

Preparation

The next question is what alcohol to prove? Should it be beer as the oldest drink? Or wine or one of the spirits? The answer had to do with what I wanted to fix, what I wanted to address. The major problem with the alcoholic drinks arises from the ethanol content, the actual alcohol in the beverage. That is the chemical that leads to most of the acute problems and all of the chronic conditions associated with alcoholic beverages. As a result it was the ethanol itself that would be proven in this study.

Michael Quinn at the Hahnemann Pharmacy in Berkeley, CA was kind enough to both prepare and provide the potency and maintain secret the identification of the proving as well as the code of which vials were verum and which were placebo. His eye to detail and ability to understand what I needed were most appreciated.

Ethanol can be distilled all the way to a 95% ethyl alcohol content, with the rest being mainly water. To make alcohol be 100% ethanol, you have to add benzene or toluene. As a result, Michael Quinn decided to take the

95 % distilled ethanol and dilute it into distilled water, such that the end result would be 1 part ethanol to 99 parts water. This was then succussed, to form a 1C potency. One part of the 1C potency in 99 parts distilled water and again succussed, produced a 2C potency. This process was repeated until the 5C potency where upon it was switched to diluting it in ethanol, just as all other remedies are. This process was repeated until the 30C potency was prepared.

The 30C dilution was then allowed to medicate or saturate blank sugar pellets. The medicated pellets came in clear glass vials, which were numbered. Along with the potentized vials there were also vials that looked identical but were unmedicated pellets. These would form the placebo arm of the study.

I would like to add a comment here. I think that the name of this remedy should probably change and probably will in the future. There may be several alcohol preparations that will be tested in the future and each one will have to have its own name. I am keeping the name as it is, because it reflects the listing in the repertory.

Procedure

Homeopaths were given a vial. They did not know the substance that the vial contained. They were told that about 10% of the participants received vials which contained placebo.

They were further instructed not to discuss or meet with anyone else who was participating in the proving. The process was the same as the one described in first part of this book. The homeopaths then found provers to take the substance in the vials. The prover took only one pellet. They were instructed to take a second pellet and then a third pellet only if no reaction was noted from the previous dose. After the third dose, no other dose would be given. (As will be observed in the records of the provers, even though the point of repetition was made verbally and in writing, sometimes there actually were reactions and yet the prover would still take a second dose. This point should be stressed in giving directions to the provers.)

I wanted the project to take into consideration different groups, different seasons and different years. This would not be one proving but a group of provings. All told, there were one hundred and fourteen people who received the vials. The proving took place with five distinct groups, beginning in 1997 and ending in 2002. Of the people who took the substance, the placebo groups showed no symptoms to speak of; their symptoms did not reach above the threshold to be included. (see below) Of the remaining people, there were twenty-five people who produced symptoms that were above the threshold to be included as probable symptoms of the substance. Of the twenty-five people, I include eighteen. The other seven repeat the symptoms of these eighteen and these eighteen have enough *overlap* amongst themselves to show a clear emerging pattern.

As a frame of reference, I went through a stack of papers near two feet tall to cull these symptoms you will read about.

If you recall the diagram from part one of the book, I illustrated several types of symptom category groups. In this proving, we only included symptoms from groups **C** and **D**. As a result, there were many people who produced symptoms(i.e. those in groups **A** and **B**, below) but their symptoms did not rise to the level of inclusion, as described before. As a result, this proving only contains symptoms from fifteen percent of the provers. The outcome, though, is the emergence of a very clean and crisp image of the remedy, with well defined symptoms. This picture does not reflect all of the symptoms in the repertory for *Alcoholus*, but it is precise and happens to fit the *materia medica* well, as well as what is seen in the office.

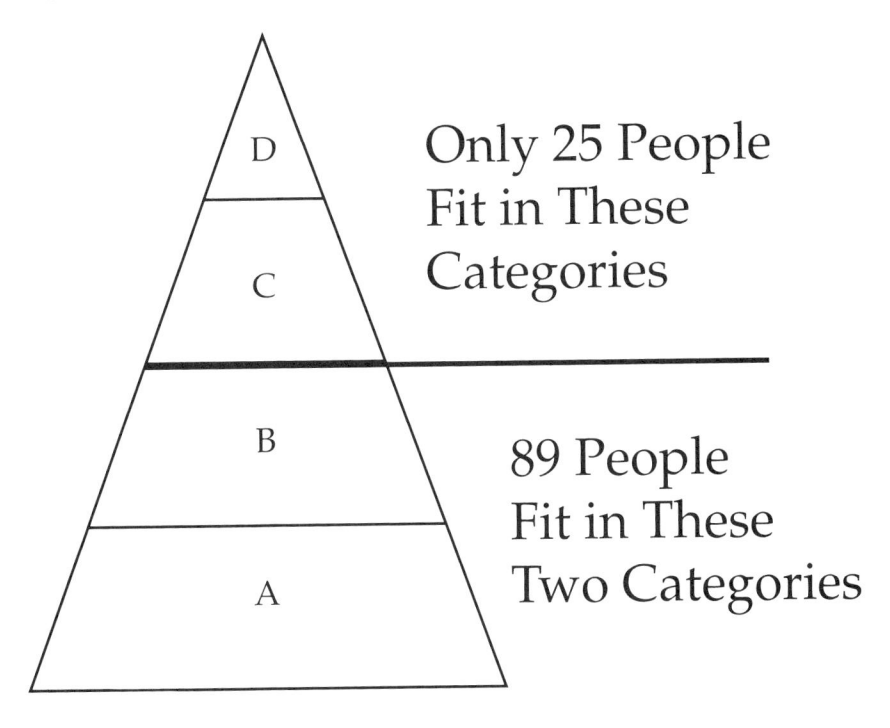

Only 25 People Fit in These Categories

89 People Fit in These Two Categories

— Chapter 10 —
Alcohol and Humans; Why the Connection?

It can be argued that the growth of our species is due in great part to the effect of alcohol. Let me explain. As you recall, up until the discovery of germs, the acceptance of germ theory and the process of pasteurization, few fully understood the role of microbes in the cause of disease. What was understood was one point clearly, drink water that was near you, near a city, and you would most likely become ill. Even now, in this year, in the places that do not have knowledge of sanitation or do not have the economic means to address these issues, the water supply is one of the most toxic aspects of the environment. Epidemic or pandemic disease runs rampant due to contaminated water.

It is with this backdrop that we consider the role of alcohol. Alcohol occurs as a natural byproduct of decay, for example, once yeast metabolizes sugars. While no one is sure how it is that people and alcohol met and developed such a strong relationship to each other, applying Occam's razor would suggest the following scenario. It begins with people liking the taste of sweets, of sweet fruits.

(This is no coincidence, of course. Genetically speaking, organisms, including people, have developed all sorts of mechanisms to help them do the things that will allow for success. With regard to that, we find pleasant the foods that build the body and unpleasant the foods that are not good for the body.)

Historically, as people collected sweets there were times when the fruit 'went bad.' There would have been times when the food, ripening and then going past ripening began to ferment. This does not take a great deal of imagination. You just have to come to my house when the children have been away for a few days. There is no way that Amy and I can keep up with all the fruit we buy for the family. We see first hand fruit going bad, beginning the fermenting process. Think how much more common this would have been thousands of years ago without any sort of refrigeration.

It is only a small step from there to the next step. Sweet tasting fruit juice would have been prized, due to the terrific taste, as well as the additional and needed calories it provided. If kept long enough, it too would begin to ferment. Now the funny thing is, that at a certain point of the turning process, when the alcohol level becomes high enough, the drink becomes more or less antiseptic or at least more aseptic. The drink still tastes good, and also it is found to have another effect. Drinking it offers a mildly pleasant feeling in the way it distorts and heightens reality. More than that, the person may have avoided illness from drinking this juice and not the water.

So began the use of alcohol by people. You had a drink that gave you calories, tasted good, made you *feel* good and that most importantly, did not kill you. It becomes easy to see why people, regardless of age, sex, socio-economic level drank alcoholic drinks as one major source of fluid. It was not water, it was alcoholic drinks. Water only became safe in the last couple of centuries. Alcoholic drinks were not used to get drunk then; they were used to get nourishment and to drink uncontaminated liquid. Alcoholic drinks were a staple of most medical treatments, and a source of both nutrition and fluid.

There are a few other points to keep in mind here. Firstly, people have an enzyme, alcohol dehydrogenase (ADH) which metabolizes alcohol. Living beings do not make things purposelessly; they do not use up unnecessary energy. For the body to produce this enzyme, it must mean that we have had a relationship with alcohol for a long time and that it must have served a constant purpose.

Secondly, in the cultures that discovered that boiling water accomplishes the same thing as alcohol, i.e., kills the microbes which make the water unsafe to drink; the gene producing ADH was not as necessary, was not selected for. As a result, ADH is severely limited in those cultures, and as a result alcohol consumption was also at a low point, until recently. Whereas the cultures that did not boil water had alcohol drinkers from childhood on for the majority of the population, the other cultures had relatively few drinkers.

Thirdly, most religions were not only tolerant of alcohol but supported its use. It was only when tea and coffee were introduced into Europe that religions began to take alcohol use as offensive. It must have been a strange set of coincidences that brought this about. On the one hand you had all the explorers going all over the world trying to find new sources of wealth. You had the reigning aristocracy trying to capitalize on their conquests and you had the local people that were conquered or that were used in trade that were drinking these teas and coffee. "Why not?" would think the aristocracy? "Tobacco, tea, coffee, why not create a market for them?"

It was as a result of the preparation of those boiled drinks, though, that the perception turned away from alcohol. As mentioned above, to prepare those drinks you boiled the water, and in the boiling of the water you killed the germs. Create a market for goods and at the same time set the stage for understanding of why it is that boiling makes the water safe. It is at this point that religions really took to being against the use of alcohol on a mass scale.

Fourth and most importantly. We are talking about alcohol in a very minute amount. We are not discussing distilled drinks. Most likely, we are referring to percentages that were less than 1 to 2 percent alcohol. The ills of alcohol, as we think of them came with the concentration of alcohol, with the percent rising to where it is now in beers 4-6%, and then to modern wines 12-13%. Once the process of distillation became known and widespread, then the nature of the relationship between alcohol and people shifted. It was no longer used to nourish or to drink as a safe liquid. Rather, they were used for the side effect of intoxication. They were used to alter one's perceptions.

Just as the process of distillation raised the alcohol content in the drink, it also raised the stakes, for good and for bad. After all, it is at the higher alcohol content that alcoholic products clean the wounds. It is at the higher alcohol levels that instruments and areas of the body can be cleaned to prepare for surgery. But it is also at these levels that the effects of intoxications and the side effects of alcohol began to destroy the body and soul.

So where are we now? Alcohol as a beneficial tool is relegated to the medical field for the most part. The most common use of it now in the day to day average world is for the purpose of intoxication. It is here, at this point, that alcohol became an evil and not an angel of humanity.

Not surprising, alcohol has become the number one drug used around the world. It is estimated that 1 in 2 people has been negatively influenced by alcohol in an intimate way. More than a third of crimes are committed while the perpetrator is under the influence. Countless car accidents are caused by someone who was driving while intoxicated. There are few people that do not know someone close, a friend, or a family member that has lost years to alcohol intoxication, let alone the poor choices made under the influence of alcohol.

Alcohol used to be called "Aqua Vitae," i.e., the waters of life for many of the reasons described above. Most of us can recall times when an alcoholic drink was just the right thing: a cold beer on a hot afternoon, or a beautiful glass of wine over a candlelit dinner, or perhaps a mixed drink at a cocktail party. When used in moderation by those who can handle it, alcohol is not by definition, evil. The rest of this book emphasizes the negative elements but it is not my intention to bring back prohibition or discourage the use of the occasional recreational alcoholic beverage.

We see how in a minor dose, alcohol has helped our species not only survive, but thrive. In the massive doses that it is commonly used today, it has turned into one of the worst drugs to plague humanity. It is by returning to this substance, in the infinitesimal dose, the homeopathic dose, that we can bring back its fuller medicinal properties.

Blood Alcohol Levels and the Brain

Alcohol amounts are measured in blood alcohol levels in milligrams of alcohol found per 100 milliliters of blood drawn, thus given in percent form. At levels up to .05, there is a generally pleasant feeling experienced by the person. As the blood levels rise that feeling is replaced as follows:

.02 – There is an increased sense of body warmth noted, with a slight lessening of inhibition. One feels relaxed and slightly lightheaded.

.05 – The person feels much less inhibited, less shy, more relaxed, warmer, but less focused. He is less coordinated. Accidents may begin to occur. The person becomes louder and bolder in their behavior, more euphoric than usual. Emotions are experienced slightly more intensely, sadness seems sadder and happiness seems happier.

.08 – The individual becomes impaired with regard to both coordination and judgement. She may think she is doing better than she really is. Speech is slurred, balance is compromised, hearing is muffled.

.10 – Reaction time slows greatly at this point. Inhibitions are totally lacking, the person begins acting out and expressing mood swings. What follows are the sorts of things that may occur—this is obviously not an exhaustive list—but it does show how alcohol can effect many parts of a person: euphoria, loudness, aggressiveness, belligerence, difficulty attaining and maintaining an erection, memory impairment.

.15 – Coordination is greatly effected in terms of balance and motion. Accidents are very likely. There is difficulty walking or standing. The person is no longer euphoric; instead they may become aggressive. Blackouts, where you can not recall what happened, may occur.

.20 – Disorientation rules here. It is hard to stand or walk at these levels. Your awareness of pain is diminished with attendant nausea and vomiting. The gag reflex does not function well, which allows some to choke as they vomit. Blackouts are very common.

.30 – One may lose consciousness. When in such a drunken stupor there is no awareness of where you are. Asphyxiation is common.

.40 – Most will lose consciousness and fall into a comatose state. Some will die from respiratory arrest or a too slow heart rate.

.50 – Many die from respiratory arrest.

— Chapter 11 —
Pathophysiology of Alcohol

Readily available and socially acceptable, alcohol remains the mood altering drug of choice for people the world over. Though many can well tolerate an occasional social drink there are many others for whom alcohol poses tremendous health and social risks. It is estimated that near ten percent of the American people suffer from addiction to alcohol. It is no surprise then, that *Alcoholus* should become an important and effective homeopathic remedy to address a myriad of physical, mental and emotional concerns facing a portion of patients today, as the toxicology of alcohol has widespread influence on the human body and soul. In this section we will briefly address the physiological and social impact of alcohol.

As a result of its popularity and its toxicity, the side effects and toxic effects of alcohol have been studied extensively and a fair amount about the topic is understood. We will touch on a few of the main points in this chapter. As is true when we study something at length we begin to see the connections between what we study and other factors. As a result of this, there is a problem in listing the symptoms of alcohol intake. It has to do with the effect that alcohol has on the absorption of other nutrients. As a result there are many symptoms that are listed as effects of alcohol, yet they are really due to the lack of a particular vitamin or micronutrient. I have tended in all such respects to keep the symptoms as an effect of the alcohol itself, since it is the interaction of the alcohol with the body that cascades eventually to the symptoms observed.

When taken in excess, alcohol impacts most physiologic systems including: gastrointestinal, cardiac and neurologic systems. Impact depends on many issues: whether alcohol consumption is acute or chronic in nature, whether there is food and what type of food there is in the system, the susceptibility of the person drinking, and the tolerance level of the drinker.

With regard to the gastrointestinal system, alcohol causes gastric irritation and gastritis and even bleeding from the stomach, engorgement of esophageal veins, peptic ulcer, poor food absorption, fatty liver, cirrhosis of the liver as well as pancreatitis. Alcohol is absorbed directly from the stomach and stays in the body until the liver metabolizes it. As a result, it damages the liver. The common symptoms of gas and bloating in the abdomen, heartburn, as well as all the symptoms related to liver disease are common in chronic alcohol use. In addition, many alcoholics sacrifice good nutrition and can be malnourished. There is a tendency to develop hypoglycemia due to inability in mobilizing glucose stores. Further, there is a tendency to develop increased stores of iron. This may explain why some of the symptoms of the remedy *Alcoholus* mirror those of *Ferrum metallicum*.

Weight loss is common in chronic alcohol use. There are several possible reasons, though one likely is that there are more energy needs of the body during its use. As a result more oxygen is used in people drinking alcohol. This may account for the symptoms *Alcoholus* shares with *Carbo vegetabilis*.

In the neurologic arena, many problems are caused by alcohol. In the short run, as a central nervous system depressant, alcohol slows down respiration and heart rate. Often seen are the following: an impaired ability to carry out complex tasks, a decrease in motor coordination, a prolonged time reaction and a decrease in speed of thought processing. Obviously, this makes it increasingly possible for accidents to occur as well as the diminution of good judgment in work, academic and social settings. A lowering of anxiety, as well as natural inhibition, is also common after the ingestion of alcohol.

There is a direct toxic effect from alcohol itself coupled with the not unusual malnutrition which together can lead to peripheral nerve damage or polyneuropathies (which may explain why so many provers experienced numbness and tingling during the proving) as well as, in the extreme, brain damage. The well known acute toxicity states of intoxication, blackouts and disorientation are replaced in chronic alcohol users by neuropsychiatric effects such as cerebellar degeneration, optic neuropathy, Korsakoff's psychosis, and dementia.

The heart may be impacted in long term alcohol use with cardiomyopathy and congestive heart failure. Thiamine deficiency, common to alcoholics, often adds to ECG abnormalities and arrhythmias.

There are many social ills associated with alcohol use. There are increased risks for both suicide and homicide; it is believed that near fifty percent of those arrested committed a crime while under the influence of alcohol. In regard to sexual relations, alcohol is blamed for decreased use of adequate birth control as well as a decreased tendency to practice safe sex. Certain red flags about alcoholism go up in families where any of the following are common: driving accidents, poor performance at work or school, isolating or antisocial behavior, violent acts, severe mood swings and self-isolation.

Alcohol and the Pregnant Woman

Alcohol should be considered a serious poison to a pregnant woman and the child she carries. Since the fetus and mother share the same bloodstream, when a pregnant woman drinks alcohol, so too does her fetus. No pregnant woman should drink alcohol, for several reasons. First, the change in nutritional levels of micronutrients make it difficult for the pregnant woman to give the fetus the nourishment it needs. Of great concern is decreased levels of folic acid, commonly found in alcoholics, as folic acid absorption is compromised in many alcohol drinkers. As a result of lowered levels of folic acid, there is a much higher incidence of midline birth anomalies such as cleft palate and spina bifida. This is particularly true in the first months of pregnancy when many women do not yet know they are pregnant.

Second is the effect of alcohol consumption on the fetus' mental ability. Fetal Alcohol Syndrome (FAS) is a syndrome of mental, emotional and physical symptoms seen in children that is directly linked to the mother's consumption of alcohol during pregnancy. Alcohol is teratogenic. There has not been any study to suggest what amount of alcohol is safe for the fetus during pregnancy. This is not from having alcohol in the past but the actual effect of alcohol use on the fetus by the pregnant mother. The diagnosis, described in 1968 and named in 1973 is very well accepted at this time. FAS is the leading known cause of mental retardation and birth defects and is present in about 1 in 600 births.

Most likely, it is not a single mechanism that causes all the negative side effects of alcohol on the fetus, it works in many locations, such as cell migration and cell development, as well as causing cell death to important areas during development. It is these cell deaths that cause the characteristic facial anomalies.

Recently the researchers in the field have discussed changing the overall way they categorize alcohol effect on the fetus based on the overall effect on the infant. The reason is that not all children who have a negative effect from alcohol develop the full manifestation of FAS, many others develop only part of the syndrome, often lacking the keynote facial features that make FAS easily recognizable. Here are some of the newer suggestions regarding classification of children who have been affected by alcohol consumption of the mother during pregnancy. This list is further defined below:

- FAS with confirmed maternal alcohol exposure,
- FAS without confirmed maternal alcohol exposure,
- Partial FAS with confirmed maternal alcohol exposure,
- Alcohol-related birth defect (ARBD). There are many defects associated with alcohol consumption by the pregnant mother.
- Alcohol-related neurodevelopmental disorder (ARND). There are many behavioral traits associated with alcohol consumption by the pregnant mother.

Diagnosing FAS

The following information has been extracted from **Ninth Special Report to the U.S. Congress on Alcohol and Health, June 1997 (RP0973)**. Free copies of this report are available from National Clearinghouse for Alcohol and Drug Information, 1-800-729-6686.

FAS is the most severe birth defect produced by in utero alcohol exposure. The terms "fetal alcohol effects" (FAE) and "alcohol-related birth defects" are used to describe individuals who exhibit only some of the attributes of FAS and thus do not fulfill the diagnostic criteria for the syndrome.

Diagnostic Criteria for Fetal Alcohol Syndrome (FAS) and Alcohol-Related Effects

Fetal Alcohol Syndrome

1. FAS with confirmed maternal alcohol exposures

A. Confirmed maternal alcohol exposures

B. Evidence of a characteristic pattern of facial anomalies that includes features such as short palpebral fissures and abnormalities in the premaxillary zone (e.g., flat, thin, upper lip, flattened philtrum, and flat midface)

C. Evidence of growth retardation, as in at least one of the following:
   - low birth weight for gestational age
   - decelerating weight over time not due to nutritional issues
   - disproportional low weight to height

D. Evidence of CNS neurodevelopmental abnormalities, as in at least one of the following:
- decreased cranial size at birth
- structural brain abnormalities (e.g., microcephaly, partial or complete agenesis of the corpus callosum, cerebellar hypoplasia)
- neurological hard or soft signs (as age appropriate), such as impaired fine motor skill, neurosensory hearing loss, poor tandem gait, poor eye-hand coordination

2. FAS without confirmed maternal alcohol exposure

B, C, and D as above

3. Partial FAS with confirmed maternal alcohol exposure

A. Confirmed maternal alcohol exposure'

B. Evidence of some components of the pattern of characteristic facial anomalies

Either C or D or E:

C. Evidence of growth retardation, as in at least one of the following:
- low birth weight for gestational age
- decelerating weight over time not due to nutrition
- disproportional low weight to height

D. Evidence of CNS neurodevelopmental abnormalities, as in:
- decreased cranial size at birth
- structural brain abnormalities (e.g., microcephaly, partial or complete agenesis of the corpus callosum, cerebellar hypoplasia)
- neurological hard or soft signs (as age appropriate) such as impaired fine motor skills, neurosensory hearing loss, poor tandem gait, poor eye-hand coordination

E. Evidence of a complex pattern of behavior or cognitive abnormalities that are inconsistent with developmental level and cannot be explained by familial or environmental background alone, such as learning difficulties; deficits in school performance; poor impulse control; problems in social perception; deficits in higher level receptive and expressive language; poor capacity for abstraction or meta-cognition; specific deficits in mathematical skills; or problems in memory, attention, or judgment

Alcohol-Related Effects

Clinical conditions in which there is a history of maternal alcohol exposure and where clinical or animal research has linked maternal alcohol ingestion to an observed outcome. There are two categories, which may co-occur. If both diagnoses are present, then both diagnoses should be rendered:

4. Alcohol-related birth defects (ARBD)

List of congenital anomalies, including malformations and dysplasias:

Cardiac: Atrial septal defects, Aberrant great vessels, Ventricular septal defects, Tetralogy of Fallot.

Skeletal: Hypoplastic nails, Clinodactyly, Shortened fifth digits, Pectus excavatum and carinatum, Radioulnar synostosis, Klippel-Feil syndrome, Flexion contractures, Hemivertebrae, Camptodactyly, Scoliosis.

Renal: Aplastic, Dysplastic, Ureteral duplications, Hypoplastic kidneys, Hydronephrosis, Horseshoe kidneys.

Ocular: Strabismus, Refractive problems secondary to small eyes, Retinal vascular anomalies.

Auditory: Conductive hearing loss, Neurosensory hearing loss.

Other: Virtually every malformation has been described in some patient with FAS. The etiologic specificity of most of these anomalies to alcohol teratogenesis remains uncertain.

5. Alcohol-related neurodevelopmental disorder (ARND)

Presence of:

A. Evidence of CNS neurodevelopmental abnormalities, as in any one of the following:
   - decreased cranial size at birth
   - structural brain abnormalities (e.g., microcephaly, partial or complete agenesis of the corpus callosum, cerebellar hypoplasia)
   - neurological hard or soft signs (as age appropriate), such as impaired fine motor skills, neurosensory hearing loss, poor tandem gait, poor eye-hand coordination

and/or:

> B. Evidence of a complex pattern of behavior or cognitive abnormalities that are inconsistent with developmental level and cannot be explained by familial or environmental background alone, such as learning difficulties; deficits in school performance; poor impulse control; problems in social perception; deficits in higher level receptive and expressive language; poor capacity for abstraction or meta-cognition; specific deficits in mathematical skills; or problems in memory, attention, or judgment.

From the Institute of Medicine. *Fetal Alcohol Syndrome: Diagnosis, Epidemiology, Prevention, and Treatment.* Washington, DC: National Academy Press, 1996.

FAS children are often born to multi-generational drinkers. As a result there are many FAE people who grew up and are now having children with FAS or FAE. Recall that part of the FAE can be addiction to alcohol and stimulants, inattention, low IQ, impulse issues. We are not talking about people who are likely to worry about a potential future fetus. These are people who are more likely to engage in risky behaviors and amongst other things become pregnant, while intoxicated, or drink during pregnancy.

I need to repeat here that the whole syndrome is totally preventable by avoiding the drinking of alcohol by the pregnant woman. It is because of this that women who are in the process of trying to conceive should abstain from alcohol entirely. The major problem is that she may not know she is pregnant until missing her first or second menstrual cycle. As a result it is possible that she would have drank alcohol before that. Because of that time delay in finding out if one is pregnant, it is prudent for the woman not to drink alcohol, if she is sexually active and attempting to get pregnant in the near future.

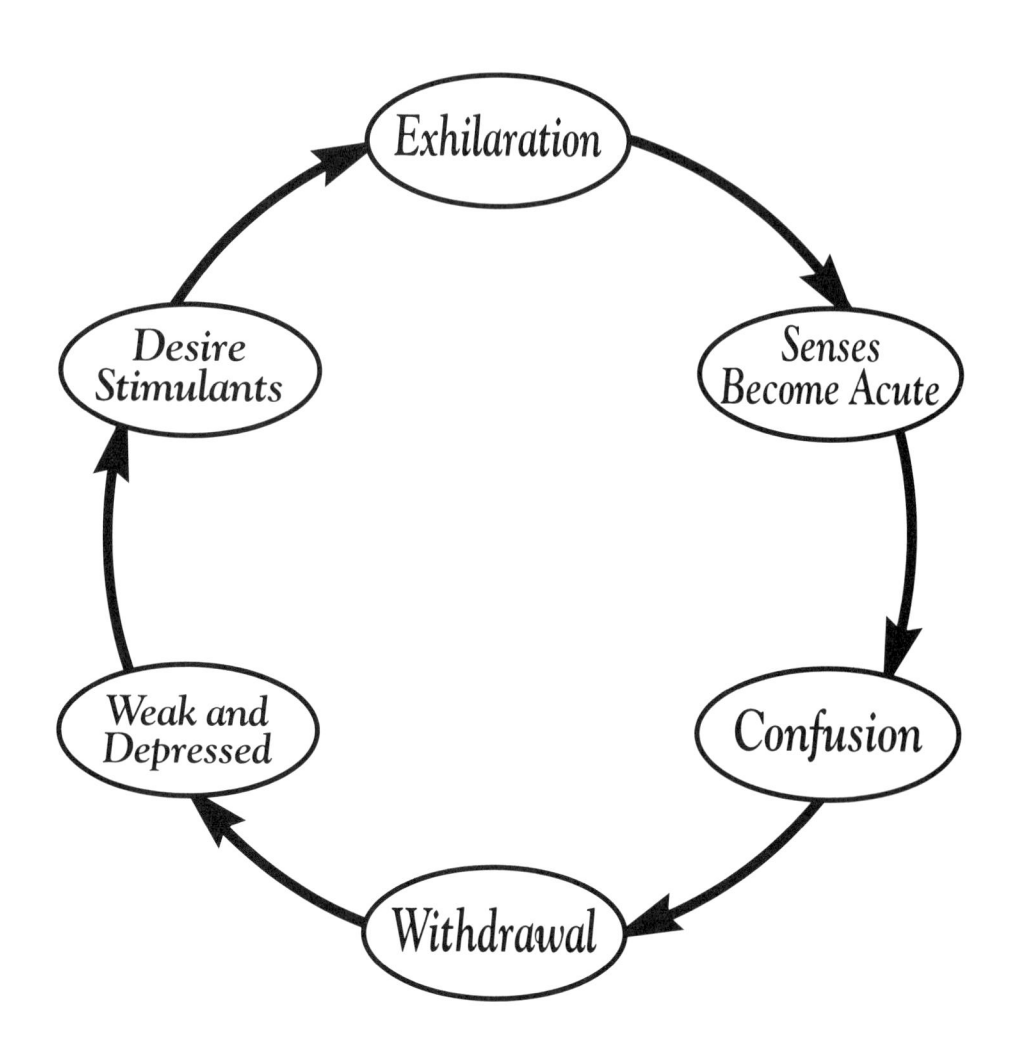

Exhilaration → Senses Become Acute → Confusion → Withdrawal → Weak and Depressed → Desire Stimulants → Exhilaration

The Alcoholus Cycle

— Chapter 12 —
Materia Medica of Alcoholus

Alcohol is known for its ability to make someone feel good initially. People are able to come out of themselves, they feel like they are floating and intoxicated, exhilarated**(1)**. When the intoxication is too much, or when they are too drunk, excessive discharges begin, including rage. The senses become acute with light, sound, taste and feeling, all becoming more vivid, often at the same time**(2)**. They get confused, there is just too much going on for them to process in a timely fashion**(3)**. In order to relieve the confusion they need to be alone or to withdraw. They close up. They do not want to have light, sound or stimulation because it irritates the system**(4)**. They become weak and depressed**(5)**. In order to get out of this down state, they want to be stimulated again**(6)**.

Mind

1. Exhilaration/Coming Out of Yourself:

One of the most striking aspects of this remedy is the excessive joy and freedom that both the provers and patients feel. A patient may experience different aspects of this *Segment*, as described below:

Loss of Inhibition

Loss of inhibition may be described in a more physical way, saying they feel a kind of **floating,** or **levitation**, or a sense that their soul is leaving, or some sort of out of body experience, just as we find in the remedy *Cannabis indica*. There can be the feeling that they are rising out of themselves.

The loss of inhibition is seen at times in their behavior in the office. The children may be goofing around. They may be **laughing a lot or talking a lot**. They may interrupt their parents' answers, sometimes contradicting, sometimes adding to their parents' comments. In any case, they tend to be many times louder than whoever else is speaking. It does not matter which of those things they do, it is the interfering and disruptive nature of their questions *and* answers that is common.

They may be hitting their parents or siblings in the interview, looking at you, egging you on. It is a kind of play they are in. They are not serious or caring about why it is that they are there, it is all a game to them.

Because of these behaviors, many homeopaths mistakenly have given this type of child *Cannabis indica* or even *Hyoscyamus*.

Deception

Deception is another aspect of the mental state. Many of these children **lie** to the parents, teachers, and to the homeopath. The concept of truth as a value is lost on them. While many children lie to stay out of trouble, the *Alcoholus* patient lies for the fun of it. They also lie to attain things. This lack of inhibition is also found in the adolescent or older teen who has been caught shoplifting or caught stealing money from her parents.

I recall one 14 year old girl that loved to shop. She was caught by her parents stealing clothes from a store. They were astounded that she would steal anything, let alone with them being in the store at the same time. When asked why she did it, she said she liked that dress. Another time she was caught stealing money from the mother. When asked why she did it, she told the parents that she wanted to buy something. There was no shame, no sense of morality, no worry of being caught, nor sense of remorse. Nothing! It didn't impact her. This lack of morality has often caused homeopaths to prescribe *Hyoscyamus*, *Anacardium* or *Morphinum* to these children.

The lack of inhibition is also seen in the need to **enjoy themselves**. This is a common trait of people needing this remedy. You can see this by how **loquacious** some of them are. They enjoy talking and do not care if someone is paying attention to them or not. They not only talk but are often very **loud**, so as to drown out all surrounding discussions. They do not seem to care about the effect they have on others in this regard.

Such children enjoy playing **practical jokes** on others. This is not the more intricate sort of joke which takes a long time to plan and to set into motion. This is the taking something and having the other person spend endless time looking for it, or the taking of an object out of someone's hand and running away and having the other person scream and chase them. This is the immature jokester who quickly becomes annoying. In fact, **this child may seem very immature to you** and the parent in many ways.

Rage

This sense of being outside of themselves leads them to seem unemotional at times. Some of the older adolescents will tell their parents whatever is on their minds, even hurtful things, without pause. Like the adults, they will not care how it is that they impact the parent with their comments. This is not done with meanness. There is a lack of awareness of who they are and how it is that they impact others. They just act without forethought or afterthought.

One of the ways that this is seen in some autistic patients is that they may become aggressive and **rageful**. By this, I do not mean that they are always mad, ready to strike out or walk around with a chip on their shoulder. Rather, they are so outside themselves that when they do things that are annoying and others try to reign them in, they strike out. It is almost an autonomic response. It is not premeditated anger. There is so little center or stability to many people needing *Alcoholus* that when someone says or does something that offends them, they immediately strike out.

At times this trait may make it seem **as if they are sympathetic**. For example, when an adolescent sees someone being mean to another person he may just step into the middle of the fray and enter into a rage. This is not preplanned. It is not a constant state of anger, rather a sense (that you or the parent feels) that he is responding to a situation without thought, a type of impulsivity.

2. Sensory acuity

Another way to see this exhilaration is to see how easy it is to get them **entranced** by sensory stimulation. Be it movies, plays, music or books read aloud, they are transported right into the story. They enjoy their sensory world. Like *Cannabis indica* children and teens, they may describe colors as vibrant, tastes of foods very clearly and with relish, and textures of clothes with superlatives. They enjoy their sensory awareness, feeling, seeing, smelling, hearing in a more profound way than others do.

Of course this acuity may also have a downside. Many of these children have the awareness, the sharpness that I just described. But instead of being transported into the beauty of it, they are disturbed by it. It is these intense symptoms of sensory integration issues that had eventually led me to prescribe this remedy for some autistic children. They are profoundly disturbed by smells, as of foods, vomiting or gagging when entering restaurants. Noise bothers them, so that they cover their ears, become confused and at times aggressive from the sensory overload and confusion it causes. Little tags on the back of shirts or socks with the seams misaligned can send them into a rage. Being hypersensitive may have its drawbacks.

So, the symptom that *Alcoholus* children have is an **increased acuity of sensations**. What they do with it is up to them. Some love it and it sends them into revelry. Others are profoundly bothered by it and it causes ongoing disturbances in their lives and the lives of their families.

In the older children, adolescents, and adults the **sexual drive increases** as well. Just as their other senses become more acute, so too does their sexual desire increase.

3. Confusion

One of the most consistent symptoms for the remedy is confusion. Some aspect of confusion will be present in every patient needing this remedy; it will often be the main complaint, or at very least, a strong symptom.

In the autistic child, as well as the child that has severe sensory integration issues, confusion will be seen in the way they **misunderstand sensory cues.** Things that happen around them will be misconstrued. They may not understand another person's intention, be it a parent, teacher, sibling or friend. For example, I recall one autistic child who would strike out scratching anyone who came near him from the side. If he could not see the person approach from the front, the child would attack him.

This confusion can be profound as well. Here we are talking about children with mental retardation at the worst and with severe processing problems.

In other children, adolescents, and adults the confusion is not as profound but is still a big problem. They do poorly in school. They are diagnosed with attention problems, with poor impulse control and/or hyperactivity. Many of these children can not do their schoolwork, and truly struggle in any self-directed work like choice times or homework. Reading is difficult, retaining what they have read is even more challenging. They come home and forget that they even have homework.

Learning new concepts is difficult for these children. They constantly make mistakes in their schoolwork, especially in spelling, writing and speaking.

Many of these children will be diagnosed with a type of processing problem. For example, one child will do poorly because of an auditory processing problem, where they hear words spoken to them but have a hard time focusing and understanding what it is that the teacher wants them to do.

Likewise, they **forget** their school supplies, forget their shoes, forget their coats and constantly lose possessions. The way I view these children is that they are so outside themselves that possessions mean very little to them. Because of these symptoms, *Alcoholus* children and adults are often confused with those needing *Cannabis indica.*

Gross motor incoordination may be seen in accidents. Having accidents is another tendency that we commonly see in those needing this remedy. We see this in the children and adolescents who stumble, fall, break things around them as well as injure themselves. We see this in children who cannot negotiate a fork and spoon, who still eat with their hands even into their teen years. We see this in the child that cannot play sports or who looks excessively awkward on the field, arms flailing one way, legs the other. We often find a disorientation in the child. Is he left-handed or right-handed? Even this he is still trying to work out. You can sometimes see the disorientation and awkwardness in his gait as well.

In adults, the accidents can be more major, such as car accidents, dropping things, falling off of bicycles, etc. It is as if their reflexes are sluggish. Their senses are still working, yet lagging behind, so that when they have to act or react, they hesitate. Interestingly enough, in the proving that we conducted, several people had dreams of car accidents as well as other types of mishaps, for the first time in their lives.

4. Wanting to be alone

The wanting to be alone comes about for two completely different reasons. The first has to do with the acuity of their senses. This can be seen in both the child and the adult. You may find an autistic child or even a more typical child who is so sensitive to the stimuli of a crowd—the noise, motion, cheering—that they want to get out of that situation. And even in the adult you may see someone who is so overly stimulated that they can not think or sleep or have peace and just crave getting home and having it all be quiet and peaceful.

The second reason has to do with the confusion. There is a whole other state in this remedy, seen in both the children and adults, that of wanting to be reclusive. This manifests differently for different people. In some, the out of body feeling, the acute senses and the confusion have led to behaviors that are so odd to other kids around them, that they can be been made fun of. They are ridiculed, taunted, and at times, physically harassed by other children at school or on the playground. As a result, the confused child may not know how or why this is happening. What he does know is that he does not want to go to school, does not want to go out to play and just wants to stay in the house. Some children never get that far. The world is so confusing that they just want to stay home.

The adults as well have this closing off, a closed and introverted feeling. Yet it is not a true introversion. It is closer to the feeling that someone who is manic-depressive would have. They had this higher feeling. They felt great and had a lot of energy and did a lot of things. But at times the energy fails. At these times they are not as happy and want to stay home. They eat less, do less, and mostly watch television or read books and take a vacation from life. We see this also in the adults that have narcolepsy and fall asleep, like those needing the remedy *Opium*.

I recall one woman who had a secret eating disorder, binging on sweets and carbohydrates—bread and cookies—when she felt unloved. Afterwards—she would feel badly about herself and not want to face her husband or the world.

5. Depression

Many times the sense of confusion, of wanting to be secluded is accompanied by sadness or depression. There is the clear sense that nothing works out, nothing will ever work out, and they do not know why. While depression is a common characteristic of the remedy, it is not a strong symptom for most. In other words, even the child that has been harassed at school, made fun of in the playground, a child that feels sad, will often be able to be gotten out of that mood by taking him to the movies or taking her out for an ice cream. I think this is because they are not all that solid. As a result, it is easy for them to fall into sadness but also easy to get them out of their depressions. It is the same with the adults in the short term. Call them, take them out to dinner and they are in a good mood. Yet in the long run, they sense that their life is not going as they wanted it to go. They sense that there is something not working right with them. It is that sense that actually gets them to the next *Segment*, looking for things to stimulate themselves.

6. Desire for Stimulation

A very consistent symptom in the adult and the child is the desire for stimulation. They want and want and want. This extends all the way into adulthood where they seek stimulants like coffee and eventually other drugs that, initially at least, have a stimulating effect. They are looking for a 'rush,' for some form of stimuli because when they get that, they feel they can function better. As is the classic case with many people that have attention problems, it takes some form of strong stress or shock or fright to get them working at an optimal pace. By listening to music *really* loudly, or driving *really* fast or taking recreational drugs, they are finally able to coalesce all their resources and focus. That is what it is like with the *Alcoholus* patient. I am reminded of the physiologic effect of alcohol on the person. If you drink spirits, like scotch, you get a kind of heat sensation that is sudden, central and rises from the stomach upward to the head, followed by a vasodilatation of the face. I think that any form of stimulation does the same thing to these people. The focus comes back into the brain. I think that part of the stealing does the same thing and may be part of this *Segment* as well. It could be that they need some type of stimulation, something like that to get a 'rush'.

Sleep

Sleepiness that is **overpowering** is consistent in the remedy, especially in the adults. This is especially seen when they are attempting to focus and unfortunately this can be seen especially while they drive.

The sleep is often **restless** due to too much noise in the dreams. The dreams of *Alcoholus* patients offer many compelling symptom, to the homeopath.

Dreams of accidents of any type are common. This can be dreams of car accidents, or of breaking things. Many times the objects are real and in the person's life.

Dreams of destruction are also common, with houses breaking, furniture moving, cars crashing.

Dreams of water. The dreams often involve large bodies of water; of the ocean or the great lakes. The nature of the dreams is unpleasant. This is the fishing trip that turned bad as a result of intense weather. Or the currents are so strong it is hard to fight them. Or the waves are so big that rescue is doubtful. Interestingly enough, this is one of the strongest symptoms listed in T.F. Allen's *Materia Medica*:

> "They think they are on shipboard at sea, and fear being drowned in the storm; they therefore throw everything in the room overboard, i.e., out of the window, into the street, or into the sea, as they think."

We have also seen dreams of being lost, either at sea or in a city or having taken the wrong road in the car.

Dreams that are sexual in nature are also common.

Dreams of people from the distant past. These are past husbands, dead relatives, old lovers, classmates from grade school. There is often no one distinctive story-line to the dreams but they are very emotive. What is interesting to me about these dreams is how they are juxtaposed by the fact that the person may have poor concentration and memory during their waking hours and yet recall old friends and happenings with detail and clarity. Also interesting to me is the fact that when many drink the crude alcoholic drink, they have a melancholic longing for the past, or have the past become quite vivid while they drink. It is a proving of the crude substance there.

The dreams are very vivid. Many times the dreams have a clear story with a great amount of detail in them, in color with many hues. Having them retell one of their dreams is similar to listening to someone tell you about their recreational drug experience; often long and with many, many details. Related to this is that the dreams may be of the day's events.

Lastly, are the dreams of suspense and deception. The patients dream that someone is playing tricks on them, wanting to steal from them or hurt them in some way and the patient is trying to get away.

Vertigo

There is a sense of dizziness or light-headedness that comes and goes. It is seen mostly when attempting to focus the mind, while driving or when getting excited. It can also be seen during menopausal hot flashes.

Head

Headaches are very common and frequent in the adults. The most consistent symptoms are:

Right-sided. It is most frequently felt on the right side of the head.

Sharp pains. While the headache may have different sensations, the most common one is a sharp shooting pain.

Sensations are also common in the remedy. The three most common ones are:

Heat and flushing sensations. The head feels hot as in a hot flash.

Heaviness. The head feels both full of more fluid but also too heavy to be held up by the neck.

Tingling. The tingling is either by itself, coming and going, or it may be associated with a skin eruption.

Eyes

The eyes experience the same **sharp pains** that are found in other parts of the body. This can be as part of a headache, or as part of a viral infection in or near the eye. The sharp pains tend to be more in the right eye.

The eye can also experience the **heat and dryness** that is seen in other parts of the body. This can be part of a general drying and heat of the body or it can be as part of an allergic reaction. The remedy has treated and cured allergies that involve the eyes with itching, tearing, heat, and a dry feel of the eye, even as it is tearing.

Visually, as mentioned in the mind section, **the sense of vision can become very acute**, so much so that they see things that others miss. The problem is that this visual acuity leads to **visual distortions especially at night.** They can easily get thrown off visually by too much light. It is as if they went to an ophthalmologist and had their pupils dilated. Their pupils can not accommodate quickly enough at night to light. As a result, too much light is coming in and blinding them. This leads to difficulties while driving at night. It is especially worse when rain causes the road to reflect the light of cars.

Ears

The symptoms of the ears are similar to those of the rest of the body. They can develop *otitis media* with **sharp pains**, especially in the **right ear**. As the *otitis* continues, it leads to a pulsating throbbing pain, with redness of the pinna of the ear.

The **hearing is often acute**, with the person hearing the slightest noises. They describe that noises bother them. The children get distracted in school by noise from other students. The adult has trouble concentrating because of the noise of the computer, or the noise of his coworkers.

Nose

Patients needing *Alcoholus* often have terrible allergic reactions overall, and that is often seen in the nose. In seasonal allergies the most common symptoms are the **tingling and itching** inside the nose, which causes them to scratch often, the clear mucus discharge, and the frequent sneezing. The nose is most **congested in a warm room** and much less congested in the cool open air. Even if the patient does not have seasonal allergies, she may still have periods of stuffiness in the nose, with the turbinates swelling, mostly in a warm room. The congestion may be associated with sinusitis, either acute or chronic.

For many people needing this remedy, the **sense of smell becomes more accentuated,** for good and for bad. While on the one hand they can smell foods and lovely smells more acutely than the general population, noxious odors are likewise more keenly experienced. This is seen most especially in the child that will hate to go out to eat at a restaurant because they do not like the smells of the place or the adult that can not use a public bathroom for the same reason. He is the child that may refuse to eat foods because of the smells or the child that acts out terribly because he dislikes the smell of the soap used to wash his clothes.

Face

The most consistent symptom seen in the face relates to the **flushing and heat** of the face. They will have the flushing that is typically seen in *Ferrum metallicum*. The flushing can be a concomitant symptom in many situations. For example, the shy person who is confused may blush easily. The woman who is going through menopause has a hot flash and her face becomes excessively red. The *Alcoholus* person's face gets warm and flushed when warm in a room. Interestingly, flushing and heat of the face is a common physiologic response to alcohol consumption.

Another symptom that is common is the **tingling**, as was mentioned above. The tingling sometimes accompanies the flushing. Sometimes the tingling is a concomitant to a viral skin outbreak, like herpes simplex.

Mouth

There are some common symptoms to the *Alcoholus* patient. First is the **dryness** of the mouth. The mouth may actually be very dry with little saliva, or it may have saliva in it with the sensation of dryness. Sometimes the mouth feels **hot**. Related to this is **a great thirst for water, most especially for cold water.**

As mentioned above, there is often a **strong sense of taste** which can be a rich experience for those that love tasty foods but can be very limiting to the child that is averse to food because everything tastes too strong.

Itching and tingling in the mouth, the palate and the back of the throat are common symptoms during hay fever or a viral infection. Viral infections of the mouth, either acute ones or more chronic outbreaks like herpes are very common. With the infections there is itching, tingling, and eventually vesicles that rupture and leave ulcers behind.

Throat

The throat shows many of the symptoms mentioned in the **Mouth** section. The same **itching and tingling** is found here, for the same reasons. During infections and most commonly during allergies, the throat is symptomatic. Some have a **scratchy**, sore throat, due to inflammation or due to a post-nasal catarrh, feeling as if they were in a smoke-filled bar all night. Others have a sensation of **swelling or fullness** in the throat that feels better if they breathe cool air. As in the ear and eye, there are sharp pains in the throat, especially when swallowing. All the sensations and **pains are worse on the right side**.

Stomach

Heartburn is a complaint in the adults. The burning is after eating and takes the appetite away. There is sometimes regurgitation of food, along with soreness in the throat. During this time, there is also gas and bloating in the abdomen.

In terms of food cravings and thirst, the **thirst is often high for cold drinks**. In terms of food craving, a **craving for sweets, coffee, spicy, salt, and meat** are common. The appetite is often diminished, while others binge on foods.

Abdomen

Gas and bloating is seen in the adults needing *Alcoholus*, making the confusion with *Lycopodium* understandable. Both remedies will have bloating of the abdomen with a disordered stomach. Both will pass flatus easily, which will relieve them. Both will have a tendency to have the discomfort be more on the right side. One place where they differ greatly is that the *Lycopodium* during this time will want warm drinks, whereas the *Alcoholus* will prefer cold.

I have noticed that both the adult patients and the provers that had a tendency towards liver symptoms, or had liver disease were more sensitive to this remedy.

Rectum

Unless there is a digestive complaint, as a severe food allergy, there is a tendency towards **constipation**. (Interestingly enough, this is opposite to what is found in acute alcohol ingestion, where alcohol may lead to type III peristaltic waves that sometimes causes diarrhea, as found in *Sulphur*.) In some there is no urge but in many there is a strong ineffectual urge and discomfort, which makes it challenging to differentiate with *Nux vomica*. Again, the desire for cold drinks in *Alcoholus* and the desire for warm drinks in *Nux vomica* helps to tell them apart.

Urinary Tract

Unlike the rectum, where there is found less frequent stools than average, we see the opposite in the bladder, where there is a frequent urge to urinate for children and adults. The adults may be waking up at night to urinate.

Male

Men needing this remedy have a **heightened sexual desire**. Just as there is the tingling in other parts of the body, in terms of sexuality, there is an easy erethism, where he becomes aroused easily.

There may be a **swelling of the prostate**, making him have to urinate more frequently, though incompletely.

Female

One of the most common symptoms in the middle-aged woman is that of **menopause**. This time of life is filled with many changes that seem to fit the remedy well. **Hot flashes** that begin in the chest and rise up to the head are common, accompanied by redness of the face and even the ears. The menses may become irregular, coming too soon or more likely too late, and she may flow less or even stop at an early age. **The vaginal tract may become dry** and sexual intercourse becomes painful.

In terms of the menses, there is a set of **premenstrual symptoms** that are common to both *Alcoholus* and *Lycopodium*, with **irritability**, **weepiness**, **sadness** and a **withdrawn** feeling. The **breasts swell and ache to the touch**. Interestingly enough, when the menses is late in a woman needing *Alcoholus*, she may dream much more than usual.

Herpes simplex eruptions are possible in this remedy. They begin with a tingling sensation in an area followed in days by sharp pains and then a vesicle erupts, accompanied by heat and burning.

Sexual drive may become strong, just as it does in men.

Chest

In terms of the chest there are two symptoms of note. One is that **the breasts will become swollen and painful before the menses**. If there is fibrocystic breast disease, then the breasts are even more painfully sore.

The other symptom has to do with **sharp pains where the ribs join the sternum.** The pains will be sharp and especially painful on motion. They can be on either side. If the liver is not functioning well, then the pains will be more right-sided.

Respiratory Tract

Allergic complaints are very common to the remedy. These may be seen in hay fever but also in repeated bronchitis and especially in **asthma**. The asthma is worse lying down, better sitting up, being quiet, open air, and cool air. It is worse from the heat and worse from allergens like pollen, smoke or animal dander. The symptoms are mostly of swelling, congestion and constriction and not so much of coughing.

Musculoskeletal

Both the spine and the extremities share symptoms in this remedy. In terms of the spine, there is a tendency towards right-sided torticollis. There is a general tendency of **right-sided back pains** that are mild and sore at times and sharp and intense at other times. They are often related to muscular stiffness and achiness but at times related to joint compressions. These pains can be in the thoracic, lumbar, or sacral area.

In the extremities the right side again is more symptomatic. There is a right-sided shoulder or elbow arthritis or pain. The hands may be arthritic and stiff.

In the lower extremities, the knee and hip and toes are commonly affected on the right side with stiffness and pain. The most common pain besides soreness is pinpoint sharp little pains.

Skin

In terms of the skin the most common symptoms have been mentioned already. There is a general **dryness of the skin**. There is an easy **flushing of the skin**, most especially the upper parts of the body. There is a **tingling** sensation in various parts of the body, though this is usually related to a viral infection or flare-up. The most common one is herpes simplex, where there is a tingling sensation in an area followed a few days later by sharp pains. Vesicles then erupt with heat and burning.

Generals

There are some very strong general symptoms to the remedy.

There is often a family history of alcohol abuse. This can be either alcoholics as parents or grandparents or the patient himself may have been an alcoholic at some time in his life, or he was conceived while the parents were under the influence of alcohol. The mother may have drunk alcohol during the pregnancy.

The miasms that the remedy belongs to are **Sycotic** and **Syphylitic**. The remedy is very strongly miasmatic. The alcohol abuse in the history seems to make the Sycotic and the Syphilitic traits erupt forth strongly. As a result, you may think of this remedy almost as a nosode. When other remedies seem to fail you, and there is a family history of alcohol abuse and the patient shows strongly Sycotic or Syphilitic traits, then consider *Alcoholus*.

The **right-sidedness** found in the remedy is very strong. Many of the complaints will be either only on the right side or more aggravated on the right side.

The **heat and flushing** is seen in many parts of the individual. In fact, the person may be **warm-blooded** in general, feeling confined, irritable, and trapped **in a warm room and wanting cool air and feeling better in the cool outside air.**

The pains found in different parts of the body tend to be **sharp and stitching**.

There is a general **dryness** to the person, seen in the skin, rectum, mouth, or vagina.

Tingling, waves, vibrations are words that many adults needing this remedy will use.

In terms of constitutional types that are similar, easily confused with this remedy, shift into this remedy or are in some way related to this remedy, we have *Nux vomica, Lycopodium, Sulphur, Medorrhinum, Lachesis, Cannabis indica, Opium, Morphinum, Hyoscyamus and Carcinosinum*. Because of these relationships it was people who needed these remedies that proved *Alcoholus* easiest.

— Chapter 13 —
A Short Case

I would like to briefly describe a young man who benefited greatly from the remedy *Alcoholus*. He is typical of one type of person who does well with this remedy. This boy was thirteen years old, in ninth grade, and the oldest of five siblings. His father described him as having the dominant 'first-born disposition' and attitude.

One of his main complaints was difficulty focusing on reading and writing endeavors. By the time he was in the fifth grade he was having a hard time focusing in school. Concentrating on schoolwork and studying for exams was very challenging tasks for him. The main problem was that when he had to focus on a paper that he was reading or one that he had to write, his mind would wander. As his mind wandered, he would stop working on his project and would eventually get up and do other more fun things. As a result, the concentration difficulty manifested as dullness while studying. Added to this, the concentration difficulty would lead to restlessness.

The restlessness was typical of other children who have concentration difficulties. However it was coupled with unique attitudes. The restlessness would often lead to silly behaviors. He would joke around, becoming very silly and immature. He would eventually act outright foolishly. This blatant joking around and foolishness would very quickly slide into inappropriate behavior for the situation he was in. He would become heedless, uncaring and impulsive, doing things that would upset parents, siblings, students and teachers. He could walk up to another child and grab him, pick him up and hoist him over his shoulders, turning him. He would make noises at inappropriate times. He spoke out in class. He would take toys, books, or other objects away from someone else, just to be funny. He would grab things from other people even in the middle of class and think it funny. He would grab food off his siblings' plates during supper just to be funny. He would act like a six year old boy goofing around. The problem was that he was thirteen years old. His teachers and parents and siblings considered him quite immature. His teachers complained of his immature disruptive behavior in school.

He could not tolerate it when he was chastised, contradicted or interfered with in any way, at any time. He would become very angry and belligerent. The anger was mostly verbal, becoming hypercritical, calling other children names such as "You're stupid," or "You're an idiot. "

He never took responsibility for anything going wrong. Things were never his fault. While this may be common to a certain type of child, this boy would blame others, lie and consistently deny any wrong doing. Even if you were *watching* him doing something wrong, he would still lie and deny he was involved. The parents never knew if the school day went well or not, as he would not tell them if he had been disciplined in school, denying that anything bad had happened. If he was fooling around and was sent to the principle, he would lie to his parents about what happened.

Interestingly enough, after chastising him, after yelling at him or disciplining him at home, he would close up, and close in. He would sit around and watch television. It was at these times that he would be most dull and most spacey. At these times he was unable to put his attention on anything; he would become so engrossed by what he was watching, you would have to tell him something three times before he would process what he heard. At these times, if you asked him to study, he would fail miserably and it is at these times that he would get up every five minutes from restlessness.

He had been given several remedies over the course of his life. When he was seven years old he fell off a bunk bed and fractured his skull. He was given *Arnica* and later *Helleborus*. He had also had amongst other remedies *Nux vomica*.

He was given *Alcoholus* 200C, in a single dose. To his parents delight, he showed signs of maturing soon after. The foolish, jesting, joking behavior and immaturity came to a halt. The aggravation from contradiction ceased at the same time. He was no longer critical or abusive. His teachers and parents had been worried about how he would fare in the next year's class. Everyone thought of him as immature and unable to keep up in his work. Within a couple of months he became a polite boy, not speaking out of turn in class, aware of others around him and not acting foolishly at all. After 18 months, he went on to another remedy but all of these complaints were a thing of the past by that time due to the *Alcoholus*.

His father, a homeopath, relates, "He used to act like the mean drunk before. He used to be hard and mean if you crossed him or stopped him in any way. Now he is polite and offers to help in the house. He really is a pleasure."

As is common in children who need this remedy, there is a strong family history of alcoholism. In this particular family, on the mother's side, her father was an active alcoholic, and on the father's side the grandparents as well as their siblings all drank heavily.

Common in the children who need this remedy is the family history of alcoholism, the difficulty concentrating, the deception, the restlessness, the sudden anger, and the jesting, as if drunk. As a quick point of differentiation with *Cannabis indica*, there is more anger in *Alcoholus* than in *Cannabis indica*.

— Chapter 14 —
The Rubrics of Alcoholus

I have debated whether or not to place the rubrics of *Alcoholus* in this book. There are many elements which trouble me with regard to the current repertory, and how people use the repertory in our times. Just as *this* book introduces a model for understanding provings, I shall, in time, address the repertory, showing how my model helps to address many of the questions and difficulties which surround the writing of, and use of the repertory. Until that time, I have been hesitant to publish or add any rubrics or additions to the repertory and offer these cautiously with the following guidelines and observations:

Firstly, I include this listing for current and future homeopaths studying this proving. These are the *only* rubrics that I have chosen. Though there were many more rubrics possible, though one could "data mine" the provings for other symptoms and rubrics, I have purposely left them out. Please do *not* include new ones and please do not assume that I wanted them in the repertory at this time. Those symptoms are left out on purpose.

Secondly, as you look through these rubrics, please note that even though the list is of 477 rubrics, many of the rubrics are similar to each other or contain subrubrics and or modalities on one symptom. In other words, these 477 rubrics can be condensed down to a **couple of hundred rubrics and really exemplifying a handful of ideas.** This proving included more than one hundred provers, over the course of several years, yet yielded this number of rubrics, in sharp contrast to some contemporary provings, which garner thousands of symptoms. With a deluge of additions to the repertory it is inevitable that an imbalance will occur in the repertory rendering it a less functional tool. I address this in another book.

Thirdly, if you look at many of the provings that have been published recently, you will find that there is a scattering of symptoms all over the repertory. One of the major problems of these provings is that the remedies are being listed in our most important rubrics. As a result, even when a proving does not have *many* symptoms, the remedies are found in important rubrics, so the remedies often come up during repertorization. As you look at the rubrics listed below, you do not see that problem. This illustrates once more, in yet another way, that this proving was analyzed clearly and that the symptoms that are included belong.

The rubrics of *Alcoholus* listed below, reflect both the provings conducted over the past number of years as well as the clinical application of this remedy. *For the current repertories,* where the rubric is listed as a 3, the symptom was proven by many people and clearly seen in practice. The rubrics listed as 2 are proven by a few people and seen in practice. The rubrics listed as 1 are proven by several people *or* seen in practice, though not as commonly as other rubrics. The grading also takes into account the balance of the repertory, a subject which has not been well addressed to date and which I shall speak to in a future discourse on the repertory.

1. MIND - ABSENTMINDED — 2
2. MIND - ABSENTMINDED - air; in open - amel — 1
3. MIND - ABSENTMINDED - dreamy — 2
4. MIND - ABSORBED — 2
5. MIND - ABSTRACTION OF MIND — 2
6. MIND - ABUSIVE — 2
7. MIND - AMUSEMENT - desire for — 2
8. MIND - ANGER - contradiction; from — 2
9. MIND - ANTICS; playing — 2
10. MIND - ANTICS; playing - children; in — 2
11. MIND - AWKWARD — 1
12. MIND - AWKWARD - drops things — 1
13. MIND - BOASTER, — 1
14. MIND - CHEERFUL — 2
15. MIND - CHILDISH behavior — 2
16. MIND - CLARITY of mind — 1
17. MIND - COMPANY - aversion to — 1
18. MIND - COMPLAINING — 1
19. MIND - CONCENTRATION - difficult — 2
20. MIND - CONCENTRATION - difficult – morning — 1
21. MIND - CONCENTRATION - difficult - air; in open - amel. — 1
22. MIND - CONCENTRATION - difficult - children, in — 1
23. MIND - CONCENTRATION - difficult - driving; while — 2
24. MIND - CONCENTRATION - difficult - studying — 2
25. MIND - CONFIDENCE - want of self-confidence — 2
26. MIND - CONFUSION of mind — 2
27. MIND - CONFUSION of mind – morning — 1

28. MIND - CONFUSION of mind - morning - waking, on 1
29. MIND - CONFUSION of mind - air, in open - amel. 1
30. MIND - CONFUSION of mind - concentrate the mind, on attempting to 2
31. MIND - CONFUSION of mind - dream, as if in a 1
32. MIND - CONFUSION of mind - excitement ; amel. 2
33. MIND - CONFUSION of mind - intoxicated - as if 2
34. MIND - CONFUSION of mind - knows not where he is 1
35. MIND - CONFUSION of mind - loses his way in well-known streets 1
36. MIND - CONFUSION of mind - mental exertion - from 1
37. MIND - CONFUSION of mind - noise - agg. 1
38. MIND - CONFUSION of mind - reading, while 2
39. MIND - CONFUSION of mind - sitting, while 1
40. MIND - CONFUSION of mind - walking - air, in open - amel. 2
41. MIND - CONFUSION of mind - warm room, in 2
42. MIND - CONFUSION of mind - writing, while 1
43. MIND - CONTEMPTUOUS 1
44. MIND - CONTRADICTION - disposition to contradict 1
45. MIND - CONTRADICTION - intolerant of contradiction 1
46. MIND - CONTRARY 1
47. MIND - CRUELTY 1
48. MIND - CURSING 1
49. MIND - DECEITFUL, sly 2
50. MIND - DELUSIONS - floating - air, in 1
51. MIND - DELUSIONS - insulted, he is 2
52. MIND - DELUSIONS - pursued; he was - murderers; by 1
53. MIND - DELUSIONS - pursued; he was - robbers; by 1
54. MIND - DELUSIONS - separated - body - soul; body is separated from 2
55. MIND - DELUSIONS - ships - storm; they are on board of a ship in a 1
56. MIND - DESIRES - full of desires 1
57. MIND - DISCOURAGED 1
58. MIND - DISHONEST 2
59. MIND - DREAM; as if in a 2

60.	MIND - DULLNESS	2
61.	MIND - DULLNESS – morning	1
62.	MIND - DULLNESS - morning - waking, on	1
63.	MIND - DULLNESS - air - open air; in - amel.	1
64.	MIND - DULLNESS - mental exertion, from	1
65.	MIND - DULLNESS - reading	2
66.	MIND - DULLNESS - sleepiness, with	1
67.	MIND - DULLNESS - thinking - long; unable to think	2
68.	MIND - DULLNESS - understand; does not - questions addressed to her – repetition; only after	1
69.	MIND - DULLNESS - vertigo; during	1
70.	MIND - DULLNESS - walking - air; in open - amel.	1
71.	MIND - DULLNESS - writing, while	1
72.	MIND - EGOTISM, self-esteem	1
73.	MIND - ESTRANGED - family; from his	1
74.	MIND - EXCITEMENT - amel.	1
75.	MIND - EXCITEMENT - desire for	1
76.	MIND - EXHILARATION	2
77.	MIND - FANCIES - vivid, lively	1
78.	MIND - FOOLISH behavior	2
79.	MIND - FORGETFUL	2
80.	MIND - GIGGLING	1
81.	MIND - HARDHEARTED, inexorable	2
82.	MIND - HAUGHTY	1
83.	MIND - HEEDLESS	1
84.	MIND - HIGH-SPIRITED	1
85.	MIND - IDIOCY	1
86.	MIND - IMBECILITY	1
87.	MIND - IMPATIENCE	1
88.	MIND - IMPATIENCE - contradiction; at slightest	1
89.	MIND - IMPERTINENCE	1
90.	MIND - IMPETUOUS	1
91.	MIND - IMPULSE; morbid - violence, to do	1
92.	MIND - IMPULSIVE	2
93.	MIND - INDISCRETION	1
94.	MIND - INSOLENCE	1

95.	MIND - INTRIGUER	1
96.	MIND - IRRESOLUTION, indecision	1
97.	MIND - IRRITABILITY	2
98.	MIND - IRRITABILITY – morning	1
99.	MIND - IRRITABILITY - morning - waking on	1
100.	MIND - IRRITABILITY - menses - before	1
101.	MIND - JESTING	2
102.	MIND - JOY	2
103.	MIND - KILL; desire to	1
104.	MIND - KILL; desire to - sudden impulse to kill	1
105.	MIND - KLEPTOMANIA	2
106.	MIND - LAUGHING	2
107.	MIND - LAUGHING - easily	1
108.	MIND - LAUGHING - immoderately	2
109.	MIND - LAUGHING - involuntarily	1
110.	MIND - LAUGHING - ludicrous, everything seems	1
111.	MIND - LAUGHING - sardonic	1
112.	MIND - LAUGHING - serious matters, over	1
113.	MIND - LAUGHING - silly	1
114.	MIND - LAUGHING - trifles, at	1
115.	MIND - LAZINESS	1
116.	MIND - LAZINESS - excitement - amel.	1
117.	MIND - LAZINESS - air, in open - amel.	1
118.	MIND - LAZINESS - sleepiness, with	1
119.	MIND - LIAR	2
120.	MIND - LOQUACITY	2
121.	MIND - MAGNETIZED - desire to be	1
122.	MIND - MALICIOUS	2
123.	MIND - MEDDLESOME, importunate	1
124.	MIND - MEMORY - weakness of memory	2
125.	MIND - MEMORY - weakness of memory - business, for	1
126.	MIND - MEMORY - weakness of memory - do; for what was about to	1
127.	MIND - MEMORY - weakness of memory - done; for what he just has	1

128.	MIND - MEMORY - weakness of memory - happened, for what has	1
129.	MIND - MEMORY - weakness of memory - mental exertion; for	1
130.	MIND - MEMORY - weakness of memory - proper names	2
131.	MIND - MEMORY - weakness of memory - say; for what he is about to	1
132.	MIND - MEMORY - weakness of memory - thought, for what he just has	1
133.	MIND - MEMORY - weakness of memory - words; for	1
134.	MIND - MENTAL EXERTION - agg.	1
135.	MIND - MENTAL POWER – increased	1
136.	MIND - MIRTH	2
137.	MIND - MISCHIEVOUS	2
138.	MIND - MISTAKES; making	1
139.	MIND - MISTAKES; making - calculating, in	1
140.	MIND - MISTAKES; making - localities, in	1
141.	MIND - MISTAKES; making - reading, in	1
142.	MIND - MISTAKES; making - space; in	1
143.	MIND - MISTAKES; making - speaking, in	1
144.	MIND - MISTAKES; making - speaking, in - spelling, in	1
145.	MIND - MISTAKES; making - speaking, in - words - misplacing words	1
146.	MIND - MISTAKES; making - speaking, in - words - wrong words; using	1
147.	MIND - MISTAKES; making - time, in	1
148.	MIND - MISTAKES; making - writing, in	2
149.	MIND - MISTAKES; making - writing, in - transposing – letters	1
150.	MIND - MISTAKES; making - writing, in - wrong - words	1
151.	MIND - MOCKING	1
152.	MIND - MORAL FEELING; want of	2
153.	MIND - MOROSE	1
154.	MIND - MOROSE - air, in open - amel.	1
155.	MIND - OBSTINATE, headstrong	1
156.	MIND - PLAYFUL	2

Chapter 14 - The Rubrics of Alcoholus

157.	MIND - PLAYING - desire to play	2
158.	MIND - PROSTRATION of mind	2
159.	MIND - QUARRELSOME	1
160.	MIND - RAGE, fury	1
161.	MIND - RAGE, fury - mischievous	1
162.	MIND - RECOGNIZING - not recognize; does - streets; well known	1
163.	MIND - RESTLESSNESS	2
164.	MIND - RESTLESSNESS - children, in	1
165.	MIND - REVEALING secrets	1
166.	MIND - RUDENESS	1
167.	MIND - SADNESS	1
168.	MIND - SADNESS - air, in open - amel.	1
169.	MIND - SADNESS - menses - before	1
170.	MIND - SADNESS - walking - air, in open - amel.	1
171.	MIND - SENSES - acute	2
172.	MIND - SENSES - dull, blunted	2
173.	MIND - SENSITIVE	2
174.	MIND - SENSITIVE - light, to	2
175.	MIND - SENSITIVE - music, to	2
176.	MIND - SENSITIVE - noise, to	2
177.	MIND - SENSITIVE - sensual impressions, to	1
178.	MIND - SENTIMENTAL	1
179.	MIND - SHAMELESS	2
180.	MIND - SHRIEKING	1
181.	MIND - SIGHING	1
182.	MIND - SLANDER, disposition to	1
183.	MIND - SLOWNESS	2
184.	MIND - SMILING	1
185.	MIND - SPEECH - confused	1
186.	MIND - SPEECH - hasty	1
187.	MIND - SPEECH - incoherent	1
188.	MIND - SPEECH - prattling	1
189.	MIND - STRIKING	1
190.	MIND - STRIKING - children; in	1
191.	MIND - STRIKING - desire - strike; to	1

192.	MIND - SUICIDAL disposition - thoughts	1
193.	MIND - SYMPATHETIC	1
194.	MIND - TEASING	1
195.	MIND - THOUGHTS - intrude and crowd around each other	2
196.	MIND - THOUGHTS - rapid, quick	1
197.	MIND - THOUGHTS - rush, flow of	1
198.	MIND - THOUGHTS - vanishing of	2
199.	MIND - THOUGHTS - wandering	2
200.	MIND - THROWING things around	1
201.	MIND - TRANQUILLITY	1
202.	MIND - UNFEELING, hardhearted	2
203.	MIND - UNOBSERVING	1
204.	MIND - UNSYMPATHETIC	1
205.	MIND - UNTRUTHFUL	2
206.	MIND - VIOLENT	1
207.	MIND - VIVACIOUS	2
208.	MIND - WEEPING - menses - before	1
209.	VERTIGO - DRIVING	1
210.	VERTIGO - EXCITEMENT	1
211.	VERTIGO - FLOATING, as if	1
212.	VERTIGO - MENOPAUSE - during	1
213.	VERTIGO - MENTAL exertion	1
214.	VERTIGO - READING - while	1
215.	HEAD - HEAT	1
216.	HEAD - HEAT - accompanied by - Face - heat of	2
217.	HEAD - HEAT - accompanied by - Face - redness of face	2
218.	HEAD - HEAT - flushes of	1
219.	HEAD - HEAVINESS	1
220.	HEAD - PAIN - Sides - right	2
221.	HEAD - PAIN - Temples - right	2
222.	HEAD - PAIN - pressing – Forehead	1
223.	HEAD - PAIN - stitching	2
224.	HEAD - PAIN - stitching - Sides - right	2
225.	HEAD - PAIN - stitching - Temples - right	2
226.	HEAD - SWOLLEN feeling	1

227.	HEAD - TINGLING	1
228.	EYE - DRYNESS	1
229.	EYE - HEAT in	1
230.	EYE - INFLAMMATION	1
231.	EYE - ITCHING	1
232.	EYE - LACHRYMATION	1
233.	EYE - PAIN	1
234.	EYE - PAIN - right	1
235.	EYE - PAIN - stitching	1
236.	EYE - PAIN - stitching - right	1
237.	EYE - PHOTOPHOBIA	1
238.	EYE - PHOTOPHOBIA - night - driving	1
239.	EYE - PHOTOPHOBIA - light - artificial light - night driving	1
240.	EYE - PUPILS - dilated	1
241.	EYE - PUPILS - sluggish	2
242.	VISION - ACCOMMODATION - defective - night driving	1
243.	VISION - ACCOMMODATION - slow; too - night driving	2
244.	VISION - ACUTE	2
245.	VISION - CONFUSED - night - artificial light	2
246.	EAR - CATARRH - Eustachian tube	1
247.	EAR - DISCOLORATION - redness	1
248.	EAR - DISCOLORATION - redness - right	1
249.	EAR - INFLAMMATION	1
250.	EAR - INFLAMMATION - Media	1
251.	EAR - INFLAMMATION - Media - right	1
252.	EAR - PAIN	2
253.	EAR - PAIN - right	2
254.	EAR - PAIN - stitching	1
255.	EAR - PAIN - stitching - right	1
256.	EAR - STOPPED sensation	1
257.	HEARING - ACUTE	1
258.	HEARING - IMPAIRED - confusion of sounds	1
259.	NOSE - DISCHARGE - clear	1
260.	NOSE - HAY FEVER	1
261.	NOSE - HAY FEVER - asthmatic breathing; with	1

262.	NOSE - ITCHING	1
263.	NOSE - ITCHING - Inside	1
264.	NOSE - OBSTRUCTION	1
265.	NOSE - OBSTRUCTION - air - open, in - amel.	2
266.	NOSE - OBSTRUCTION - warm - room	2
267.	NOSE - SMELL - acute	1
268.	NOSE – SNEEZING	1
269.	NOSE - SNEEZING - frequent	1
270.	NOSE - TINGLING	1
271.	NOSE - TINGLING - Inside	1
272.	FACE - DISCOLORATION - red	1
273.	FACE - DISCOLORATION - red - excitement	1
274.	FACE - ERUPTIONS - herpes	1
275.	FACE - ERUPTIONS - herpes - Lips	1
276.	FACE - HEAT - flushes	1
277.	FACE - TINGLING	1
278.	MOUTH - DISCOLORATION - Tongue - white	1
279.	MOUTH - DRYNESS	2
280.	MOUTH - DRYNESS - sensation of	2
281.	MOUTH - DRYNESS - thirst, with	2
282.	MOUTH - ITCHING - Palate	1
283.	MOUTH - NUMBNESS – Palate	1
284.	MOUTH - TASTE - acute	1
285.	MOUTH - TASTE - bitter	1
286.	THROAT - CRAWLING	1
287.	THROAT - FULLNESS	1
288.	THROAT - HEAT	1
289.	THROAT - ITCHING	1
290.	THROAT - PAIN - right	1
291.	THROAT - PAIN - swallowing	1
292.	THROAT - PAIN - sore - extending to - Stomach	1
293.	THROAT - PAIN - stitching	1
294.	THROAT - PAIN - stitching - right	1
295.	THROAT - PAIN - stitching - swallowing, on	1
296.	THROAT - SWELLING	1
297.	THROAT - TINGLING	1

298.	EXTERNAL THROAT - TORTICOLLIS	1
299.	EXTERNAL THROAT - TORTICOLLIS - right; drawn to the	1
300.	STOMACH - APPETITE - diminished	1
301.	STOMACH - DISORDERED	1
302.	STOMACH - DISTENSION	1
303.	STOMACH - DISTENSION - eating - after	2
304.	STOMACH - ERUCTATIONS - eating - after	2
305.	STOMACH - ERUCTATIONS; TYPE OF - food	2
306.	STOMACH - NAUSEA - food - smell of	1
307.	STOMACH - NAUSEA - mental exertion, from	1
308.	STOMACH - PAIN - burning	1
309.	STOMACH - PAIN - burning - eating - after	1
310.	STOMACH - THIRST	2
311.	STOMACH - VOMITING - food - smell of	1
312.	ABDOMEN – RUMBLING	1
313.	ABDOMEN - DISTENSION	2
314.	ABDOMEN - DISTENSION - flatus, passing - amel.	1
315.	ABDOMEN - DISTENSION - menses - before	1
316.	ABDOMEN - DISTENSION - painful	1
317.	ABDOMEN - FLATULENCE	1
318.	ABDOMEN - INFLAMMATION - Liver	1
319.	ABDOMEN - INFLAMMATION - Liver - chronic	1
320.	ABDOMEN - LIVER and region of liver; complaints of	1
321.	ABDOMEN - PAIN - Liver	1
322.	ABDOMEN - PAIN - Sides - right	1
323.	ABDOMEN - SWELLING - Liver	1
324.	RECTUM - CONSTIPATION	2
325.	RECTUM - CONSTIPATION - chronic	2
326.	RECTUM - CONSTIPATION - constant desire	1
327.	RECTUM - CONSTIPATION - ineffectual urging and straining	1
328.	RECTUM - CONSTIPATION - stool - remains long in the rectum with no urging	1
329.	STOOL - BILIOUS	1
330.	STOOL - BLACK	1
331.	STOOL - HARD	1

332.	BLADDER - URGING to urinate - frequent	2
333.	BLADDER - URINATION - incomplete	1
334.	PROSTATE GLAND - SWELLING	1
335.	MALE GENITALIA/SEX - COITION - enjoyment - increased	1
336.	MALE GENITALIA/SEX - COITION - enjoyment - prolonged	1
337.	MALE GENITALIA/SEX - EJACULATION - thrill prolonged	1
338.	MALE GENITALIA/SEX - SEXUAL DESIRE - increased	2
339.	MALE GENITALIA/SEX - SEXUAL DESIRE - wanting	1
340.	FEMALE GENITALIA/SEX - COITION - enjoyment - increased	1
341.	FEMALE GENITALIA/SEX - DRYNESS - Vagina	1
342.	FEMALE GENITALIA/SEX - ERUPTIONS - herpetic	1
343.	FEMALE GENITALIA/SEX - HEAT	1
344.	FEMALE GENITALIA/SEX - MENOPAUSE	2
345.	FEMALE GENITALIA/SEX - MENSES - irregular	1
346.	FEMALE GENITALIA/SEX - MENSES - late, too	1
347.	FEMALE GENITALIA/SEX - MENSES - scanty	2
348.	FEMALE GENITALIA/SEX - PAIN - Vagina - coition - during	1
349.	FEMALE GENITALIA/SEX - PAIN - burning	1
350.	FEMALE GENITALIA/SEX - PAIN - stitching	1
351.	FEMALE GENITALIA/SEX - SEXUAL DESIRE - increased	2
352.	LARYNX AND TRACHEA - HEAT - Larynx	1
353.	RESPIRATION - ASTHMATIC	1
354.	RESPIRATION - ASTHMATIC - air - open air - amel.	1
355.	RESPIRATION - ASTHMATIC - hay; from (= hay-asthma)	1
356.	RESPIRATION - ASTHMATIC - warm - room	1
357.	RESPIRATION - DIFFICULT	2
358.	RESPIRATION - DIFFICULT - air - cold, in - amel.	1
359.	RESPIRATION - DIFFICULT - air - open, in - amel.	1
360.	RESPIRATION - DIFFICULT - lying - while	1
361.	RESPIRATION - DIFFICULT - sitting - amel.	1
362.	RESPIRATION - DIFFICULT - smoke, as from	2

363.	CHEST - CONSTRICTION	1
364.	CHEST - HEAT - flushes	1
365.	CHEST - HEAT - flushes - extending to - Face	1
366.	CHEST – OPPRESSION	1
367.	CHEST - PAIN - motion - agg.	1
368.	CHEST - PAIN - Costal cartilage	1
369.	CHEST - PAIN - Mammae - menses - before	1
370.	CHEST - PAIN - Sides - right	2
371.	CHEST - PAIN - Sides - motion, on	1
372.	CHEST - PAIN - Sternum	1
373.	CHEST - PAIN - stitching	2
374.	CHEST - PAIN - stitching - motion - during	1
375.	CHEST - PAIN - stitching - Ribs	1
376.	CHEST - PAIN - stitching - Sides - right	1
377.	CHEST - PAIN - stitching - Sides - motion, during	1
378.	CHEST - PAIN - stitching - Sternum	1
379.	CHEST - SWELLING - Mammae - menses - before	1
380.	CHEST – TINGLING	1
381.	BACK - PAIN - Cervical region - right	1
382.	BACK - PAIN - Dorsal region	1
383.	BACK - PAIN - Dorsal region - Scapulae - right	1
384.	BACK - PAIN - Lumbar region	1
385.	BACK - PAIN - Sacral region	1
386.	EXTREMITIES - AWKWARDNESS	1
387.	EXTREMITIES - AWKWARDNESS - Hands	1
388.	EXTREMITIES - AWKWARDNESS - Hands - drops things	1
389.	EXTREMITIES - AWKWARDNESS - Lower limbs - stumbling when walking	1
390.	EXTREMITIES - CRAMPS - Lower limbs	1
391.	EXTREMITIES - CRAMPS - Thigh – right	1
392.	EXTREMITIES - CRAMPS – Leg	1
393.	EXTREMITIES - CRAMPS - Leg - Calf – right	1
394.	EXTREMITIES - CRAMPS - Foot – right	1
395.	EXTREMITIES - HEAT – Foot	1
396.	EXTREMITIES - HEAT - Foot - burning - uncovers them	1
397.	EXTREMITIES - INCOORDINATION	1

398.	EXTREMITIES - INCOORDINATION - Upper limbs	1
399.	EXTREMITIES - INCOORDINATION - Lower limbs	1
400.	EXTREMITIES - PAIN - Shoulder - right	2
401.	EXTREMITIES - PAIN - Elbow	1
402.	EXTREMITIES - PAIN - Elbow - right	1
403.	EXTREMITIES - PAIN - stitching - Knee	1
404.	EXTREMITIES - PAIN - Foot – Heel	1
405.	EXTREMITIES - STIFFNESS - Hand	1
406.	EXTREMITIES - STIFFNESS - Fingers	1
407.	EXTREMITIES - STIFFNESS - Lower limbs	1
408.	EXTREMITIES - STIFFNESS - Hip	1
409.	EXTREMITIES - STIFFNESS - Knee	1
410.	EXTREMITIES - STIFFNESS - Knee - right	1
411.	EXTREMITIES – TINGLING	1
412.	SLEEP - DEEP	1
413.	SLEEP - SLEEPINESS	2
414.	SLEEP - SLEEPINESS - air, in open - amel.	1
415.	SLEEP - SLEEPINESS - indolence, with	1
416.	SLEEP - SLEEPINESS - mental exertion	1
417.	SLEEP - SLEEPINESS - overpowering	2
418.	SLEEP - SLEEPINESS - riding - car	2
419.	SLEEP - SLEEPINESS - sitting	2
420.	DREAMS - DESTRUCTION	1
421.	DREAMS - ACCIDENTS	1
422.	DREAMS - ACCIDENTS - car; with a	1
423.	DREAMS - AMOROUS	1
424.	DREAMS - ASTRAY, going	1
425.	DREAMS - DANGER - water, from	1
426.	DREAMS - DECEIVED; BEING	1
427.	DREAMS - FRIENDS - old	1
428.	DREAMS - INTRIGUES	1
429.	DREAMS - LOST; being	1
430.	DREAMS - MANY	1
431.	DREAMS - MANY - menses, before	1
432.	DREAMS - SEA	1
433.	DREAMS - SEEING AGAIN an old schoolmate	1

434.	DREAMS - SHIP	1
435.	DREAMS - STORMS - sea, at	1
436.	DREAMS - VIVID	1
437.	DREAMS - WATER	1
438.	SKIN - DRY	2
439.	SKIN - ERUPTIONS - herpetic	2
440.	SKIN - ERUPTIONS - herpetic - burning	1
441.	SKIN - ERUPTIONS - herpetic - itching	1
442.	SKIN - ERUPTIONS - herpetic - stinging	1
443.	SKIN - ERUPTIONS - vesicular - burning	1
444.	SKIN - PRICKLING	1
445.	GENERALS - AIR - open air - amel.	2
446.	GENERALS - AIR - open air - desire for	2
447.	GENERALS - COLD - air - amel.	2
448.	GENERALS - DRY sensation - Internal parts; in	2
449.	GENERALS - FAINTNESS	1
450.	GENERALS - FOOD and DRINKS - alcoholic drinks - amel.	1
451.	GENERALS - FOOD and DRINKS - alcoholic drinks - desire	1
452.	GENERALS - FOOD and DRINKS - coffee - amel.	1
453.	GENERALS - FOOD and DRINKS - coffee - desire	1
454.	GENERALS - FOOD and DRINKS - cold drink, cold water - desire	1
455.	GENERALS - FOOD and DRINKS - meat – desire	1
456.	GENERALS - FOOD and DRINKS - pepper - desire	1
457.	GENERALS - FOOD and DRINKS - salt - desire	1
458.	GENERALS - FOOD and DRINKS - spices - desire	1
459.	GENERALS - FOOD and DRINKS - stimulants - desire	1
460.	GENERALS - FOOD and DRINKS - sweets - desire	1
461.	GENERALS - FORMICATION - External parts	1
461.	GENERALS - HEAT - flushes of	1
463.	GENERALS - HEAT - flushes of - menopause, during	1
464.	GENERALS - HEAT - flushes of - extending to - upwards	1
465.	GENERALS - HEAT - sensation of	2
466.	GENERALS - HEATED, becoming	2

467.	GENERALS - PAIN - stitching	2
468.	GENERALS - PAIN - stitching - right side	2
469.	GENERALS - PAIN - stitching - inward	2
470.	GENERALS - PRICKLING - Externally	2
471.	GENERALS - SIDE - right	3
472.	GENERALS - SYCOSIS	1
473.	GENERALS - SYPHILIS	1
474.	GENERALS - TOUCH - agg.	1
475.	GENERALS - VIBRATION, fluttering, etc.	1
476.	GENERALS - WARM - room - agg.	2
477.	GENERALS - WAVELIKE sensations	2

The Proving Journals

The following pages contain the journals of 18 provers. The symptoms listed are the ones that may be attributed to the remedy *Alcoholus*. I have included some old symptoms for context only; these are not included in the *materia medica* or repertory. They vary in style and length. We have kept the individual style of every document as we received it. The difference in length and symptoms between the provers illustrates well the nature of provings. Some people have enough sensitivity to produce symptoms, yet not enough to produce many symptoms, thereby producing a short proving. Others have a greater sensitivity, yet one that matches mostly the physical symptoms, as is found with prover #18.

Prover #18's papers, in some ways, were the ones that I had most difficulty with. In many respects, it was the easiest to contend with. The symptoms were very clearly delineated. However, the shear size of the document was enormous. What you see here is a tiny percentage of the total document. She was very aware of many of her symptoms. I had a choice of a few different ways to deal with this document. For example, I could have listed a particular symptom and then just referenced all the other days that the symptom was seen.

In the end, I decided to keep all the symptoms attributed to the remedy. I did this for two reasons. First, to give a flavor of what it was like to have a proving of the physical symptoms on a day by day basis. Second, to give a sense of what it was like to go through all the documents, all the levels of detail that are inherent in all the documents. All the provers had documents with many pages and with a great amount of detail. However, their sensitivity was such that only the pages presented here belong. With prover #18, there were a few symptoms that kept on recurring and so you have that as an example of a lengthy journal.

Prover #1

Prover #1 is a 45 year old man. He is a former dancer with a thin and graceful body. His chronic symptoms place him near the *Phosphorus*, *Cannabis indica* and *Anhalonium* group of remedies. These are the types of remedies he had taken before and is sensitive to. Also, he had taken hallucinogenic drugs in the distant past, using them in the context of spiritual seeking, rather than as recreational drugs. His symptoms show that his sensitivity was mostly in the mental and emotional realms. His symptoms matched precisely the mental and emotional elements of the *Cycle* of *Alcoholus*. Interestingly enough, the recollection he had on November 15 is very similar to the one striking symptom mentioned in *Allen's Materia Medica* and is one that was repeated in other provers.

Wednesday, November 14, 2001
5 minutes after Prover (P) took the remedy:

Prover (**P**): "I definitely feel something interacting with my field..."

Homeopath(**H**): Noted that **P's** face was flushed red–mostly his cheeks and nose.

Within another minute:

P began analyzing the dog in highly descriptive language. "That dog would stand out in a crowd, she has a *definite* personality. I'm seeing more deeply into her."

P: "I definitely feel spacey...Well maybe not spacey, I'm in an altered state."

H notes that **P** has a HUGE smile, and is leaning back in his chair.

P: "I can really go into things."

H observes that there is a light or glimmer in his eyes, and easy laughter, and he is still smiling.

P: "I have such a desire to look at things. I just want to walk in your yard, look at the trees, see the subtle colors of the season...I want to go for a walk. I want visual stimulation."

P: "I don't feel like eating, I don't want music on – it's more about visuals." **H** had her child's photo album on the kitchen table. **P** grabs it and starts to look through it. "I feel like I could just whip through this!"

H makes some comments about what it felt like to be pregnant, to have another life growing inside her. She notices that **P's** eyes are opening wider and wider.

H notes that **P** still has the HUGE smile on his face. She asks, "Do you think you could stop smiling right now?"

P: Laughs, "I think that would be hard to do."

P: "I'm starting to feel a little impatient. Do you have any art books?" **H** brings out a pile of art books which **P** excitedly, yet somewhat discontentedly begins to peruse.

H observes that **P** is still waxing on in superlatives, being very descriptive, standing, gesturing.

P: "I'm mentally stimulated, yet there is an impatience." **P** picks up a book he has been reading the last few days, and brought along to show **H**. He tries to read a passage, and says, "My comprehension seems to be less than normal. I couldn't watch Ingmar Bergman's *Wild Strawberries* right now. For now, it's television, with a remote in each hand!" (By this he is indicating a short attention span.)

P and **H** discuss contemporary sculptors briefly.

P: "It's still not easy to stop smiling." "It's hard to hear you talk seriously about something. Everything seems funny. How am I going to drive home? I'm going to have to stop for stimulation."

P: "Feelings are still really marked, but it's starting to mellow a bit."

P: "The color of the chair and [**H's** toddler daughter's] pushcart look particularly rich to me with the sunlight upon them. I see beautiful little tableaus going on all over the room."

P: "Do you have blocks?" **H** brings out a big box of children's wooden building blocks. **P** sniffs the blocks. (He says this is not really a weird thing for him. He tends to like to sniff things.) **P** plays with the blocks on the floor, asks **H** what type of wood she thinks they are made of.

P: "They smell sour, like oak." **P** starts building a high tower.

H offers **P** a cookie.

P: "No."

P finishes his block tower and knocks it over. "I don't enjoy that stage as much." "I'm trying to make the blocks not be so 'blocky.'"

H notes that **P** is being fussy, particular, indecisive. (After describing this scenario to the students in the NESH class, **P** and **H** suggested that this was also a kind of 'discontentment'.)

P is still handling the blocks. "I can't really start...It would be challenging to have a sustained conversation about anything."

P: "It might be fun to draw together...That's the first time I've suggested that to a woman I wasn't trying to sleep with!"

H notes that **P** puts all the blocks back in the box in a very neat and orderly fashion.

P and **H** sit at the kitchen table to draw. **H** notes that **P** clears the crumbs from his area before accepting paper. **H** offers **P** a pen.

P: "Do you have crayons?"

H takes out some large blocky crayons. **P** smells them.

H finds an unopened present left over from her daughter's birthday party a day before.. "I found another present, do *you* want to open it?"

P: "YES!!!" (He answered very enthusiastically, eyes wide open.)

P gets up to help himself to some water. **H** suggests he use the water filter feature on the faucet, and notes that **P** was a little confused by the way the filter operated.

P: "I'm surprised the water comes out *here*…"

H offers **P** something to eat.

P tries a cookie. In a joking tone he states, "I feel like the cookie brought me down."

At this point about an hour has passed and **P** mentions that he is "not feeling as high."

H and **P** begin to draw together.

P: "Drawing is really very satisfying."

After just one exchange, **P** would rather draw by himself. "Now I feel like I can stay with it."

P picks up his book again to see what his comprehension is at this point in the proving.

"I'm still having a little problem concentrating on the text, but it's better than before."

P mentions that he still has the desire to 'get into things, aesthetically.' (He is continuing to draw on his own.)

P mentions that he wants 'resolution' with his drawing. He doesn't want to leave it 'unfinished'.

H notices that **P** is not smiling so intensely anymore. He is concentrating on his drawing, holding it up admiringly.

H suggests going up to her new house site to show **P** around. **P** is interested, but says that he 'is not ready to leave'. He wants to 'work on this area of the drawing' some more. **P** holds the drawing up to inspect it and says, "I like that…I would like to do 12 variations on this theme…"

P and **H** leave the house, and head up to **H's** new house site which is under construction. In the car **P** says: "I feel completely wide open, the day feels free." **H** asks if **P** had felt that way before starting the proving. **P** answers that he hadn't been feeling that way at all lately. Even if he has a free day (no work scheduled), he hasn't been feeling this 'open.' **P** adds, "Do you think this is a drug remedy?"

P and **H** arrive at the house site. **H's** husband takes **P** into the house, and describes the floor plan to **P**. **H** notes that **P** is engaging with **H's** husband, asking pertinent questions, and responding appropriately. **H** asks **P** if he is indeed interested in the conversation. **P** says that he 'can listen to it' and is 'interested'.

H: The group moves outside to the garden. Everything has frozen already a few times, and is starting to decompose. **P** is intrigued by a rotting watermelon. He picks it up by its' crispy vine, and smells it.

H and **P** get back in the car to head home. **P** mentions that he is 'still feeling a little stoned', and that he's starting to feel like 'being alone.' Upon entering the house **P** asks for and eats a date. "I'm definitely down from the high. Emotionally everything isn't so funny. I feel like being quiet, not feeling social."

P asks to borrow the crayons he had been using. He picks up the crayons and smells them again.

P says his good-byes and sets off out the door. **H** notices that **P** has forgotten all his belongings: his book, large satchel, and the crayons he just asked to borrow. **H** runs out after him.

About 1 hour later:

H receives a message on her answering machine from **P**, in which **P** describes the details of his drive home. Apparently, **P** felt very 'spacey' while driving, and ultimately began to fall asleep at the wheel. He woke up to find himself in the oncoming lane of traffic. He had caused a bus to swerve and skid in order to avoid hitting him. "I almost caused an accident! I should not have been operating heavy machinery!"

P and H spoke on the phone at approximately 5:30 pm that evening:

P: "I don't really feel like interacting. I'm in more of an interior space, more melancholic." **P** mentions that he had accepted a dinner invitation for this evening, but was now feeling like he would rather stay home.

Thursday evening, November 15th. P and H meet at P's apartment for dinner:

P reports that after he and **H** spoke yesterday in the early evening, he continued to feel melancholic, "…literally *heartache,* sadness, lonely… I don't have a love in my life." He also felt, "tired…didn't want stimulation …didn't want to read or listen to music… Just want to relax and keep quiet, it's like a stasis." At that point **P** just sat on the couch and 'did nothing'.

H: A few hours later **P** did put on some 'spacey, ambient music' and found it 'enjoyable'.

P also kept his dinner engagement that evening. He found it interesting that the topic that night at his friend's house was 'ephemera'. In general there was a 'spacey' quality to all their conversation. **P** notes that these are not people who are ever given to this kind of conversation. **P's** godchild was talking about how she sees objects in the air, and **P** recounted to them all a hallucination he had during a fever when he was 12 years old, **(First time he thought of this in years):**

P: "I was sick for a few days with a fever and chills. The fever had climbed during the night when I awoke needing to go to the bathroom.

I discovered my bedroom was completely under water up to the ceiling. My bedclothes and my pajamas were wafting in the underwater currents. I had no thought of drowning and was not in the least bit distressed. I got up out of bed and made my way slowly, under water, to the door. When I opened my bedroom door the water from my room poured out the doorway and flooded the upper hallway; I watched it swirl around the banister and cascade down the stairs. I walked through waist deep water across the hall to the bathroom. When I turned on the bathroom light I saw that the water had all drained away now, but the ceiling and walls were dripping wet. The bath mat was soaked and sloshed water as I stepped on it. At this point my mother must have heard me moving about and had gotten up out of bed to come and check on me. When she came into the bathroom I asked her, "Where did all the water go?"

H: This morning (the 15th) **P** had woken up with thoracic, upper mid back soreness and stiffness. The stiffness felt better with motion. The soreness continued all day, and was worse touch. The pain was mostly on the right side.

By 6:00pm (when **P** and **H** saw each other) **P** said he 'feels exhausted', yet no longer 'as spacey or forgetful'.

H's observations: **P** seems more subdued than usual, down a few notches. Hair messier than she had ever seen it. Not as animated as usual. Operating on a lower frequency.

P and **H** sat down to eat. **H** had brought along a bottle of wine, and after initially refusing a glass, **P** changes his mind and drinks about 2 glasses over the course of dinner. They both note how much **P** is eating. Afterwards, **P** says he feels 'better after eating'. **H** notes that he has also livened up a little and is more engaging after eating.

Friday, November 16th, 12:50 pm, message left on H's machine:

P reports waking at 4 am, and not being able to get back to sleep for a while. In general though, he was feeling much more himself, his energy was better, and he had a nice workout that morning. He had had a consultation this morning during which his client spoke of the sexual abuse she had experienced as a child. **P** noticed that while the woman shared this information with him, tears began to fill his eyes. He felt that that was a little unusual for him. While he is always empathetic, this was definitely a more intense reaction than he normally has.

H was travelling away from home for the Thanksgiving holidays, and since **P** felt that things had pretty much plateaued, he was comfortable keeping notes for himself until he and **H** met again in person. **P** promised to call **H** if anything unusual came up.

Wednesday, November 28th – P and H meet in person for a follow-up:

H went over **P's** initial case. Together they noted:

P's music taste has changed. **P** has been enjoying rock and roll more, and a more 'intense' and 'concise' music.

H: "You mean less drifty-wafty stuff?"

P: "Yeah."

H: Also, **P** used to be able to sleep in many positions, but has now noticed that he is sleeping more on his left.

P: "The scales have tipped towards the left side."

H: Most notable has been that **P** is feeling more anger. **P** said this began around the 25th. **P** is having 'angry fantasies'. **P** will "wake up in the moment and fantasize about telling someone off." While **P** was watching a movie that had some form of injustice done to a character (the character was being oppressed), he imagined what he would do if that injustice were being done to him. He began to have a 'violent scenario' in his mind. He felt that since such an injustice were being done, it, "would've felt good to release in that violent fashion."

P also mentions getting a, "more vicarious thrill from violence," and feeling, "an anger wanting to be expressed when alone…When I catch myself in one of these fantasy scenarios, it seems unproductive–like there's some discontent in me that's being expressed unconsciously. I'm flowing with it, but something feels amiss."

P and H speak again approximately December 1st:

P states that the anger scenarios have continued, but since the 30th of November they have changed into feelings of, "perceived attacks." **P** finds himself, "thinking about what people think of me and say behind my back." Thoughts such as, " Does _____ (a close friend) really like me, or is he just pretending?" **P** notes that this kind of suspiciousness is very unusual for him.

Friday, December 7th, P and H present their proving to their NESH classmates, as well as Drs. Paul Herscu and Amy Rothenberg:

H: During this weekend **P** declares that just by talking about the proving with the class, he feels under its' influence once again. Feels really tired and a bit spacey. He even walked into the ladies bathroom accidentally (when heading for the men's bathroom), during a class break.

In an email to H dated December 18th P reports, eleven days after finding out that the remedy was *Alcoholus* **30C:**

"…still feel under the influence of *Alcoholus* **30C**"

"…still notice my having to be more watchful and mindful when operating the car, things can seem like they are happening more quickly around me, like my reaction time is slowed."

"…A little drunken at times. Balance is more challenging first thing in the morning or upon getting up in the middle of the night. Have to hold wall sometimes to stand and use toilet."

"…Notice a marked increase in sensitivity to alcoholic beverages."

Prover #2

Prover #2 was a 77 year old man, who practiced veterinary medicine. Constitutionally, he seemed like a person who would do well with *Sulphur*, in terms of his chronic symptoms. The remedies he had responded well to in the past were *Lycopodium* and *Carbo vegetabilis*. He too produced many of the symptoms of the various *Segments* of *Alcoholus*, though in a slightly different color to Prover #1. Most interesting to me is the fact that there were both the *Segment* of *Weakness* as well as the *Segment* of *Heightened Senses* within the same person. Also interesting is the dream on day one, of old acquaintances, and on day 4 which was essentially an identical dream to T. F Allen's description in the *Encyclopedia of Pure Materia Medica*.

Also of note is the fact that I would not have chosen a 77 year old man to prove a remedy. Just as there is an age requirement of 18 years old there should also be a requirement on the other side. While the 18 year old requirement fits the legal restrictions on medical testing, people who are advanced in age may be more at risk of developing too strong a reaction. Here, the fact that he responded well to *Carbo vegetabilis*, historically, should have been a big clue to exclude him from the proving.

Given the above statement, there is an interesting event that happened here. The reaction the prover had is the type that is seen in the most sensitive of provers. In the diagrams that I drew in Part one of the book, I would place this prover as one of the most sensitive. He is the type that experiences the proving as an acute illness, with a near complete syndrome shift. It is as if he is going through a severe acute ailment. These provers are always the easiest to spot, yet their reactions may, at times, be too severe.

Day 1 - 7/23/97

    8:00 am Took the first dose of remedy. He read some. He had a loose stool.

    8:30 am Laid down and took a nap. He had two weird dreams.

Dream #1

    Walking in a jogging suit in old neighborhood and seeing a stray dog with rope around his neck; this was a brown, shaggy, puppy. He picks up the dog's rope, which is his old rope. He is self-conscious, being in the neighborhood, barefooted with the dog. He walked up to his old house and the door was open. Two women were in the house. One of them might have been his ex-wife. The dog was their old dog. The dog had left a trail of loose stool all the way down the street. He asked the women what they wanted to do with the dog.

Dream #2

He visited this apartment and an old friend's roommate is there. The old friend is gone, but his jacket is on the chair. The friend has a hood of a car, tools, cans and trash all on the floor. He stepped on glass vial and apologized for breaking it. Also, he is barefooted in this dream. There was a hole in the floor with liquid coming out and he was trying to clean up the liquid and stop it from coming out of the hole.

P had no certain feelings towards these dreams. He never dreams about his ex-wife. He feels these are two weird dreams. The glass vial is like the vial he uses for floating up stool samples and was full of brown/red liquid. He wonders if both dreams are related to the proving. Both are new dreams. Both have liquid, barefooted, past people/places.

H: Dream #1 may relate to **P's** life with his first wife. I think the dream is about guilt. I know **P** feels very guilty for things not turning out well with his first wife and their kids. He was and is always self-conscious about what others think about him, which he dreamed when he was in his jogging suit, barefooted in his old neighborhood.

11:35 am Took 2nd dose of remedy.

1:30 pm P naps but no dreams this time.

2:30 pm P: "When I got up from nap I noticed that my hearing was more acute. The air conditioner sounds louder. Television sounds louder. Voices seem louder."

8:00 pm H: Hearing continues to be more acute. Things seem louder. More acute in left ear.

Day 2 - 7/24/97

8:00 am H: Hearing back to normal.

H: Not sure if he feels less achy. His chronic right knee pain is not as bad.

9:30 pm H: His lumbar and thoracic spine as well as his right knee, are less achy.

Day 3 - 7/25/97

3:00 pm P: "There is a sharp, sticking pain in his back above the right kidney, lasting one minute." It is a moderately intense pain, feeling like the size of a needle. It occurred while he was driving.

6:30 pm H: He got out of the car and started walking and became light-headed. He had to stop and hold on to a nearby vehicle, lasted for about one minute and then it passed. It seemed to begin while we were discussing his symptoms.

9:00 pm H: He complains of a definite low energy for the last few days. He thought at first it was due to the rainy weather and having to stay inside. He usually prefers to work outside daily. When he felt this way in the past, he would take *Lycopodium* and it would all go away in a few hours. He had no initiative. He stated he did not know how long he could put up with this.

Day 4 - 7/26/97

5:00 am P: "Woke from a dream. There was mass destruction, like an earthquake or tsunami. My wife and I were on a ship full of people. We were shipwrecked on a sea coast. There were dunes, rocks, and sea cliffs. There was lots of chaos. My wife was hurt and I was carrying her. I was trying to get off the ship and away from all the chaos. There were people dead and missing. We needed specific medicine and we did not have it. I was looking for a jar to put some drinking water in. The roads were impassable or non-existent. I found a suitcase with coins in it and took two silver dollars and other people took the rest of the coins. There were two giants (men) there that everyone was afraid of. I was glad when they left. We were looking for clothes to put on. There were clothes all over the place. There was a big sea animal or machine there too. I tied ropes to it to pull my wife and I out of the area. It did pull us out.

H: He had no idea what the dream meant. During the dream he felt he wanted to get out. Said he was in a hell of a mess and wanted out.

H: A few hours later he tried to describe his emotional state.

P: "Hard time describing how I feel...I don't like this feeling... It feels

I have lost my direction…I usually have things lined up to do. Now I feel like "to hell with it." Can't take calls or work like this. Where is this going to lead? I feel all knocked out. I have no energy…I don't care about doing anything…Rather just stay in bed with wife."

H Put call into NESH. **H** is afraid he will go into *Carbo vegetabilis* state, like he did 4 years ago.

Paul Herscu says to stop proving and take *Lycopodium* 200c.

Day 5 - July 27

9:30 am P: "I worked in the garden today. I feel better…My energy is coming back. I even killed a copperhead snake in chicken house."

Day 6 - July 28

7:30 am P: "I feel good today. My energy is back."

Prover #3

Prover #3 was a 42 year old woman. She was constitutionally similar to *Medorrhinum, Sulphur* and *Lachesis*. Prover #3 shows more of the symptoms of the remedy, more fully exemplifying the confusion seen in this remedy. She too had similar dreams to Provers #1 and #2.

Day 1 - July 14, 1997
Took the first dose at 13:30

13:40 H: Tingling in head, radiating upward to crown from both temporal areas, accompanied by laughing.

13:45 P: "The left-sided neck pain that I woke with just shifted to posterior of neck and it is more right-sided…Now my entire head feels lighter. There is a buoyant feeling with lightness in my shoulders."

14:00 H: More color and slightly flushed. Her outer ears feel hot. The feeling of pain switched from the right side of her neck to the left side of neck for the past 10 minutes.

14:02 P: "Tingling of face and head now more centered on both ears. In right leg, ever since my first pregnancy, off and on, I've had a feeling that my blood doesn't return up, but rather lodges in my right leg, there causing a feeling of dullness and pain—an achy pain. That is usually exacerbated by weight gain or salt intake and relieved by elevating the right leg. Over the last six months, it has been worse and even worse over this last month. I just felt a new sensation there. It was a sharp, transient pain at the inner side of my right ankle, followed by a tingling of my entire right foot. (I think I have a bad vein in my right leg.)"

14:15 P: "I am experiencing tightness behind my right calf and it continues to feel slightly tingling around the entire right ankle."

14:20 H: The tingling of head and ears stopped now.

14:50 H: Pain behind right heel is minor but constant.

15:00 H: Right leg still feels dull and slightly swollen.

Day 2 - July 15, 1997

The most significant thing of this day was a very vivid dream last night. When I awoke, the dream stayed with me. (In fact, almost a month later she still felt the dream.)

"In the dream I found myself walking through a house in the country, that had been recently discovered by our family. It seems that it had once belonged to our great-grandfather and had somehow gotten lost over the years until just recently. As I moved through the house I felt alone and saw no one else but knew there were older relatives of mine nearby. The purpose of being in the house was to choose belongings that we could claim as our own. The house was an old, rambling three-story farm house with curved narrow staircases with an open central stairway. I toyed with the idea of picking up several small items, but they didn't seem to really call to me. On the third floor, I found an old quilt — white and red gingham borders, which I immediately knew was for me. I picked it up and made my way to the second floor and found several bags of fabric lying on the floor. They also were for me, but instead of carrying down the tight staircase, I decided to throw them over the banister to the first floor. When I descended the stairway, I could not locate any of the bags —they were not anywhere to be found.

"I looked up the stairwell, but was startled when I could not see the third floor! I ran up the stairs to the third floor and looked over the banister and could see the first floor! I ran down to the first floor looked up and still could not see the third floor. Perplexed, I gave up worrying about it and looked around the living room. I found several pieces of fabric on the couch and gathered them up into my arms. On a shelf I found a small vase in the shape and color of a clump of purple grapes and felt immediately attracted to it. I grabbed it and wrapped it in my quilt and headed out through the dining room. Suddenly I found myself sitting at the dining room table with other unknown people and looking at a decaying old wooden cupboard with cobwebs hanging over them... I then woke up."

10:00 H: Very fitful sleep due to heat and humidity. She was slightly groggy until 10:00 am, then becoming more alert.

15:00 P: "I cat-napped during a lecture in a chilly, air-conditioned room. In between nodding off and waking during this time I had a weird 10 second vision of jarring, of a near-accident (like a "day-mare"), that would come into my mind suddenly, then vanish before I had a chance to think or react."

15:00 H: Right calf slightly painful and dull feeling without throbbing.

21:00 P: "While watching a movie in a theater, I felt warm and fuzzy from both ears with an energy radiating upwards. I experienced a feeling of lightness or airiness, kind of like I was smiling with my mind. This feeling lasted about 30 seconds and slowly faded. This occurred without other symptoms. At first I thought it was a reaction to the special effects in the movie, but as I did a mental inventory, I realized that the feeling was reminiscent of the initial feeling of head energy when I started the proving the first day."

22:00 H: Increased energy until bedtime. Able to feel energized throughout the evening and sexually aroused.

23:30 Slept until 5:30 next day.

Day 3 - July 16, 1997

Woke up at 5:30.

06:00 "Menses started this morning. Probably explains hormones last night. I tend to become amorous just before menses and just after it."

Day 4 - July 17, 1997

17:30 "I have mind fatigue. I'm exhausted from taking care of a 12 year old quadriplegic at work. It is emotionally very difficult for me. I am now trying to relieve this fatigue by sitting down and writing."

"Energy low at this and I feel hot, flushed."

"Slight headache; will be relieved once I drink a small cup of coffee."

"Feel fatigued around my eye area."

"Feet feel very sore and tired, achy on the bottom. I would like a good long soak in a tub to relieve them, but unfortunately I have about 6 hours of work before I can do so."

Day 5 - July 18, 1997

04:00 "Menses stopped by midnight. Short menses-2 1/2 days, which has become normal for the past year."

"Slept 23:15 to 03:45. Woke up easily but felt sleepy until about 09:30. Without dreams, but when I dozed off during prayers (on and off occasionally for a few seconds), I would have vivid and sharp visions of strange occurrences. For example, I would see something startling like an almost car accident that would cause me to jerk back and then I would wake up. Again, these small "visions" lasted 2-3 seconds."

Day 6 - July 19, 1997

"Went to sleep at 22:30 and woke up at 03:45. When I first went to sleep I woke up with a sudden jerk when I thought that I visualized a car slowly veering off the road. Took a while to get back to sleep; every little sound kept me awake for about a half an hour. Woke up at 02:30, chilly and had to get up to pee. Then I covered up with a blanket, slept soundly until alarm went off."

"I've noticed that since taking the remedy I've been reversing letters in words when I first write them down and have had to cross out my words. I'm used to writing on a computer so my hand writing skills have declined, as evidenced by this journal, but I feel that I have gotten worse (in reference to switching letters, especially vowels)."

15:00 "Mild confusion and perplexed after attending a seminar and finding myself with a lot of questions."

22:00 "Itchy, red, blotchy rash on inner thighs found during bath. Somewhat relieved by scratching."

Day 7 - July 20, 1997

06:00 "Feeling fuzzy in my mental clarity this morning."

13:30 "My mind feels clearer, but still a fuzziness remains, even my ears feel a little fuzzy, without hearing difficulty though."

"Body still slightly sluggish."

"Sharp, sudden headache in both temples, relieved by eating lunch."

"Itchy rash remains on inner thighs, but just started feeling itchy about 13:30."

21:00: "Continue to feel slightly sluggish in the mind, not fatigued, just a vagueness like I need to shake my mind out of cobwebs but can't."

"Persistent headache, encompassing entire top of head in circular fashion above my ears. It had lifted in early afternoon, but returned about 17:00 and stayed. I forgot to take Tylenol."

Day 9 - July 22, 1997

06:00 "Feeling generally annoyed at husband for no obvious reasons. I'm in a good mood so I'm perplexed why he annoys me. I feel more alert today than I did yesterday."

17:00 "Annoyed at work when a patient arrived without announcement, but quickly shrugged it off because patient was interesting and needed attention."

Day 10 - July 23, 1997

"Sharp pain down left buttock to top of posterior left thigh, lasted about 2 minutes with residual pain while sitting for about 10 minutes. Relieved with movement, sustained movement. Joints, looser today, cracking noted around wrist. Joints without pain."

06:00 "Slept well and woke up before alarm and quietly woke up to the sounds of gentle rain and birds singing. I usually need an alarm to wake up."

22:00 "Still feeling distant and annoyed with husband. But very happy seeing my son who I haven't seen in 1 1/2 weeks. Irritated at work by events out of my control concerning my patient. Frustrated by this but felt better after venting frustration to anyone who would listen at that time."

"High energy until bedtime at 23:30. I was too busy at work to keep journal."

"Intermittent headaches that hit my temples sharply and stayed for less than one minute, but came and went until bedtime for a total of approximately 4 times since this afternoon."

23:30 "Gums bleeding after flossing, but feel better with it."

Day 11 - July 24, 1997

06:00 "Sluggish this morning, but had to wake up to get to work. Worried about having rain on my vacation (starting tomorrow). Still annoyed with husband who seems bewildered about my indifference to him."

Day 13 - July 26, 1997

09:00 "Upbeat, organized, but relaxed about vacation and getting to the beach. Feel like going with the flow and not rushing around. Calmer."

14:00 "Dull, sustained headache while driving to beach. Not used to being a passenger and I keep nodding off (falling asleep) and waking up."

23:10 "Feeling sexual, but left unsatisfied because husband is sleeping. Hopeful that tomorrow will be more conducive to sex. I felt annoyed at husband for falling asleep while I was taking a bath. Relieved by letting him sleep on couch to wake up to wonder where I was."

Day 14 - July 27, 1997

08:00 "Feel contented due to having good sex with husband upon waking. I feel lazy today. Just want to go with the flow of the day."

08:00 "I feel rested by good sleep despite the small bed. House at beach overlooks a small pond with birds singing all the time, very uplifting and my body feels good near the water. Cool breezes into the house."

"Without appetite, ate because I should."

17:00 "Sitting at beachside. Mind lulled by the waves, drowsy, content. Body feels thick."

Day 15 - July 28, 1997

10:00 "Feeling lazy, both with mind and body. Not feeling any pressure to do anything. Cloudy, hot day."

17:00 "Had a very hard day emotionally after yelling at my ex-husband. I was relieved by crying and venting frustration at my husband. Felt much better after swimming in 63 degree water. Felt rejuvenated and tingling all over."

Day 16 - July 29, 1997

"Slept well even though I had to urinate twice because we ate a late dinner. Woke after sexual dream in which I was making love to a man who I was once close to but no longer have a deep friendship with."

"Sexual drive has kicked into overdrive. When we have time, such as a vacation and not exhausted, I can't wait to make love to my husband. I prefer night sex, but he prefers morning sex, so far it's been only in the morning, but I plot to keep him awake later today!"

15:00 "Occasionally I am frustrated by my inability to slow my rapid thoughts down to match the lazy pace of our vacation."

Day 18 - July 31, 1997

18:00 "Great day today. Spent entire few days at beach and feel relaxed, clear, satisfied, complete."

18:00 "Positive energy, like my battery completely recharged. Body achy slightly from no exercise, but I feel inwardly good. Beach day, blue, clear water. Slight warm wind. Hot sun and sand."

Day 20 - August 2, 1997

10:00 "Feeling fuzzy after sleeping too long."

Day 23 - August 5, 1997

09:00 "Very sleepy for drive home . Had to stop and buy popcorn to eat on the way home."

Day 27 - August 9, 1997

"Feeling sloppy, disorganized."

Prover #4

Prover #4 was a 43 year old man. His general constitutional symptoms pointed to *Lycopodium*, *Staphysagria*, and *Medorrhinum*. While he exemplified further the confused aspect of the remedy, he also experienced the heightened senses. Again, the dream on day 5 is almost straight out of T.F. Allen's *materia medica*.

Day 1 - September 19, 1997

Took the remedy at 10:00am

10:20 am: "I have a floating feeling, a lifting out from my norm."

10:25 am: "I have a slight physical nervous sensation, a slight tremor all over my body. It resembles a sugar buzz."

10:26 am: "My mental function feels more sharp-edged. If someone said something or a surprising event happened, my attention would get to it more quickly…I feel like I would startle easily. It feels like some adrenaline is moving through me. I feel an overall heightened state of awareness and alertness. It feels like I took about half a hit of pot (*Cannabis indica*)."

10:26 am: "My hearing is more accentuated. I am more conscious of room noise. I feel like a slight ache in my right eardrum. (It went away by 10:45.)

10:35 am: "Floating feeling is subsiding."

10:45 am: "All of the feelings are subsiding a bit…The pain in the ear is gone…the room noise is less accentuated…the heightened sense of awareness is diminishing… I was having trouble concentrating on controlled writing, like I had too much caffeine, during the heightened state of alertness, and floating sensations. Lasted for 30 minutes."

10:55 am: "Symptoms have lessened but still present, the sharpness in sensory acuity…I have a feeling of extra cautiousness about driving. My senses have been altered, I feel less focused, and I need to be more careful. Again, it is as if I had taken a half a hit of marijuana and feel like I am in a vigilant state about driving."

Noon: "Feel increased sexual desire for 10 minutes."

5:15 pm: "Some floating feeling still."

"Energy very high and positive…Increased sexual desire…A slight feeling of adrenaline…my creativity is high."

11:00 pm: "Floating feeling remained. My mood stayed exceptionally great. Now I have suddenly gotten tired and sleepy. Years ago I took Prozac. This whole experience is the same general sensation I developed on Prozac, only sharper."

Day 2 - September 20, 1997

5:15 am: "I woke up at 5:15, which is much earlier than usual. Dream: Awkward, weird, but very vivid dreams. Dreams of conflicts with people. I was at work and no one would get me a bite of food (first time dreamed of food). Old musicians were there. The Rolling Stones were at the radio station to perform live. The Doors were there too. I had some sexual content to the dreams as well."

5:15 am: "My sensory awareness is lighter. For example, I am more conscious of the taste in my mouth, of the tastes of food, of the fact that my sleep was not as restful as usual. During sleep I was aware of all the tossing and turning…I am still very aware of room noise, even in my sleep. I thought my upstairs neighbor was blasting his television. I am more aware of the temperature in the room. I put earplugs into my ears and went back to sleep. Again, more vivid dreams and again about food. Again I awaken being sexually aroused."

"After discussing my state with homeopath, the following points are clear. I have increased attention to visual detail yesterday and today. I was more likely to take note of smaller details I would normally overlook. My vision was not clearer but my perception and attention to it was. I would notice the way someone's eyes looked or their expressions or body language."

"When I came home last night I was much more aware of the different smells in my building, in the hallway, and in my apartment."

"I was more aware of my 'morning mouth' when I awakened this morning. It was not abnormally anything, not more bitter or sour, but I was more abnormally vividly aware of it."

"During the night, I was more sensitive to temperature changes, and as a result the air conditioning unit never got the temperature just right."

"I woke up groggy and craved coffee. This resembles how I feel in the morning after I smoked marijuana the night before. I feel in a heightened and dull state at the same time. The floating feeling remains…I feel a little crabby with the groggy feeling. This is not the usual state that I wake up in."

"I have had trouble with gas and bloating since the proving began."

3:30 pm: "Most symptoms diminished. I don't feel floating feeling any longer."

9:15 pm: "I am fatigued and sore and feel like I am getting sick. All my muscles are sore, especially the feet, the right knee, and lower back on the right side. I have a slight sore throat. My feet feel warm…the floating feeling has returned as has the accentuated sense of smell."

Day 3 - September 21, 1997

2:00 am: "I woke up for 30 minutes, which is very unusual for me. My mind was very active and it was hard to settle it. Eventually, I fell back to sleep."

6:30 am: "I had a very vivid dream last night. It was about some young adults, alluring and beautiful, interesting and compelling. They had a lot of games and odd theatrics to draw me in. They used mostly illusions to be compelling. They would not respond to any direct questions. They would only come up with a new illusion. In the dream I became a lover or confidant of one of them, but it turned out to be a black widow sort of thing. This one lover would kill any of the people I was attracted to. As I tried to hide and get away, the lover tracked me down and tried to kill me. The dream was very vivid, detailed and sharp edged in a way that my dreams are usually not."

"My physical condition is much improved over last night. My muscle fatigue is mostly gone, with only a slight pain in my right knee…The floating feeling is still there but I did not notice the degree of accentuated sensory acuity as I did the day before. Sound seems normal to me now."

9:30 pm: "I had a craving for salt and spice earlier so had barbecued potato chips."

Day 4 - September 22, 1997

"I slept really well last night, the air was cold and I was bundled well, my preference. My mood is great the past few days, much better than usual, more confident. Interestingly, I have had much less gas and bloating in my stomach and abdomen in the last few days than I did at the beginning of the proving and before it."

Day 5 - September 23, 1997

"I had a strong, vivid dream that I never had before. I woke up from it very sad. The dream was that I was visiting a friend from my past and he said he had a movie of my life, a sort of flashback of my life, the parts that I have lost and were not accessible to me any longer…there was a lot of water in the dream. Lots of flooding water. It kept me from getting where I needed to go. I was stranded by the water and then by snow. I tried walking in the snow with my sneakers and I had to change to different shoes. It was at a high elevation and the weather was damp and oppressive.

"I was visited by lots of people from my past in the dream, my 'guides' if you will. The dream was somehow affirming of who I was, that I was okay. In the dream he showed a video of me, at different ages in my life. I was very sad watching it, and I began to cry almost immediately. I do not recall the details but only that there were lots of details of my childhood, of my possessions. The memories were flooding in and it was overwhelming. There was a melancholic sweetness to the dream.

"At one point of the dream I was on Rollerblades as a kid. (I was watching the video.) I was shirtless and happy. I was in my early adolescence, probably around 13-14 years old. I was surprised at how sexual I seemed. Confident, cocky, vulnerable and scared…I caught up with myself, I put my hand on my 14 year old head and told myself to take care of me. The 14 year old looked up at me and said "I will." The 14 year old didn't understand, but accepted it. It was like a visit from another dimension. I was the older wiser me looking out for my younger self, before all the hurt of my life came crashing in.

"But it was so, so sad, and I was bawling with tears in the dream. Then I woke up…this dream was the most powerful dream I have ever had in my life. When I woke up I felt so sad, but somehow unburdened by something big in my life. This dream seems like such a gift, such an intervention in my life somehow. It was not about the details of my life, as much as an intense emotional feeling held deep inside me."

Day 6 - September 24, 1997

"The good feeling and high energy did not last. Today, I feel much more lethargic and depressed. My attitude is predominantly negative and I want to isolate myself."

"I have been craving salt and spicy foods."

Day 19 - October 7, 1997

"The level of vivid dream has finally diminished. In the last few days, I had my normal dreams again. I noticed that a lot of my dreams were vivid and meaningful to me. One of the common threads in many of the dreams had to do with water. It was prevalent in many dreams. It was everywhere, like oceans. It wasn't a drowning sort of thing in the dreams, but it was deep, and made problems that were tough to overcome."

"I have noted two things that are better in my life since taking the remedy. First, the gas and bloating that I have tended to in my life is much reduced, remarkably so. The other thing is that my allergies were greatly reduced from what I usually experience. My fall allergies usually begin in the morning, with sneezing, itchy nose, snuffles, post nasal drip, redness of the eyes, and low energy. I had some of these symptoms, but to a much lesser extent than anytime in the past."

Prover #5

Prover #5 was a 25 year old woman who was in good physical shape. She is an Olympic medallist. She was a *Nux vomica/Calcarea carbonica* constitution with a strong family history of alcoholism. What was most interesting to me about this proving was that she lost her coordination during the proving, which was a lot to say for an Olympic medalist. Also interesting was that her menses were delayed, a symptom unusual in one her age, and yet common in the proving.

Day 1 - August 7, 1997 - From the Prover's own journal.

(NOTE: Menses started yesterday with normal "blahs.")

6:00 pm first dose.

6:28 pm "I feel light-headed with head rushes."

11:12 pm "I have a throbbing headache behind my eyebrows & cheekbones."

"I feel groggy, limiting my ability to focus and concentrate."

Day 2 - August 8, 1997

"One weird dream. I can't remember the content, but it seemed surrealistic."

9:45 am "Same head condition resumes."

10:30 am "Very runny nose and lots of sneezing."

11:45 am "The headache and lack of clarity continue on."

1:10 pm "I went for a bicycle ride: I was very disoriented and unfocused during the bike ride, almost crashed and struggled for energy."

10:00 pm "I went into a hot tub and had a severe compression headache."

Day 3 - August 9, 1997

11:30 am "After a run, I felt sick, "fluey" with sinus pressure behind cheek bones and a sore throat caused by a post-nasal drip, lasting for 4 hours. This is very unusual as I am usually much better after I exercise."

I chose to end the test by drinking coffee and taking another homeopathic remedy.

"Interestingly enough, I used to be achy and feel tight in my muscles all the time. This was better during the proving.

My sex drive was decreased during the proving."

Further recollections about the first two days of the proving:

"My mind was so groggy and unclear, I couldn't concentrate or focus. It was hard to distinguish what was going on around me, or in my body. Even talking on the phone was difficult. It was more like I couldn't fully comprehend or hear what was being said, rather than not being able to form my words."

"I was annoyed, freaked out (more of an anxious and confused feeling, not like a focused fear) on the bike ride. I was drifting off the trail. It was hard to keep the handlebars straight. I had slow reaction time."

It is now late September and the menses are three weeks late, which is very unusual.

Prover #6

Prover #6 was a 37 year old woman who had responded well to *Sepia*, *Tuberculinum*, *Nux vomica*, **and looks like she may need** *Lycopodium* **at some point. There is a history of liver complaints with elevated liver enzymes. Prover #6 illustrated the confusion and lack of confidence clearly, reflecting the relationship of this remedy with** *Lycopodium*. **Also interesting is a Herpes simplex eruption that flared, common during this proving.**

Day 1 - July 22, 1997
Time of Doses: #1 - 10:10 am, #2 - 1:20 pm, #3 - 4:40 pm

10:30 am "Felt flushed from shoulders up to head, lasted only about one minute and dissipated. Felt like a wave of heat."

(At the same time her face becomes red and slightly puffy. She tells me that there is a rawness in her throat and a tickling, a feeling of choking and she begins to cough, 4 times, her face becoming redder during this time.)

10:30 am (20 minutes after remedy) "Flushing as noted above accompanied by face turning bright red (per observer). Had post-nasal discharge and loose cough, no phlegm. Felt briefly as if I was choking. Aggravated by talking. Coughed about four times, no phlegm, dry but felt like choking, hawking—like cough to clear mucous."

10:40 am "Felt stuffy; craving open air. Breathing pattern less regular snd rhythmic, more aware of breathing. Breathing also more shallow and alternating with sighing, more frequent sighing. (These symptoms were very subtle and confirmed by supervisor. This lasted until 11:00 am.)

1:30 pm (10 minutes after remedy #2). "Felt stuffy and warm, better with an open door and fresh air. This is not like an air hunger, but more because of the heat."

(Rumbling in the abdomen. Had this after taking the first dose as well. Her face is very flushed with these episodes as well.)

2:35 pm "Felt sensation like a lump in throat."

2:50 pm "Phlegm in back of throat, feels 'stuck'; coughing to clear throat. Accompanied by facial flushing and warm sensation. Feel like a "plugged" sensation. No amelioration with cinnamon candy. (This occurred while I was driving.)"

3:00 pm "Right posterior thigh cramping noted after sitting in car driving, relieved by shifting weight. Lasted several minutes."

3:50 pm "Right posterior thigh cramping, like a squeezing, better by walking around and worse by sitting. This recurred at 5 pm, 8:30, and 9pm, while driving a car."

6:00 pm "Slight blurring and fuzziness of vision (both eyes) while reading in outside glare. Very brief (less than 10-15 seconds). Symptom stopped after looking away from page."

9:00 pm Paroxysms of coughing due to post-nasal discharge with hawking and gagging for about 20 seconds and then resolved. I recently had a cold, but these symptoms were more regular and intense."

9:30 pm "Physically and mentally very tired. Reading in bed. Fell asleep by 10:30 pm. Normally I am up until 11-11:30 pm. Felt like I can't do another thing. Feeling mentally fatigued. Unsettled about an article I read in homeopathy journal which caused me to question my confidence in both homeopathy and my ability to practice it. While this is a chronic problem, I felt it much more intensely, doubting my decision to pursue homeopathy."

Day 2 - July 23, 1997

5:30 am: "I heard my husband's alarm, which I usually sleep through but not alert enough to get up."

6:30 am: "My alarm went off for first time (usually it goes off three times before I get up) and I got up out of bed right away.

DREAMS:

#1 - Homeopathy class hanging around at break; then go into an auditorium where there is a rehearsal in progress for *Oklahoma*. Recognized some people from high school. (Significance of dream—I have upcoming high school reunion, was in Oklahoma. It was a change for me to recognize people in my dream.)

#2 - Had conversation with classmate from high school (very vivid and clear); actually had a coherent conversation with her. Significant is upcoming reunion. Strong feeling of guilt stirred up with this dream because I haven't kept in touch with this friend and we were close.

"Noted certain times that my energy was low and feeling sluggish physically and mentally first noted at approximately 9 am when I was in a car. It didn't matter if I drove or someone else drove. Yawning frequently when getting in car (concomitant with driving). Better getting out of car."

"Nasal stuffiness with minimal clear discharge. Clearing throat several times from post-nasal discharge. No modalities."

MENSES: Due in several days. Noted mild breast tenderness when pressure applied, i.e., when removing bra. (This is an old symptom of mine but it had resolved with a previous remedy.)

"Chewing left lower lip on way home from work; small bump (not ulcer) developed in area. Not sure of why doing this."

"Appetite good, ate three meals. Craved meat at dinner; had Caesar salad with chicken. (Normally eat vegetarian.)"

RECTUM: "Slight abdominal gurgling and gas before bowel movement."

Around 8:00 pm sensitive to loud music and husband talking in a restaurant. Having trouble concentrating on husband's talking. Lasted about 5 minutes."

"Hard to stay awake 9-10 pm, when trying to read…Concentration is difficult. Foggy; felt like someone drugged me. Went to bed 10:15 pm.

Day 3 - July 24, 1997

"Woke up for no reason at 4:15 am. Went back to sleep until 4:45 am…Restless, but went back to sleep. 5:40 am husband's alarm went off (usually I don't hear)…6:00 am out of bed right away with alarm."

DREAM "Felt like I was observing this scenario from outside. Large group of people attending a conference, they were waiting for buses to arrive and take them to dinner. I recognized a good friend of mine, but I was going through the crowd with luggage and trying to remain anonymous. Some foreign guy was going among people and being very obnoxious by physically touching women in a sensual way. Women were dressed very provocatively. Then saw this guy going up stairs and looked like Alice Cooper, with blood coming out of his skull. (Unable to link any of this.) Felt disturbed by dream; pretty weird and very vivid."

"Not craving chocolate; I normally crave it before my menses as I am now."

"I had a lot of energy in the morning. Went for a run in the heavy rain. Normally would have dismissed running due to weather, but felt like getting out."

"Craving meat; specifically hamburger with bacon and cheese. This is very unusual for me since I gave up meat two years ago and do not usually crave it. I ordered a bacon cheese burger at a drive in restaurant and ate the whole thing and it tasted great! Very satisfying."

"Mild breast tenderness after removing bra."

7:30 pm Experienced yawning again when in car, but not as fatigued as yesterday. Felt sluggish on way home (worked 11:00 am-7:00 pm), but not as much as yesterday.

Day 4 - July 25, 1997

"Restless between 4-5 am, but quickly back to sleep. Didn't hear first alarm (husband's 5:15 am), but 2nd alarm 5:30 am stirred me. Feeling very tired; still desire to sleep. 6:00 am out of bed."

"Menses begins today on time."

2:00 pm "Energy level was fine until I was in my car. I was driving, rarely yawning."

3:00-4:00 pm "Feeling sluggish and progressed until I was so tired could barely keep my eyes open! I had to have husband drive. Slept for about an hour to an hour and a half and felt better. Able to drive later in the evening."

11:00 pm "Eyelids fluttering observed by others while I was talking about homeopathy. I was not aware of this. Lasted several minutes. No other symptoms."

"I am concerned and resentful about how low my energy level is with this remedy. I yearn for my previous energy level."

"I feel a loss of control. I feel behind in my work, overwhelmed, confused. Too many demands of me."

Day 5 - July 26, 1997

2:00 am "Woke briefly, went right back to sleep. 6:30 am woke brief, right back to sleep."

2:00 pm-4:00 pm "Energy level fine until 2pm, when I became sluggish. Felt like I could nap, but instead watched a movie."

Day 6 - July 27, 1997

"Decreased concentration and dull senses. I feel like I could fall asleep easily. I have less ability to concentrate when I have this decreased energy. It isn't related to what is happening at the time either. For instance, I can be occupied with something versus driving in car or just sitting still, I feel the same way."

"Very frustrated by decreased energy. I don't feel in control and also not able to keep up with my normal routine (for example, my exercise)."

"Very dull, mild headache in temporal area mostly, on both sides though mostly on the right side, first noticed with low energy symptoms, not related to food intake. This symptom persisted intermittently and changed to only the right side, moderate intensity like a throbbing. It is better applying light pressure. It is worse lying down especially on the left side. Still noted upon going to bed (11:30 pm)."

Day 7 - July 28, 1997

"Sleep was restless and stirring frequently."

DREAM: "I was living on the street as a bag lady and was helped by a king who was actually trying to make me his mistress and I was always resisting his advances."

"Afternoon while driving in car-very sluggish. Better for walking around, but still lower energy than normal."

"Passenger in car, husband driving, long trip. After being in car 20 minutes, I couldn't keep my eyes open. Napped for almost an hour and slow to wake up. Better for getting out of car."

ABDOMEN: "I had large ice cream cone which was very satisfying. Better for sweets, especially in the evening; cookies, chocolate. Feel it may be "comfort food" as I am at my parents' house, discussing their future."

RECTAL: "Some gas throughout day especially after eating; mild bloating. Bowel movement after dinner, which is unusual for me, as I usually have one in the morning."

Day 8 - July 29, 1997

"Good energy level until getting in car for ride home. Tried very hard to stay awake. Had some tea and cocoa in am for caffeine to see if it affected energy, without any major change. Drove around 2 hours, got sleepy and then husband took over. Didn't sleep right away but within 1/2 hour, napped for about 1/2 hour-45 minutes."

"Had some stiffness when first getting out of car, especially right lower extremity. Some cramping of right upper leg, better for moving around and shifting weight."

5:30 pm "I still have some mental slowness or dullness. I am slower to respond and it is now difficult to recall some names."

Day 9 - July 30, 1997

Dream: "I have had a similar sort of dream in the distant past. The person in the dream is not me, at least not this time. (In past dreams it was me.) The person is being sabotaged with a car that breaks down frequently and thus prevents them from getting to where they need to go. The person setting them up is acting as a friend, maybe even a lover. But deception is obvious to me as the observer but not to the person in the dream."

Day 10 - July 31, 1997

Slept from 11 pm-7:00 am. Woke up briefly for alarms. Feel more like my normal sleep/wake cycle. Slow to get going in the early am, then good energy. Ran about 3 miles, weather pleasant.

1:30 pm "Onset of feeling mild constriction in the head…diffuse but then settled in on left side. Headache was temporal and throbbing. Was pretty stressed before and during the headache, but also attribute to running, possibly because this has happened previous but usually if hot and humid and usually only right after the run, not this much later. Felt sluggish at work around 2 pm and remained sluggish most of the evening. Felt anxious about headache in middle of day, worried about my ability to continue to work if it intensified. Again had dullness of mind with sluggish episode and headache. Headache intensified by 2:30 pm and I had some difficulty with concentration. Ate lunch around 2 pm with no change. It was better if I rested with head still and eyes closed and worse motion. Feeling tired. Headache did decrease in intensity enough that I could carry on with work. At bedtime, noted mild throbbing in the right temporal area. (I am lying on that side.) Then fell asleep."

Day 11 - August 1, 1997

Slept from 11 pm-7:00 am. Woke up pretty easily. Feel like, "I am back to my normal sleep/wake cycle."

"Very occupied with thoughts of discontent about my career, my house and my husband's lack of organization. Feeling like things are not in order, or as I would like them to be."

"Over a disagreement with my husband, I became very upset and cried hysterically with violent sobbing, uncontrollably, which is very unusual for me. This lasted about 20-30 minutes. I continued crying even when my husband came to console me. I was very much comforted by his hugging and soothing words, but continued sobbing."

Day 12 - August 2, 1997

Three millimeter flesh colored bump on inner medial aspect of third finger of left hand (closer to nail). Not sure how it got there; could have been with gardening. Slightly tender if touched. Otherwise doesn't bother me.

Day 13 - August 3, 1997

Dream: "Husband was very distraught about being insulted by a business associate. Was supposed to meet me at a restaurant where I had even ordered for him but it hadn't come yet. He was very late arriving and was drunk. I was very upset by this and left the restaurant. Then dream ended."

"No episode of sluggishness, even with driving in car."

Day 14 - August 4, 1997

"Craving salt at lunch. Someone brought in potato chips, normally don't eat these."

"Was sluggish from noon until 4 pm and then perked up a bit knowing only one more hour of work. More energy late in evening after rainstorm, better cooler weather."

"Having trouble concentrating on studying after 10 pm. Spoke with husband on phone and mind stayed preoccupied about our communication which was very good but which made it difficult to study."

Day 15 - August 5, 1997

"Gorgeous weather, low humidity with warm heat, in the 70's, gentle breezes. 11:30 ran in park 3 miles. Felt very energized. Felt sluggish 3 hours after run; yawning, similar to previous days of decreased energy."

"Feeling very scattered and overwhelmed by all that I want to get done. Disorganized. Could not stay focused on task. Went from one thing to another. Feeling pressure and almost defeated by amount of work to do to still catch up. Feeling lack of confidence and a depressed mood."

2:30 pm "Left-sided throbbing headache, mild intensity. It is better lying still and worse from motion, especially bending forward. The pain is accompanied by some sluggishness which actually preceded it"

4:30 pm "Pre-occupied with left-sided headache. Inability to concentrate going from one thing to another. Unable to complete tasks."

Day 16 - August 6, 1997

"Actually woke up before alarm, but in bed until alarm went off and then got up. Went to bed on left side and woke up on right side. (Have noticed this more consistently recently.)"

4 pm "Gas and bloating and lower abdominal gurgling (ate 2-3 pm) …No bowel movement this morning so feel as if things are "backed up." This sensation over by 8 pm."

Day 17 - August 7, 1997

"Dream centered around moving furniture and clothes from one house to another house…It was a real effort to do this move, had to travel great distances…In the dream I felt as if it was an almost impossible effort. I felt frustrated and uncertain in my dream."

"Right lower pelvic pain (similar to ovulation) like a rather sharp, constant pain; lasted 10 minutes; occurred right after a bowel movement. Abated within half an hour. No further episodes."

"The small bump on left third finger still there. It doesn't bother me unless I rub it which I'm tempted to do sometimes since it's on the inside. It's mildly tender with rubbing hard."

10:30 am "During car ride to work, feeling very drained of energy and also depressed, as if there is a numbness about me. Driving more slowly than I normally do. My mind is very occupied with things I'd like to change about my life (job, husband's messy tendencies). This feeling and mood is better with company and better out of the car."

"Desires sympathy, but reluctant to talk to anyone except my husband about my feelings. Resent the fact that my husband had to travel this week (normally I'm okay with his travel). Talked on phone a lot with various friends and family to keep myself occupied since I'm feeling alone without husband."

Day 18 - August 8, 1997

"Bump on finger persists. Slight depression in center."

"Very hungry by dinnertime, ate at restaurant. Great food, loved the interesting flavors and spices. Very satisfying, but ate too much."

8:00 pm-9:00 pm "My eyes are itching and irritated bilaterally, attribute to some smokers nearby, better taking contact lenses out and scratching eyes. This is more noticeable than in past with smoking exposure."

Day 19 - August 9, 1997

DREAMS "I was in a scenario with a car and several people trying to get somewhere and took wrong turn, not sure if we ever got there."

"Eyes became irritated again in evening. Was in environment where people around were smoking. Eyes felt irritated, dry, and again better from rubbing them."

"Nodule on finger flattening out, spreading out so not sticking out as much. Central core getting a little darker."

"Noted lower abdominal gurgling, loud at times with increased motion and infrequent passing of flatus (no odor). Had rectal pressure at end of anus which lasted only briefly. No urge to move bowels at first upon awakening. Then fleeting urge which didn't result in any stool."

Day 20 - August 10, 1997

DREAM "I was faking that I was in a comatose state, yet I was actually aware of things going on around me. People were talking about how sick I had been and the progress of my medical state. I almost felt a sense of satisfaction for having fooled them. This was rather a vivid dream which is new for me."

Day 21 - August 11, 1997

"Bump on finger getting smaller, central core darker in color."

Day 22 - August 12, 1997

"High energy-even with studying. Much better and sharp contrast to one week ago."

"Humid, cloudy with occasional breeze. No air conditioner in house. Felt great being outside or with breeze or air circulating."

"Bump on finger decreased in size by half; still has central core which is slightly darker."

"Ate dinner out with husband and business associate. Had some wine (I have avoided up to now.)…Made me sleepy."

"Good focus and concentration. Mind more calm (in contrast to last week). Studied for 4 hours (homeopathy). Felt productive."

Day 23 - August 13, 1997

DREAM "relatively vivid."

"Weather cloudy and very muggy (humid). Not really affecting my mood…Better for being in air conditioning or cooled by air circulating.

"No bowel movement in morning again, no urge to defecate. The timing of the bowel movements has definitely changed. I used to have bowel movements in the morning, and now they happen any time, including the evening and I feel bloated, crampy, and pass flatus on those days…Between 5-6 pm loud stomach grumbling and passing flatus. At 7:30 PM ate pizza and had loud stomach gurgling shortly after. No urge to defecate."

"Very agitated by being misled about my car repair by a local service station. Feel as if I was treated unjustly."

Day 25 - August 15, 1997

DREAM

Husband and I in bed. He was on phone with my nephew. Tall man came into our bedroom and husband didn't respond. I panicked, fearful of my life. Man tried to attack me. I got a knife and tried to stab man in back. Husband still not doing anything to help, still on phone!!! Man went down with blow from knife and then got up. Dream ended. (Never had similar dream, but in distant past do remember some dreams of being stalked. I was very frightened in this dream and angry that my husband wasn't responding.)

Day 27 - August 17, 1997

"Eyes feel dry at times, especially at day's end. Feels like my lubrication (ocular) isn't as good. Vision gets slightly blurred or lacks clarity. Sometimes if inside and lighting is low, have to look at something in distance."

"Loud gurgling in abdomen after eating in evening."

"Mild breast tenderness with feeling of fullness and fluid retention. (She is before the menses.) This had disappeared with *Tuberculinum* in the past."

Day 28 - August 18, 1997

"Small bump a bit scaly in center; size unchanged."

"Had conversation (with husband) about where I am with my studies …He was very surprised by my feelings of inadequacy and frustration with myself for not being further ahead."

Day 32 - August 22, 1997

"Mild left-sided breast tenderness, worse if pressure applied. Menses begins with slight dark vaginal discharge."

Barely perceptible right sided frontal headache; mild throbbing with moving head. At 11:30 am, noted this right sided headache very faint again, except more in temporal region; occurred with turning head and then abated.

"Ate minestrone soup for lunch. Within 1 1/2 hours, I noted lower abdominal rumbling, bloating and gas. This persisted into late afternoon and evening eventually with some cramping, not relieved with anything except passing gas."

"Middle portion of left finger bump becoming more indented, size slightly smaller."

Day 34 - August 24, 1997

11:45 am "While sitting in class noted very dull diffuse frontal temporal headache on the right side worse than the left side. Symptoms only lasted several minutes and repeated on several occasions over next 1/2 hour."

1:00 pm "Headache is still noted as dullness; more constant. While in restaurant headache intensified with feeling of warmth. The headache was bilateral, throbbing and felt like a band across my forehead. It was worse heat and motion."

1:00 pm "Went to restaurant and felt very warm all over (almost flushed) upon entering room. Continued to feel this way and between 2-2:15 pm, a sensation of being very warm, desiring open air intensified. (Others did not feel this much warmth.) Felt better going out into open air."

1:00 pm "Feeling mildly panicked about the headache…felt better talking to others."

2:30 pm "Slightly better in open air, but then when returned to classroom at 2:40 pm headache still very much present. It is better closing the eyes and keeping the head held still. It is worse lying down with head on table. The headache is accompanied by an inability to concentrate and anxiety. Inability to concentrate in class, the mind is dull. Feeling very irritable by headache and lack of control over body. Concerned about ability to drive 6 hours home. Feeling persisted until 4 pm when I feel mint antidoted remedy and since headache abated."

2:40 pm "Feel very warm and stuffy in classroom (not like a suffocation). Feel better fanning myself."

3:10 pm "No change in headache. Accompanied by yawning several times and feeling sluggish."

3:15 pm "Took two 200 mg Advil out of concern that I can't drive home with these feelings."

3:45 pm "The heat is somewhat better by open air and air conditioner in car."

3:45 pm "No change in headache. Feeling as if it must be related to remedy. Suffering too much. Ate large peppermint mint patty. Headache gone completely in 5 minutes. Other symptoms improved as well."

4:00-10:00 pm "No irritability. Felt in control and in good spirits."

Day 38 - August 28, 1997

"Herpes simplex virus beginning to erupt. It is located in a new place, in the right perineum, near the anus. By September 10th the right labia majora is tingling, red, and has vesicles develop as a quick onset. By September 11th, the area is ulcerated and painful. By September 13th, the right side is less painful but persists, but now the left side is red, itching, and small vesicles develop. By September 14th, the viral outbreak is diminishing. The right was worse then the left side. My herpetic eruptions had gotten much better and have become very infrequent since *Sepia* was taken two years ago."

Prover #7

Prover #7 was a 32 year old woman who responded very well to *Nux vomica* constitutionally. She too, explains about the confusion. She took only one dose of the remedy as she felt symptoms right away. While she experienced many, many symptoms, the majority of them were within her usual steady state and were therefore discounted. There were some, though, that were different.

H: Within the first minutes there was nothing out of the ordinary. The conversation was normal. On the three hour follow-up, when she was evaluated to see if she should take a second dose, she changed her story about what she had felt originally. On the three hour follow-up she said, referring to the first few minutes, "I had a real problem comprehending things right after taking the remedy. Even though we were talking and everything seemed normal to you, I was actually having a tough time understanding what you were telling me. It was all so confusing…I felt slow in understanding."

H: She was slow in motion as well when she walked out of the house. She said that she felt lightheaded later that day, "Like how I feel when I am flying and I am jetlagged." "I feel like my brain is swollen." She felt slow in motion as she operated her car.

The only other symptom of note was that she developed a sensitivity to noise that lasted into her tenth day.

Prover #8

Prover #8 was a 42 year old woman. Her chronic symptoms, with a tendency to develop asthma, place her around a *Sulphur*, *Medorrhinum*, and *Nux vomica* constitution. She has a strong family history of alcoholism, as well as she herself being alcoholic in her 20's. Her symptoms vacillate between the dull side of the remedy and the active, energetic aspect.

DAY 1 - December 15, 1997

STOMACH: "After the dose I seemed to not want to eat as much. Some change in awareness of stomach. Felt full quicker. For the rest of the evening, I was aware of slight pressure (difficult to describe) not painful at all. The closest thing I can compare to is slight indigestion in my esophagus and stomach areas."

RESPIRATION: "About 2 hours after first dose, I became aware of increased secretions/phlegm in my airway. I had the feeling of needing to clear my throat and to swallow. I felt one or two wheezes when I exhaled."

DAY 2 - December 16, 1997

MIND/EMOTIONS: "Dreading appointment I made this morning …Feeling very blue throughout morning…Negative thinking and very poor concentration, worse than usual variations of normal. It took me 45 minutes to pick up a few items at the store…In the afternoon, I had extreme emotions, sadness and tearfulness, then anger for several hours. There was no identifiable cause. I had some strange violent thoughts, for example, of shooting my cat."

GENERAL: "Low energy…Low motivation. I have a lot to do but procrastinating doing them."

STOMACH: "Good appetite. I ate three meals with a little snacking (of cookies) in between but not as driven to eat as in past weeks. No change in types of foods I desire."

RESPIRATORY: "My airway felt clear today except when I went for long walk of one hour outside. The temperature was about 35 degrees and I felt a little wheezing for the first half of the walk but it went away without going into a coughing fit, I had to clear my throat a few times."

DAY 3 - December 17, 1997

Took a second dose at 5pm.

MIND/EMOTIONS: "Enjoyed activities that were solitary and creative. I needed to refocus myself often. Some decrease in concentration. I felt calm, with no extremes of emotion today."

STOMACH: "Appetite was more normalized today."

SLEEP: "Asleep within 15 minutes. I slept all night. I recalled snippets of dreams of a bank robbery involving a young man pulling a heavy desktop off of the desk."

DAY 4 - December 18, 1997

MIND/EMOTIONS: 8am "Concentration very poor. I had trouble organizing myself to dress and gather things to go out. In the midst of this fogginess I had a little explosive episode; kicking a drawer shut that wouldn't close. Later in the day I was vacuuming, feeling okay, not aware of feeling angry but became frustrated with some little thing and had impulse to throw something and did throw a metal vacuum tube at a door. It was very surprising to me. It was like a feeling of anger and power exploding suddenly out of me. When my son came home from school we had a disagreement and I had to exert great self control to keep from yelling. I kept some distance from him for a while. This was at 3pm. By 4:30pm I felt like I was back to normal. I had had feelings like this in the past but very rarely in the past 6 years. A walk outside helped my mood."

STOMACH: "My eating is more connected to my appetite. It is not as driven as before my menses. I noticed that same feeling as on day one of the proving of pressure in stomach and esophogeal area."

RESPIRATION: "Noted in mid-morning (started then) the feeling of secretions in airway along with some wheezing. This was noticed throughout the day. This is not a tight, constricted feeling. It is more like bubbles popping in the airway, little wheezes at random times."

DAY 5 - December 19, 1997

MIND/EMOTIONS: "Good concentration. No impulsive actions, I feel calm and positive."

RESPIRATION: "Airway feels clear. There is no longer wheezing or bubbling feeling in chest."

GENITOURINARY: "In the evening, I had a sharp intense knifelike pain which felt like a bad menstrual cramp, though it is not my menses. The pain went from the uterine area down to the labia."

SLEEP: "I fell asleep within 15 minutes. I was aware during sleep that I was dreaming and that the dreams were brighter, with more movement and with a lighter feeling than earlier in week."

DAY 6 - December 20, 1997

MIND/EMOTIONS: "Calm…In good spirits. I have good concentration. Feeling social and positive thoughts in general."

GENERAL: "Good energy level. Stayed present and alert even though had to be indoors working."

STOMACH: "I am back to snacking frequently, mostly cookies, cheese, crackers and pickles."

DAY 7 - December 21, 1997

HEAD/EMOTIONS: "Feeling calm. Good concentration. Brief feelings of sadness missing people who are dead."

DAY 8 - December 22, 1997

MIND/EMOTIONS: "In fairly good spirits. Somewhere in between being very task oriented and enjoying what I was doing. I am feeling a little driven. Alert. Good concentration. I noticed a little bit of the explosive feeling again while vacuuming. I felt like the vacuum and I were too big for the space and as I bumped into things I had brief desire to kick and hit things. I didn't act on it, except to yank the vacuum around but eventually the feelings passed."

GENERAL: "Good energy level. Busy. The best energy level is when I am outside."

STOMACH: "Continuing to snack frequently. Eating at times when not hungry."

SLEEP: "Slept all night. Dreams were fun and about having a good time."

DAY 9 - December 23, 1997

MIND/EMOTIONS: "Alert, good concentration. In fair spirits. A few periods of irritability and impatience with others, when I felt they ought to be doing something."

GENERAL: "Good energy level. Took a long walk and enjoyed outside, it was 30 degrees outside."

RESPIRATION: "Noticed a little congestion and phlegm in my throat when I walked outside."

DAY 10 - December 24, 1997

MIND/EMOTIONS: "Not as present in body due to sedentary activity and low stimulation. Feeling dull and lethargic."

GENERAL: "Lower energy. Inside working all day with low stimulation."

STOMACH: "Snacking frequently on cookies."

SLEEP: "Aware of dreaming but unable to recall it, felt like active and enjoyable dreams."

DAY 12 - December 26, 1997

STOMACH: "Eating lots of holiday 'junk food' though not hungry."

GENITOURINARY: "Increased libido (I am mid-cycle)."

SLEEP: "Awake on and off though didn't really awaken completely but I was aware of restlessness and light sleep through the night."

DAY 13 - December 27, 1997

MIND/EMOTIONS: "Impatient at times. Tended to withdraw at these times."

GENITOURINARY: "Increased libido. Some sharp mild pelvic pain on right side, feels like ovulation pain."

SLEEP: "Slept all night, longer than usual, 9 hours, but had a hard time waking up. Drowsy in the next morning."

DAY 15 - December 29, 1997

MIND/EMOTIONS: "A lot of questions in my mind. Thinking a lot about habits and patterns and had some big insights into areas I had felt stuck. Felt relieved after this around mid day."

HEAD/EYES/EARS: "Woke up with dull headache. Felt very heavy headed. Eventually took Tylenol. Subsided around noon."

GENERAL: "Energy level low in the morning, better in the afternoon related to moods above."

STOMACH: "Decreased appetite today. Less snacking, maybe related to my emotional insights."

DAY 16 - December 30, 1997

MIND/EMOTION: "Irritable at times. Focused on getting things done. Did enjoy a few activities like cross country skiing."

MUSCULOSKELETAL: "Ongoing awareness of tensions in neck and shoulders."

DAY 17 - December 31, 1997

MIND/EMOTIONS: "Worrying more. Somewhat obsessing about things. It is very cold and gray outside which seemed to increase my low mood. Felt better after a walk. Tolerated cold temperatures outside."

DAY 18 - January 1, 1998

MIND/EMOTIONS: "Feeling some pressure and task orientation. Some anxiety about the future. Not feeling much pleasure in activities. The gray sky seemed to aggravate my low moods."

STOMACH: "Ate more than appetite warranted in evening."

DAY 19 - January 2, 1998

MIND/EMOTION: "Anxious. Not enjoying activities very much. Heavy gray sky seemed to aggravate low mood."

DAY 20 - January 3, 1998

MIND/EMOTION: "Enthusiastic, looking forward to fun activities planned for day. Enjoyed these activities."

GENERAL: "Energy level is very good. Enjoyed outdoor physical activity."

DAY 22 - January 5, 1998

MUSCULOSKELETAL: "Muscle aches after pushing a tractor yesterday."

SLEEP: "Slept longer than usual. Very difficult waking up."

DAY 23 - January 6, 1998

MIND/EMOTION: "Had to push self to get up. Wanted just to stay in bed all day. More initiative by mid-day. Some irritable periods in evening. Wanted to have more physical and emotional space from others."

GENERAL: "Very low energy in morning. Better by late morning."

HEAD: "Headache in am. Took Tylenol in the morning and it resolved."

SLEEP: "Slept all night. Very hard time waking up."

DAY 25 - January 8, 1998

MIND/EMOTION: "For last several days, very low motivation and groggy in the morning. Pushed self to do necessary tasks, low mood; pessimistic thoughts entering mind often."

GENERAL: "Very, very low energy in the morning. Went back to bed after being up for 1 hour. Slept 1 hour more. Energy increased some as day went on. Aggravated by heavy gray weather."

HEAD: "Woke up with headache. Took Tylenol. Headache gone by 10 in the morning."

DAY 26 - January 9, 1998

MIND/EMOTION: "Poor concentration and memory and difficulty expressing thoughts due to lack of sleep."

GENERAL: "Tired, low energy."

DAY 27 - January 10, 1998

MIND/EMOTION: "In good spirits. More alert than yesterday. Enjoyed social activities. Felt better associated with sunny weather."

GENERAL: "Energy level better than yesterday."

DAY 28 - January 11, 1998

GENERAL: "Energy level fair especially considering interrupted sleep pattern of last 3 days (working nights) seemed to have more energy with sunny weather today."

DAY 29 - January 12, 1998

MIND/EMOTION: "Fairly alert."

MUSCULOSKELETAL: "Sore everywhere after playing basketball yesterday."

Prover #9

Prover #9 was a 64 year old man who appeared to be in good health. He is tall and looks to have a *Phosphorus/Sulphur* constitution. He too, describes the dichotomy between acuity of perception on the one hand and the mental confusion on the other.

Day 1 - August 7, 1997

H and P: NOTE:-In order to calm my prover's concerns, I took a dose of the remedy at the same time. Here are my symptoms:

6:30 pm "I am lightheaded and "spacey"…There is a heavy feeling at the right forehead…I have difficulty thinking and concentrating. For example, my wife told me three telephone numbers to write down and it was very difficult to recall them and write them. My coordination was fine."

6:40 pm "I have tingling over both triceps bilaterally, on the skin of my upper arms."

6:45 pm "There is a loud ringing in my right ear."

7:10 pm "I have a heavy pain in my right shoulder and neck which radiates to the right jaw."

(At this point I was worried because I had a lot of planning and management to do related to my mother's recent stroke and nursing home placement, so I went to Starbucks and got a Grande coffee of the day to antidote.)

Day 2 - August 8, 1997

"I awoke and recalled dreams of floating in water on rafts, and being pursued, but not fearfully, more like a competition and some races."

"I noted that my life-long tendency to crusts in my nose and the desire to pick them had disappeared."

"Note: Two months later, crusts are now starting to return."

Prover #10

Prover #10 was a 46 year old man. He has a history of using recreational drugs in the distant past and has an allergy to alcohol. He tended to develop sinusitis or congestion in his nose. Constitutionally, he looks mostly like *Sulphur* and *Nux vomica*. Prover #10 illustrates the acuity of the senses.

August 16, 1997

08:45 Took the first dose.

09:00 "I'm starting to feel light-headed as I am sitting around talking. Everything around me seems lighter in a visual way. Everything is a little clearer visually-has a sharpness to it."

09:10 "I am feeling a tingling feeling at the top of my head. It is like pins and needles, but quite pleasant."

09:30 "I have to leave to drive to a tennis match. I am feeling energized. I am experiencing a restless movement with my arms and hands while I am driving. (I am touching my face, ears, my one arm is touching the other.) My thoughts are racing some, no particular content other than a slight concern that I will be late for my tennis match."

09:45 "I am still driving to my tennis match. I feel a sensation of excitation in my chest, it is a little heavy feeling. Also I feel a slight tenseness around my eyes, but it is not uncomfortable. I feel my mental concentration is more intense, but not strained. In fact, I feel a contented relaxation in the midst of feeling energized and somewhat excited."

10:00 "I arrived at my tennis match. I still feel excited and there is a fluttering in the pit of my stomach and a radiating sensation in my chest near my breast bone rising up to my neck which is a pleasant feeling."

11:15 "I played an hour of tennis. I am feeling a little jittery in my arms. It is a tremulous sensation in my forearms and hands. It is very hot and humid outside. I am now sitting in the shade. There is still a tingling tightness in my chest, right between my pectoralis muscles which is rather pleasant. I am also continuing to experience a slight sense of excitement."(His tennis game was more focused and he played better than usual.)

14:30 I am at my in-laws swimming pool. They had food for lunch that I didn't like. I ate some but am still hungry.

Head, Ears, Eyes, Nose and Throat: "Visual acuity seems improved—vision is clearer, sharper. My head is feeling a little pressure at the top. It is a pleasant sensation, kind of like a hat is on my head." (The sensation on the scalp then gets described as if it is a tightness, like wearing a hat.)

Chest: "The most unusual sensation I have been experiencing is in my chest. I feel a tingling sensation. Still mostly about six inches across in the mid chest. It is a pleasant feeling that is accompanied by a low level excitement. This radiated from the mid chest outward" (There was also a lifting sensation in the chest and diaphragm.)

Skin, Hair, Nails: "Just the tingling sensation on my skin in my arms, hands, legs, feet and chest."

Mental: "My mind is more clear and focused." (He had waves of relaxation and drifting in and out of sleep in the afternoon. He describes a sensation of sleep washing over him but then he becomes alert again.)

General State: "My general state is relaxed, with a slight feeling of excitation. I also feel calm, contented and focused." (He is more relaxed with less anxious than usual. Almost exhilarated. Generally all symptoms are noted to be mild and pleasant to the prover.)

22:00 "I am feeling very tired. I am in bed and about ready to go to sleep."

Head, Ears, Eyes, Nose and Throat: "The pleasant tightness is gone. My visual acuity is still clearer and sharper than normal."

Chest: "Still some subtle tingling."

Skin, Hair, Nails: "I still have a tingling sensation in arms, hands, calves, feet and chest that is in part a sensation on the skin."

Emotional: "I am feeling very contented more so than usual."

Mental: "Clear and focused, but relaxed."

General State: "I am tired at the end of the day, but pleasantly so. The tingling sensation in my body has evolved into feelings like my body is vibrating. It is subtle and I usually notice it only when I am in a quiet place or attending to my body specifically. The vibrations seem to be going outward, but are strongest in my feet, calves, arms, hands and chest."

August 17, 1997

03:00 Dreams: "I had two vivid dreams so far. In one the woman I was with had a car accident. She went swerving off the road to avoid hitting an animal. Something to do with a skunk and then the police came."

"The other dream involved going to a show to see a woman I wanted to sing with, on stage. She was singing and there were a number of people in the audience. I knew one guy who was giving me a hard time about something but in a friendly way, joking with me."

"I woke up with a lot of intestinal pain on my left side. I expelled a lot of gas. (I ate ice cream before going to bed and have lactose intolerance.) The pain was particularly intense. I then had a bowel movement which was pretty explosive and the explosiveness is unusual for me. I also felt a little nauseous which is likewise unusual for me."

(New is that he slept on his right side with right arm extended. He did not want to sleep on his abdomen, as usual, because it felt too closed down, too closed in. He says that he wants to stay open.)

August 18, 1997

08:00 Head, Ears, Eyes, Nose and Throat: "My visual acuity is still noticeably clearer and sharper. My head is clear. My sinuses feel clearer today, I have not blown my nose since last night. My ears are okay, except for my left ear being a little itchy. My throat is okay."

Chest: "I still have a slight sense of excitation in my chest right where my sternum is. It is now a little tight and heavy feeling, but again, not unpleasant."

Skin, Hair Nails: "My arms and hands still feel different but now it is like a pulsating feeling as the blood courses through my veins there."

Emotional: "I feel rested, relaxed and content."

Mental: "My mind is clear and focused."

General State: "I have a bitter dry taste in my mouth this morning. My tongue in particular feels very dry and the saliva in my mouth is kind of thick. As I wake up more I am beginning to feel the vibrating feelings in my legs and feel like yesterday."

09:00 "I just finished meditating. My sinuses are stuffy again and I am blowing my nose again. I am feeling intense hunger."

"I noticed during my meditation that my hearing and sense of smell seemed more acute."

Head, Ears, Eyes, Nose and Throat: "My visual acuity is still clearer and sharper than normal. My hearing and sense of smell are also somewhat more acute. In my head there is a tightness around my eyes and a dull pain especially above the left eye-feels a little like a hot poker. My sinuses are clear now. However I have been coughing up phlegm today every couple of hours."

Chest: "My chest is clear, but I still have a vibrating feeling between my pectoralis muscles and sternum."

Stomach: "I was feeling some intense waves of hunger at times today which is new to me."

General State: "I still feel a vibrating sensation throughout my body, but most intensely in my extremities-arms, legs, hands and feet."

23:30 "I am in bed and ready to go to sleep."

Head, Ears, Eyes, Nose and Throat: "My visual acuity is still clearer and sharper than normal. My ears are okay. My sinuses are pretty clear. I am still blowing my nose a fair amount (every 1/2 hour). My throat has cleared up. My head is okay."

Chest: "No radiating feeling anymore."

Emotional: "I feel pleasantly weary from the busy day and very content."

Mental: "Clear and focused."

General State: "The vibrating feeling in my body has subsided some. The tingling is still strongest in my feet and in my calves especially on the right side."

August 18, 1997

04:45 Dreams: "I was driving in the country with some guy (he could have been my father, he was a fatherly figure). Just before that I had been at a store buying some tools. When I stopped in the road with this guy I had to compare the way I was doing things with how he was doing things. We were looking for some festival or event. I stopped the car on a dusty road."

Mouth: "I have a very bitter taste in my mouth and my saliva is very thick. My mouth was wet, but my tongue was dry."

08:00 Dreams: "I was in a store. There were long cords that needed to be stretched and tied to hooks in order to keep the door open. I was having a difficult time finding the hooks on the wall. Someone helped me to find them on one side of the wall. I was in what seemed to be a grocery store. Before that I was in an elevator and it seemed like something dangerous was happening, but I can't remember clearly. Then a phone rang and I picked it up and the person on the phone said it was Ian Fleming, but I had to hold a button down on the phone in order to talk. The voice on the phone sounded like a person I know in real life who calls fairly often and is very difficult to talk to. The general tone and feeling of the second dream was of being deceived."

Sleep: "My sleep was more restful and refreshing than usual."

General State: "I am in bed. I just woke up, got out of bed, defecated and am back in bed writing. The most noticeable sensation is still increased visual acuity which is sharper and clear, as is hearing. My mouth still has a funny bitter taste, with my tongue very dry and my saliva pasty and thick."

Head, Ears, Eyes, Nose and Throat: "See above for eyes and ears. In addition, I feel a heaviness around my eyes, but it is subtle. Especially around the right eye, just above the right corner of my eye brow. I also feel a pleasant pressing between my eyes that is like a bridge between my eyes. My sinuses are clearer today-I don't feel I have to blow my nose yet today. Throat is okay-no mucus today."

Emotional: "I feel very content, relaxed, alert and well rested."

Mental: "Clear and focused."

17:00 General State: "I am at home after a fairly relaxing day. I went to brunch with my visiting relatives, then to visit my in-laws. Afterwards, I went home and saw two patients in my home office. Amazingly enough, my body still has that vibrating sensation. It is stronger than it was this morning. (I did inadvertently have some caffeinated tea this afternoon as my father in-law's; he misunderstood my request for herbal tea.) I can even feel the vibrations in my face which I hadn't felt before. In general, things continue to go well and I feel relaxed, alert and contented."

Head, Ears, Eyes, Nose and Throat: "Sinuses are pretty clear, although I have been blowing my nose every hour or so. My throat is okay. Visual acuity and hearing persist being clear and sharp."

Chest: "Still feel the radiating sensation in my chest at the sternum."

Lower Abdomen: "I have a throbbing sharp pain in my lower abdomen, on the left side that feels like a hot poker. The feelings are annoying but not intense." (The pain was in the left lower quadrant, just above the iliac crest. It was worse from sitting and better standing.)

Emotional: "I am still feeling generally relaxed and content."

23:30 General State: "I am in bed ready to go to sleep. I am feeling tired after a relaxing evening at home with my family. The vibrating feeling is quite faint and only present in my arms and hands."

Head, Ears, Eyes, Nose and Throat: "My sinuses are stuffy. My eyes are itchy and red as I am experiencing a flare up of my allergies. However, my visual acuity and hearing remain sharper and clearer than I remember before taking the remedy. My head is okay as is my throat."

Chest: "No real vibrating sensation in my chest now."

Lower Abdomen: "I feel a slight fluttering sensation. It is like a line is stretched across my belly just below my navel. It feels like a string that is a little tight and is being twinged or plucked like a guitar string."

August 19, 1997

Dreams: "The first dream I can remember was about some mafia style gangsters. One guy was trying to put something over (deceive) on some other people. The Mafia types created a roadblock and were just shooting men of a certain age to make sure they got the guy they were after. Then one guy who got shot in the head, shot the guy who shot him. He also shot him in the head and then they just kept shooting each other."

"Another dream I remember was where I was with my daughter and another daughter (in real life we have only one daughter), we were all put in a cellar type place. First we were separated. Then I was down in the cellar and then all the kids were dropped back in through a hole in the ceiling or brought in. My daughter was doing okay, but her younger sister was having a difficult time and I was trying to comfort her."

"The last dream was where a voice like John Wayne's announced that there was a "Lalapolooza" coming. We were eating breakfast at the time. The whole group ran outside and we were in the mountains on a farm. There was a huge storm approaching. The storm contained funnel clouds (tornadoes). I was obviously visiting the farm. Everyone who lived there was well trained and began to engage in emergency actions to get all the livestock to safer ground. Then a semi-trailer truck which was towing a tow truck and a pick up truck to higher ground sped off. We got to the shelter just in time, not everyone went in but the funnel clouds just passed over us and then touched down on an adjacent farm and destroyed it. We were all relieved we had been spared."

"These dreams had deception and danger in them. Gangsters deceiving and killing each other, being thrown into a dungeon, and a storm that ravages the farm next door. The dreams were disconcerting and upsetting."

General State: "I feel the vibrating sensations in my body very slightly, mostly in my arms and hands."

Head, Ears, Eyes, Nose and Throat: "I have some twitching in my facial muscles this morning on the left side just above my lips. I had this during the night as well. (This is not a new symptom, but I haven't had it for several months and it is relatively uncommon.) My visual acuity and hearing remain sharper and clearer. My sinuses are fairly clear this morning. My throat is okay."

Neck: "My neck is not stiff at all."

Chest: "I still have the vibrating sensation again right above the sternum."

Stomach: "I feel both a mild hunger and a mild nausea this morning. The feeling is on the right side below my rib cage. It feels like a churning wave."

19:00 "I don't feel much of the vibrating feelings in my body now. Mentally I feel a little scattered and emotionally I feel tense and keyed up."

23:00 General State: "I feel a slight vibrating sensation in my ankles and feet."

Head, Ears, Eyes, Nose and Throat: "My visual acuity and hearing are still sharper and clearer than normal. My sinuses are quite clear and I haven't blown my nose in several hours. My throat has been clear since 6:30 pm."

Emotional: "Okay except a little apprehensive about our car that broke down when my wife was driving earlier today (the engine may be broken)."

Mental: "Somewhat concerned about what is wrong with the car, but still alert and focused. I seem to be less concerned or affected by stress than usual."

August 20, 1997

09:00 General State: "I do feel a slight tingling in my hands and feet and head, but nowhere else."

Dreams: "I only remember one dream. A woman got in our car and drove it up the driveway. I was happy it started, but was concerned that she would damage the car. She got out at the top of the driveway, but wouldn't tell me who she was or how she got the key to the car."

Sleep: "I slept very well. My sleep is still better than usual. An alarm woke me and I went back to sleep. The baby woke me, I put her back to sleep and went to sleep."

Head, Ears, Eyes, Nose and Throat: "My sinuses are fairly clear. I do feel some pressure in my sinuses above my eyes, especially at the bridge of my nose. It feels like something is pushing on the bridge if my nose like a vise, but not very hard. I did wake up in the morning with a slight bitter taste in my mouth. Throat is okay. My vision and hearing are still more acute than usual."

Chest: "No radiating feeling in my chest today."

Mental: "My mind is clear and alert. A little less focused than the previous few days as I have been a little distractible. (At one point I forgot where I put a section of the newspaper.)"

22:00 Head, Ears, Eyes, Nose and Throat: "My eyes and ears are still sharper in their perceptions. My sinuses are clear and I have been blowing my nose less today. My throat is clear. My head is okay."

Skin, Hair, Nails: "A little tingling sensation in my feet."

Emotional: "I am feeling a little drained emotionally after a long and stressful day, but also satisfied that tensions at home have been defused. My wife had tensions and stresses about going to work and I did not get sucked into that at all. However, I am drained, fatigued, and slightly sad tonight."

August 21, 1997

08:30 General State. "I have a sharp pain in my upper right arm. It is just 4 inches below my shoulder in the middle of the outside area of my upper arm. It is like a white hot needle piercing the skin, the sensation is intermittent. About every 5 to 10 minutes I feel this poking sensation. I didn't pay much attention to it originally, but it started yesterday evening, I just didn't attend to it much as it has been more intense and persistent this morning."

Head, Ears Eyes, Nose and Throat: "My visual acuity and hearing are still slightly clearer and sharper. My throat is clear. No bitter taste in my mouth this morning."

Skin, Hair, Nails: "The vibrating sensation is still subtly present in my lower legs and feet, but not really anywhere else."

23: 00 Head, Ears Eyes Nose and Throat: "My sinuses are a bit stuffed up especially the right side, but no pressure or headache. My eyes and ears still have some increased acuity."

Neck: "My neck is little stiff. Some pain on the right side from my shoulder up the right side of my neck-it is kind of a dull shooting pain."

Skin: "Not much in the way of tingling or vibrating sensations in my body. A little in my feet and solar plexus, just below my umbilicus."

August 22, 1997

Dreams: "I don't remember much in terms of dreams. I did dream and one dream was very sexual and had to do with sexual photographs of a woman. It was a famous woman and there was some scandalous controversy about the pictures."

07:30 Head, Ears, Eyes, Nose and Throat: "My visual acuity and hearing still seem clearer and sharper than before I took the remedy. My sinuses are okay, the right nostril has a little mucus in it. My throat and head are okay."

Chest: "There is a slight radiating feeling in my chest at the sternum."

Skin, Hair, Nails: "There is a slight tingling feeling in my feet which is a pleasant sensation."

23:00 General State: "I did have that strange white hot needle sensation in my right upper arm again. It happened around dinner time. It lasted about 1/2 hour and occurred 4-5 times for a couple of seconds each time."

Head, Ears, Eyes, Nose and Throat: "Still a sense of increased acuity in vision and hearing."

Skin, Hair, Nails: "I do have a vibrating, tingling sensation in my feet, but nowhere else in my body."

August 23, 1997

Lower Abdomen: "I had some distress in my lower abdomen at 7:30 a.m. as I ate very hot spicy sausage last night. The feeling was like a dull pain that had a churning sensation associated with it, like a hand grabbing my intestines and squeezing them as the fingers moved around gripping the intestines. This lasted for 20 minutes or so. I have had this happen three other times during this proving."

Skin, Hair, Nails: "I have a vibrating feeling in my lower legs and feet, but nowhere else to speak of."

22:00 Stomach: "Still full from dinner. I have a satisfied feeling there—pleasantly full, a kind of warm glow just below my rib cage on the left side."

August 24, 1997

06:00 Dreams: "I dreamt I was flying a small propeller airplane in an area that was snow covered and a ski area. At one point I jumped out of the plane and down the mountain. There were a lot of trails and at one point I was a little worried about getting lost. Then the trails lead to a subdivision of houses. Then I was sitting next to the leader of the spiritual retreat I went to yesterday and was telling him stories. Then I was back in the plane and getting ready to jump again, but the door was in front of the propeller so I decided it was not a smart idea."

Head, Ears, Eyes, Nose and Throat: "My visual acuity and hearing still seem sharper than before the remedy."

Skin, Hair, Nails: "No tingling anywhere in my body to report."

August 25, 1997

10:00 Sleep: "I slept pretty well. I wonder if the effects of the remedy are wearing off some. I don't feel the tingling sensations much anymore and my sleep is not quite as restful the last couple of nights."

22:00 General State: "It was a fairly productive day. I am in bed ready to go to sleep. I did play very good tennis today. My concentration and focus were quite good and it seems like my tennis game has been better in the last week. I feel fairly organized and that my life is currently enjoyable and manageable."

August 26, 1997

08:00 Dreams: "I remember one dream in which a woman from work who just had a baby and is on maternity leave had a threat against her life. I somehow was in charge of protecting her. I had a very organized plan that I was explaining to other people. Again, there was danger and deception."

23:00 "I have been craving something sweet tonight which is unusual. I ate a half bar of chocolate. I am not really tired, but I have to go to sleep as I need to get up early tomorrow (6:30)."

August 27, 1997

06:00 Dreams: "I only remember one dream. In that dream I was driving in a car and my mother was with me (my mother has been dead for several years). We were trying to get away from something dangerous. At some point a police car started to follow us, but it was old and beat up so we sped up, made a U-turn at a turnpike type exit and lost the police car. The dream seemed to be about danger, deception and safety."

Stomach: "Gaseous and a little bloated, as I have been for a few days."

Lower Abdomen: "Also gaseous. I had a bout of diarrhea this morning. My abdomen feels crampy with a churning uncomfortable sensation."

17:00 "My stomach is gaseous. I have pain in my abdomen associated with the gas. It is short bursts of pain radiating up from my lower abdomen to higher up. Laying down helped make it less intense."

23:45 Lower Abdomen: "Still some residual pain, similar to early in the evening with shooting pains radiating in little bursts but this time from higher to lower in my abdomen, but less intense. Lying down still helps relieve the pain to some extent.

August 28, 1997

09:00 General State: "At 3:10 am I still had some gastrointestinal (GI) distress and defecated (semi-formed stools which were a little explosive). I felt better when I went back to sleep. I woke up feeling better GI-wise and had another bowel movement and then felt much better still. My arms are tingling this morning as are my feet and my face (not intensely, rather subtle and pleasant). I feel really good this morning despite the reduced hours of sleep I had. I feel content and am looking forward to not working again until next Thursday, after today."

23:00 Head, Ears, Eyes, Nose and Throat: "My vision and hearing remain sharp and clear."

Emotional: "I am relaxed and feel content, except I forgot a book at work. I have to drive an hour for no other reason than to go back and get it tomorrow. So I am slightly irritated with myself for that."

Mental: "I was a little forgetful today as I forgot my umbrella at one point in the day and then later a book that I needed to take home."

August 29, 1997

08:15 Dreams: I had several dreams one only I can remember clearly. I was in a bakery and I wanted to buy a round pastry that was covered in chocolate like a donut, only bigger. The woman serving me gave me a credit card receipt covered in chocolate (instead of the pastry) and I reluctantly paid her the $1.59 counting out the 59 cents in change, 2 quarters, 1 dirty nickel and 4 pennies. I then objected and asked for the pastry I had seen others get instead of the chocolate covered credit card receipt that she gave me and then I woke up. Again a dream of deception."

General State: "I have a dry mouth this morning and a bitter taste in my mouth. I must have slept in a funny position as both my hip joints hurt, the right more than the left. It helped to walk around as the stiff soreness seemed to lessen considerably after walking."

Mental: "I feel a little groggy as I am still waking up and it takes me a little longer than usual. (I usually wake up alert and focused.) My mind feels kind of thick and slow."

August 30, 1997

10:00 Back: "A slight pain in my upper back below my scapula when I turn to the right. It is a sharp, short lasting pain."

Mental: "My mind feels a little sluggish this morning."

Prover #11

Prover #11 was a 40 year old man. He illustrates the way the dullness and confusion are exemplified in the physical realm. He also describes this feeling in the ears that is similar to flying, a common finding in the proving.

P took 3 doses of the remedy, as he did not feel anything with the first ones. While there were many symptoms the first day, they were not different from his normally experienced ones.

Day two

H: P woke up with a numb palate, at the roof of the mouth.

At the same time, he developed pressure in his ears and in the eustachian tubes. He said it was, "like when I am underwater or landing in an airplane." The pressure and congestion were better if he pressed his nostrils together and blew in to clear them, as in a *Valsalva* maneuver. He did this when he was in pain or really congested. It would relieve both sensations quickly but they would come back again, soon after.

His voice was weak the whole day.

He has become restless, like he usually does when he has low blood sugar.

Day three

H: He had a restless sleep the night before, waking up often and finding it difficult to fall back asleep. He is very tired this morning, which is unusual for him as he is usually a morning person. He felt weak all day.

He had a painless diarrhea, which is unusual for him.

Today he had pressure in his eyeballs, similar to the pressure in his ears the day before. His sclera were really red.

He said his skin of his face felt strange. "The skin of my face feels dry and tense."

Day four

P: "Life is back to normal today."

Prover #12

Prover #12 was a 41 year old woman. Her chronic complaints are arthritic pains and allergies and it was these symptoms that flared up the greatest. She too mentions an airplane in describing her congestions and dreams.

Day 1 - July 13, 1997

7:15 am P: "I just took the first dose. Shortly afterwards, my chest felt heavy as if I had just walked into a smoky room. This lasted for five minutes."

H: During the first 5 minutes, there was a marked red flushing of the face.

Day 6-7, July 18-19, 1997
Took another dose today

H: Pain in metatarsal areas is much worse than usual. There are no new spots, the pain is in the same old locations, the pains are unchanged in all ways except in intensity.

P: "I had a weird dream last night. I was on an airplane that had rows and rows of seats, with lots of windows. We were flying, but there was no one flying the plane, and on the outside there was fog that was so thick it was like smoke. We were about to land through this smoke, and then I was transported somewhere else."

Night 2-3 am H: Her allergies were greatly increased today. She is really stuffy tonight, waking up in the middle of the night between two and three in the morning. Her nose is discharging clear mucus and she can not stop sneezing. She is feeling pressure in her head. She takes Benadryl and goes back to sleep.

Day 14 - July 26, 1997

H: She developed an itchy boil on the cuticle of the middle finger of her left hand. It looks vesicular, fluid filled, lasts for four days, and then recedes, leaving behind a small pinpoint indurated area. The next day, the same thing repeats on the fifth finger of the same hand.

Day 23 - August 4, 1997

H: Triangular reddened coloration to the central area of her face. Her fingers are also redder and she flushes when she speaks.

H: She has needed no anti-inflammatory drugs for a few weeks. It has happened in the past that the arthritis may quiet down but it is noticeable now that it is clearly better.

P: "There is something odd about my comprehension and focus. I am more prone to accidents…my memory is confused and my addition is full of miscalculations…I usually have an excellent memory but now I am forgetting many words that are common, such as 'window' or 'chair'. This is very unusual for me."

Day 42 - August 23, 1997
She took another dose at 8:30 am today.

8:30 am H: Her nose becomes very stuffy, and at the same time her heart begins to race.

8:35 am H: The stuffiness in her nose has increased, with drainage clear which is usual for her. But the nasal congestion is the worst it has ever been. It is worse lying down.

8:40 am H: There is almost a complete blockage of the nose…her voice sounds nasal. She can not inhale through her nose, her eyes are slightly glassy and wet.

H: Her toes have been much better, with less pain, less often, with long periods of comfort. This is very unusual for her chronic arthritis.

H: She reports that last week, she noticed a white and red discoloration on her face.

P: "I have noticed one other major difference in my life. I am having a lot of difficulty with spelling. I never had a problem before in my life. I used to win spelling contests. This comes and goes episodically sometimes at work and other times when applying my mind."

H: Something very different is that she giggled or laughed after each statement or answer.

H: She had an occurrence that was very unusual to her. She developed stabbing pains in five different locations all within five minutes of each other, all lasted a minute or so. The first one was three inches to the right of her umbilicus, the second one was in her right nipple, the third one was deep in her right ear, near the tympanic membrane, the fourth one was the right side of her throat, and fifth at the right temple.

Prover #13

Prover #13 was a 56 year old man. He too describes the same type of congestion as mentioned by other provers. We had to antidote the proving because the symptoms were worsening.

Day 1

7:20 am P: "I immediately felt a pressure of my tongue against the soft palate. It was more a dryness then a swelling…I could not swallow the feeling away. I drank water and the symptom went away after 30 minutes."

10:30 am H: After a second dose, three hours later, he experienced a tartness in the mouth and felt the same dryness of tongue against the soft palate as he did before.

10:53 am P: "I felt a momentary light-headedness when I turned around too quickly."

H: This was followed immediately by a mild chill.

2:50 pm P: "I feel more tipsy today. I feel off balance, as if to fall to my left side."

3:00 pm P: "The back of the soft palate has a scratchy throat feeling."

Day 2

6:00 am P: "I feel really more serene than usual on a workday…I feel really good."

8:00 am H: P experienced a two second spurt of rapid heart rate which is new to him.

Day 4

8:00 pm P: "I feel quite worn out tonight and am having trouble clearing the congestion in my nasopharynx…I am also coughing."

Day 5

5:00 am P: "I was restless and wakeful several times during the night, with congestion, like a lump in my throat too high to swallow."

8:00 am P: "My throat has a full feeling and scratchy in the soft palate area, in the same place where it first occurred when I took the remedy."

H: He went to get a hot drink which felt soothing. He is also having a runny nose on the right side and is still coughing.

9:10am P: "I feel pressure in the sinuses in my forehead…It takes effort to concentrate on work…I want to go to sleep…I feel chilly."

9:35 am P: "I had a headache across my forehead-it felt like a passing wave."

Noon H: He has become sensitive to abrasive noises and loud voices.

2:30 pm P: "My head feels clearer now…It is easier to breath, but my throat still feels full and scratchy."

6:00 pm P: "I have become indecisive…My impaired decision making is evident in my writing. I am making mistakes writing."

Day 6

7:30 am P: "Difficulty swallowing woke me up the pharynx area is still clogged and full…The most brilliant yellow mucus I'd ever seen and very thick is discharging…Hot drinks are the only things that soothe the throat."

9:54 am H: Chores aggravated all his symptoms.

11:10 am H: P has developed a rattling cough that is productive.

Day 7

6:20 am P: "I had strange but very vivid dreams last night."

6:20 am P: "I am very clogged up…swallowing is difficult…my voice is affected…I can't clear my ears." He still had a thick sounding cough.

9:30 am P: "I am feeling very low today. I don't feel good. The things I have to do today seem a large effort."

10:20 am H: He developed a tender, swollen gland on the right side of his jaw... He feels chilled…He describes an aching feeling in his back, near the right kidney area.

6:12 pm P: "I have an ache in my right ear which is worse swallowing tea."

Day 8

12:38 am P: "I am restless…it is hard to sleep…I am too warm and there is the aching pain in my back."

5:30 am P: "The back is still achy on the right side. The back feels stiff also."

7:51 am H: P experiences an enlarged right-sided submaxillary gland which is tender. The right-sided maxillary arch, the cheek bone, is also tender to the touch.

8:55 H: The left side of the neck has become tender and a gland is swollen there. The discharge from nose is a paler yellow.

11:31 am H: P develops a headache, with pressure above eyes, at his eyebrows.

12:15 pm P: "My eyes are burning."

Day 9

6:00 am H: the neck aches, the glands are still swollen, his voice is hoarse. Added to these, his right thumb has become really stiff.

10:15 am P: "My head is heavy and it hard to keep my eyes open."

10:25 am P: "I feel light headed upon standing up."

12 37 pm P: "I have the chills slightly. My neck glands on the right side are swollen a lot. The last time I remember these glands swollen like this was when I was 8 years old with mumps."

1:30 pm P: "I could have fallen asleep during lunch. My eyes are like burnt holes in a blanket." His temperature is elevated by 1 degree.

5:55 pm P: "I am coughing a lot and felt a bitter taste in the back of my mouth."

6:45 pm H: P is having a chill every 3-4 minutes.

Most of the day and evening H: P is constipated during the chill and the respiratory tract infection. **P** tells, "I usually have 5 bowel movements a day and now I have only one a day."

Day 10

5:20 am P: "Chills begin again. With the chill, I feel weak and slow and want to go back to bed." This is very unusual for this person.

All day H: The proving writing in the journal has become sloppy with mistakes in spelling.

9:15 am P: "I have an ache above the inside of the left kneecap, as if moving too abruptly would cause it to go out from under me. This only happens when I walk, and only intermittently so."

9:30 am P: "I am still feeling chills."

10:50 am H: P experiences a right-sided back pain, extending up under ribs, which is worse when sitting down.

12:03 pm P: "My eyes begin to burn."

12:23 pm H: P reports a coughing fit followed by chills.

4:40 pm P: "The skin became tender on my arms. Contact or friction feels like a burn to me. I feel aching extend down over both hips now."

5:54 pm H: The aching is beginning in both thighs.

Day 11

H: P slept on his back to alleviate the coughing fits. He normally never sleeps on the back.

H: P awakened with a cramp in the top of the right foot, pulling his big toe up (dorsiflexing the toe).

H: P hears ringing in the ears, which he sometimes hears, but this is more than usual.

P massages Vic's Vapo-rub (a mentholated lotion) to antidote remedy. Most of the symptoms stopped soon after this. By the next 2 days all the symptoms of the past 11 days were gone. But he said "after the Vic's, I feel well again inside myself."

Prover #14

Prover #14 was a 24 year old woman. Her chronic symptoms fit *Medorrhinum*, *Carcinosinum*, and *Ignatia*. She had asthma and allergies. Though both conditions were stable, they got worse during the proving, demonstrating the same congestion as others had, but now in the lower respiratory tract.

Day 1 - September 28, 1997
Took remedy at 10:05 am

10:10 am: "My breathing has become more shallow, and more difficult within 5 minutes of taking the remedy." (Objectively, homeopath saw that the breathing was more shallow. She can hear a slight inspiratory wheeze. Tells her about the tightness of chest, and begins to take deep breaths because of slight air hunger. Feels tingly and light in head and chest. Feels anxious with the breathing. She went outside but the breathing was not better.)

10:15 am: "Feeling tingly and lightheaded. There is tingling in the whole body, but especially in the chest. A flighty feeling like my mind isn't totally clear and it doesn't feel completely normal."

10:30 am (She is beginning to go into a fuller asthmatic attack. She wants to sit still, straight up and pull her shoulders forward to protect her chest. The struggle is to get the air in, not out. She sighs occasionally, which helps her breathing.)

10:45 am: "My mouth is very dry. Also, the roof of my mouth feels itchy, never had that before in my life." (She drank some water and the itching and dryness felt better.)

11:00 am: "My breathing is totally fine now…The asthma attack I just had began with a constriction, a tight feeling, in my lower throat (about 2 inches above her suprasternal notch) and then it moved down into the chest behind the sternum."

11:15 am: "Mouth still dry."

8:45 pm: "I am feeling warm and also drowsy. This feels like a cloudy mind and a relaxed body. I am still thirsty and drinking water on and off the whole day…My breathing has been shallow in the last half hour, with tightness in the lower chest, with difficulty moving air in and out of the lower part of my throat, though not as bad as this morning."

9:15 pm: "Shallow breathing continues, worsening, with the throat and chest tighter and breathing in more difficult."

10:15 pm: "I took an inhaler for the asthma attack."

Day 2 - September 29, 1997

8:15 am: "I am still thirsty and my mouth is still dry."

11:15 am: ""I felt a sharp pain in lower sacral area (middle and right side). Pain lasted a few seconds. It seemed to be from the inside out and it was noticeable when I was walking."

2:45 pm: "I again have a pain in my low back, on the right side, while sitting, a heavy firm feeling this time, not a sharp pain."

2:45 pm: "My mind is foggy and tired. I am feeling sleepy and disconnected from people around me." (She did not feel like being engaged by others…was in her own private world.)

3:30-4:00 pm: "I feel more giddy, more calm inside. It is not that the energy level is higher, as much as *different* inside. I feel freer inside my mind. This is so different from a couple of hours ago when I was inside myself, not wanting to communicate with others."

6:00 pm: "Talked to my mother this evening. I am in a hyper giddy state, almost unaware of other sensations…very bubbly, laughing and full of stories. This state continues as I interacted with roommates and housemates."

6:00 pm (I notice that she is smiling, almost smirking now, and when I mention it she says it was like that today, she smiles and laughs easily today.)

"I feel like if I open my mouth I'm going to just start smiling."

6:00 pm: "Throbbing pain in top of sacrum area, sharp, like it needs to be stretched or like I pulled something out of alignment. It is worse on the right side but it is in both sides."

"Mind and head feel light in a clear way. It's hard to explain." (She giggles. The prover was so smirky tonight I found it hard not to smile and then we both start laughing. It was really contagious. I asked her, "Are you sure you didn't smoke some marijuana before meeting me?" as she seemed drunk or stoned to me. She said that she had not.)

Day 3 - September 30, 1997

8:25 am: "Mouth is still dry and I am still drinking water."

"The feeling of giddiness I had yesterday was real for me. My mind was clear in the evening, it was like being high on marijuana. It was more uplifting. I smoked marijuana in the past, it was a similar beginning, yet with marijuana it would later become a downer, depressing me. This state yesterday was different, it got better and better and it was uplifting at the end, not depressing."

10:05 pm: "Headache on the right side of my head above the ear. It was dull and occasionally sharp. It began after a telephone conversation."

Day 4 - October 1, 1997

"Energy level better than it had been for the past few days. I am coming back to my normal energy."

6:00 pm: "I am very confused and stifled by my day. It has been stressful at work for the past few days. I feel frustration, uncertainty, anger and fear. All of this makes me feel trapped, mostly in my abdomen and chest…I was asked to work extra in the next few days and at the same time my own class schedule picks up…I don't feel like I can clearly communicate my feelings to others…I feel overloaded and will fail at what I want to do…I need to feel my freedom."

Day 5 - October 2, 1997

"Dream about old friends. In the dream I was giving up some possessions that I was strongly attached to. I felt like that symbolized my feelings of freedom that I am dealing with now. The dream was also about letting go of a boyfriend that left months ago. I can finally let him go without all the emotional sadness that hounded me before. Inside my dream I consulted different people with different personalities. I think they represented different aspects of myself, the practical side, the emotional side, the silly side, the angry side, the needy side, the independent side. It seemed important, in my dream, to honor each part of myself."

Day 6 - October 3, 1997

"Another dream about driving my mother all over the city. We got very lost."

Day 7 - October 4, 1997

"I made major decisions in the last couple of days about my career, my housing situation, my studies, in short, my whole future. I can not believe how easy it has been to make these decisions. My mind has been very clear about them. It has been much easier than before in my life. I seem to be more in touch with my thoughts and emotions."

Day 10 - October 7, 1997

"Headache on the right side above the ear just the previous ones. It lasted 20-30 minutes."

Day 13 - October 10 1997

3:00 pm: "I just had a strange sharp heart pain. It was a bit shocking and overwhelming and lasted about 30 seconds. I have never had anything like that before in my life."

(The pain did not radiate anywhere. She had to be still with the pain. She covered the pain with her hand. When asked to show me where the pain was, she pointed to the head of the 4th rib.)

(Over the next days, her anxieties, ambivalence and decision making went back to how they used to be, difficult to know what to do with her life, her relationships, her housing situation, her work.)

Prover #15

Prover #15 was a 25 year old woman. Constitutionally, she fits Sulphur and Medorrhinum. During the proving there was a flare up of an old tendency toward Herpes simplex.

Day 1 - February 19, 2000 - Took remedy at 9:33 am:

9:41 am "Very dry in the mouth, 'extra dry', especially the roof of the mouth. Drank some water but it doesn't help."

10:10 am "Mouth still dry."

10:22 am "My mouth is so very dry! Roof of mouth is dry and itchy, like a tickle."

10:45 am "Ate apple to see if it will help with the dryness. No change."

10:50 am "Tip of tongue dry, but roof of mouth not dry any more."

10:50 am "I feel like I'm getting a little sore in my mouth. There is a small pimple-like, round bump inside mouth on right cheek, in the middle…Feels like a canker sore, but it doesn't hurt."

10:55 am "Tip of tongue not dry any more. Teeth feel 'filmy,' like thickened mucous, lasting only 5 minutes."

12:00 pm "After eating pasta for lunch, developed another little white bump above the first one, at gum line of upper teeth, on cheek, about the size of a pencil eraser."

12:30 pm "I took a walk and my mood was better than normal. I'm usually in a good mood anyway, but I was extra happy, appreciative of how beautiful everything was. I was also excited about taking the remedy."

4:00 pm "Had a bowel movement, normal amount of stool. Unusual as she has only one a day in the morning, after drinking her Metamucil the day before." (If no Metamucil can be constipated for 10 days, ever since she was a child.)

Generally "Not very hungry today, ate just a little soup for dinner."

7:30 pm "Eyes became watery, some pooling, and a few tears, first left eye, then about 10 minutes later, both eyes. Both eyes a little itchy during this time…Stopped at 10 pm."

9:00 pm "Warm food/drink makes the first bump in mouth that she got feel a little raw."

10:00 pm "Another small white bump appeared under bottom lip on the inside, left side of center of mouth."

Dreams: "Had a vivid dream I was in a haunted house. There was a man on this pendulum and I was trying to get the pendulum to move so he would fall off and die. I actually dreamed about a human and didn't dream about animals!" (All of her dreams are about animals prior to remedy.)

Day 2 - February 20, 2000

Morning: "When I awoke this morning, the upper bump on right cheek was about half the size as yesterday; the first one on the bottom right cheek feels a little raw and sore."

"Face feels extra dry this morning." (She usually uses lotion in the morning, but dryness felt more so than normal, used more lotion.)

"Mouth feels dry still, comes and goes, cheeks feel dry, and top of tongue, not edges or tip, dry mouth, better by drinking room temperature water, hot tea doesn't help or orange juice or apple juice or fizzy water, just room temp water helps just a little bit. Dry mouth most of the time all day."

"Went over 6 hours without eating, but felt fine and didn't get cranky!"

12:00 pm: "Took a two hour walk, felt really good to be outside, everything fresh, felt like the "zippity-doo-dah" gal!"

3:30 pm: "Had an afternoon bowel movement, second one today, very unusual, first was at 8am, my usual time for a bowel movement."

9:00 pm: "The bottom of my feet feel a little sore and tired, toes felt a little stiff, couldn't really stretch them out; and lower back a little sore."

Day 3 - February 21, 2000

2:30 am: "I woke and drank 3 large glasses of water as mouth was dry (like I had licked a salt block!)."

5:30 am: Woke second time and couldn't get back to sleep. Throat felt sore and dry; gargled with salt water at 6:30 am."

(Tired today, had to drive 45 minutes away and don't like to drive, from 3:30 on, just wanted to go to bed.) "My little sore throat lasted from 5:30 am to 8 am."

"Mouth still dry, most of the day. When awoke this morning second and third bump were gone. First one is half the size, about the size of a pencil tip, not sore or raw, pink colored. Other ones were white too, then pink, then went away."

3:30 pm: "Arms and back very tense and stiff from driving, I hate to drive."

4:30 pm: "While driving, had a 'foggy' feeling like, "I can't do this any more, I have to go home now," lasted about 10 minutes… Great thirst today, all day."

Day 4 - February 22, 2000

6:30 am: "The last sore on bottom lip gone."

6:30 am: "The skin behind ears not as itchy." (Flaky skin and itchy behind ears an old symptom which she had before taking remedy.)

6:30 am: "Dull aching pain all over body (husband has flu symptoms and sore throat that started over the weekend), lower back, shoulders, neck, upper thighs…feels like I've been hit by a car and I waddled away."

"I was very tired and unfocused all day, my mind is numb, not angry, not anything, too tired to be anything."

"Sore throat, glands sore under chin toward neck, both sides, got worse as the day went on, hurts to swallow saliva, food, not made better by hot or cold liquids."

2:30 pm: "Headache, top of head, center, inside my head, with pain also at base of skull at top vertebrae, worse at 5 pm, and better by 6:30 pm, so I went to bed."

"Thirsty all day, drank lots of water, little sips, about 12 glasses; thirst increased approximately 4:30 pm. No appetite all day, had green Jello and tea for dinner, tasted good."

Day 5 - February 23, 2000

"Woke achy, still no appetite, same as yesterday."

"More confused today than the unfocused feeling yesterday, didn't understand what others said, no train of thought, I couldn't follow a conversation to save my life! At 4:30 pm, felt I was on autopilot with no control of my body. Autopilot going home, that's the only way I got home because I have a homing device in me that lets me go home."

1:00 pm: "I ate lunch and it felt like shoving glass down my throat; sharp, sticking pains."

1:30 pm: "I had one sheer moment of bliss when a woman at the office told my coworker (who prover does not like) to shut up, and I thought 'oh, she's fighting back, yeah' and then I was back to feeling dull. Just wanted to sleep under my desk, everything took too much effort."

"Dull headache most of the day (on middle top of head and base of neck), home from work at 4 pm, took an aspirin and felt better by 6 pm."

3:30 pm: "Itchy watery eyes for 30 minutes (usually get watery eyes when sick) in past if get bad headache, eyes will start watering, headache area on top of head is altered, usually get them in temples."

Day 6, - February 24, 2000

"Throat still sore, body tired, eyes itchy and watery, still sick."

10:30 pm: "New sore inside mouth, right side, lower underneath where first one was, size of an eraser tip, bloody red color, can see veins on the bump, no pain."

1:30 am: "I awoke and drank two glasses of water."

Day 7 - February 25, 2000

"When I awoke sore on right side of mouth has doubled in size, sore and raw feeling, all day, sensitive to salty food and anything hot, hurts, made me want to cry! Had some potato chips and sore hurt, eating an orange is like sheer hell! I noticed white mucus covering over lower half and raw, and a little bloody on upper half, bled a little when I brushed my teeth in the morning."

6:00 am: "Itchy skin on stomach, left side, is gone; it had been itchy for a few months now."

7:30 pm: "Three more white bumps appeared on the roof of mouth behind front teeth, in a row along teeth line."

Day 8 - February 26, 2000

8:00 am: "Sore on lower right side of mouth now coated with mucus, larger, now the size of a dime, still sore; still sensitive to salty food and anything hot. Three bumps behind front teeth have disappeared. There is a new eraser size sore on right side of roof of mouth which appeared at 8:30am, behind front right side tooth. Both bled when I brushed my teeth and they hurt, were raw and sore."

"When I awoke noticed I scratched my left ear during sleep and woke with a sore on top of left ear, pillow had a little blood on it. Scalp has a thick, scaly appearance behind left ear and in front of head on scalp, skin looks to be 1/4" thick, scales, itchy and scratched at my head until the scales were gone, scalp felt raw."

Day 9 - February 27, 2000

"Sore on lower right side of mouth still there; it is the size of a dime with mucus coating. Sore on right side roof of mouth has decreased in size to size of a blunt pencil. They both are sensitive to citrus fruit, sad that I cannot eat any fruit without pain."

"Throat felt dry and scratchy in the morning."

"Nickel size scab on left ear at top is sore. Scalp has little raw scabs around both ears and back of head, I think I scratched in my sleep, scalp not getting better with dandruff shampoo, itchy."

"Not much appetite today, only ate a potato at lunch with salt. Didn't get cranky!"

"Hands, feet, and upper chest felt cold in the afternoon, around 4pm and lasted all night. Had a hard time staying warm."

Day 10 - February 28, 2000

6:00 am: "When I woke, sore at right side of roof of mouth was gone. Sore on lower right remained size of a dime with mucus coating, still raw and sore. Mouth felt raw and sore in general."

"Hands and feet cold all day."

"Scalp has little raw scabs around both ears behind the ear and scalp there, in hair along scalp line, itchy and thick, gross. More hair than usual falling out when I washed it, 20 or 30 hairs instead of 4 or 5, distressed because I don't want to go bald!"

4:00 pm "Noticed little sores on left side of tongue, on the edge, like dark reddish-black, sensitive, felt like they'd bleed if I eat something acidic."

"Not hungry, I don't remember what being hungry feels like! Food doesn't taste good, don't want to eat. Mouth is also too sore to eat anything enjoyable. Everything tasted bad, tastes bloody and mucusy and the touch of all that stuff in my mouth makes it sore, and then I'll have to swallow it, so I didn't eat, but I also wasn't hungry. Normally I wouldn't make it through the day and I'd have to eat, but it didn't happen. Had spicy Indian food and almost died because sores hurt from the spices."

"No bowel movement again today."

"Hands and feet cold in the morning and early afternoon."

Day 11 - February 29, 2000

"No bowel movement again."

"Bumps on left side of tongue still there, dark red, and sensitive to citrus."

"Mouth feels a little less raw and sore today. Sore on lower right side of mouth decreased in size and not as tender and raw feeling today, looks whitish, round, about pencil eraser size."

6:00 am: "Took shower, hair is falling out, handful of hair in the shower, on the pillow and in my hairbrush, I'm going bald! May be due to new shampoo which was pretty strong; stopped using it."

6:00 am: "Scalp still has little raw scabs around both ears and back of head and thick, brownish colored scales on top of head, doesn't itch." (Homeopath looked at scalp and saw very small 1/16 inch little reddish mark on top of left ear, didn't see scales, skin behind the ear slightly thickened but hardly noticeable.)

6:00 am: "Normal appetite and thirst today."

6:30 am: "Menses began today, normally."

Day 12 - March 1, 2000

6:00 am: "Sores on lower right side of mouth and sores on tongue are gone."

Scalp looks 100% better, as does the scab on the ear. Skin behind the ears is still itchy and crusty."

Prover #16

Prover #16 was a 52 year old woman, who has the constitutional tendencies of Lycopodium and has responded well to Cocculus indica. She has a history of recreational drug use in the distant past. In addition she has the return of an old viral symptom of Herpes simplex, during the course of the proving. It is interesting that during the proving, many developed infections or had their allergies flare up, even though it was the wrong time of year. Some had their summer allergies to pollen develop in the winter.

Day 1 - October 21, 1997
3 hours after first dose report:

"Immediately following taking remedy I felt a tickle in the rear of my throat behind and below the uvula. It went away…I am thirsty for water."

"Sensation of spaciness as soon as I took the remedy. I feel very deeply relaxed, as when taking magnesium."

"I feel somewhat detached from objects on wall, pictures (on the wall) seem to float in space. My depth perception seems off."

"I am more sensitive to noises and find them intrusive. I am sensitive to someone's clogs walking on the floor; I am very aware of them. I am hearing things I never heard before here."

"In the dining area I felt that I wanted to be around others. Not wanting to visit with them but be around people."

(She described this as a "herding" instinct.)

"Felt like separated by a glass wall; cut off from others." (She had this sensation when depressed many years ago. It was much more pronounced when depressed "like in a bell jar.")

" I feel a dreaminess...like spaciness…feel languorous…detachment from present reality…I can read, edit and write but feel like I am not totally involved, not totally immersed…as if sleepwalking through what I am doing…It started as soon as I took the remedy and continues."

"My sense of time seems slowed down. I am not impatient but I don't have a sense of how slow or fast time is passing."

(She had this sensation once after taking LSD, a long time ago. She usually has a good sense of time.)

"Food tastes really good. I am very cognizant of each individual taste… more inclined to eat slowly and savor food. I am usually a fast eater."

Physical symptoms: "Sense of body really relaxed after taking the remedy, felt as if like body is limp, like anesthetized."

"Bending over brings a rush of blood to the head."

"Felt a brief stitching pain on right side of my *latissimus dorsi*, outside of rib cage midway between waist and armpit which lasted a few minutes at most."

"Have had some transient pains after lunch (2 hours after remedy)… slight throbbing sensation on both temples as if coming down with headache but didn't get a headache."

"Warm flush during lunch. Seemed stronger than usual. Left the forehead moist."

Nose started running briefly, both sides affected with a clear and thin discharge.

"Felt tingling sensation in very tip of right big toe. Had left leg crossed over right. Then tingling spread to sole of right foot as if bubbles rising up against sole of foot. Tingling in right hand. All of these symptoms are transient."

"Very thirsty one hour after lunch and still feel thirsty…Mouth not dry (has plenty of saliva) but feels dry…As if I ate a lot of salty food but I didn't." (Drinking lots of water and herb tea.)

"When walking I get a shooting pain in right big toe from old injury."

"I have a real urge to have a bowel movement but I am not successful (usually not a problem in public bathroom). Slight flatulence before urge for stool."

(The face is ruddier than usual.)

"I am craving sour and savory more pronounced than usual. Had hot soup which created pain in lower left molar.

"Sensitivity to noises continues, hearing heating system go on, muffled voices."

(At this time, 2:15 pm, we left the store and drove out to my house in the woods. Prover drove her car.)

5 pm: "Hearing definitely more acute. Sounds that I would not ordinarily notice, like car noises, are easy to hear."

"Separation feeling; still like sleepwalking…Going through the motions but not really being there…Still feeling somewhat outside environment…It is not an unpleasant sense of spaciness or dreaminess, but I am concerned that my driving might be affected…Had to pay more attention driving car…No anxiety involved with spaciness."

"I was sleepy at 3:15 and have to concentrate extra hard to read…Words and paragraphs don't seem to be registering on my brain…Took nap for 30 minutes." (She usually does not take naps.)

"No typical stiffness in neck after nap even though napped in awkward position."

"Thirst not as strong but still present."

"Sense of time still somewhat disoriented…Time passed slowly when taking a walk but quickly at other times."

"Hot flash around 3:30 and feel the heat of the room more strongly."

(After this, prover left to drive back home out of state. She called me at 9 pm to say she had made it home safely. She still feels spacey and still has increased thirst. She will send me a complete journal, which she taped as she drove home in car. We will talk later this evening.)

Day 2 - October 22, 1997

"Driving last night, I was blinded by car headlights and couldn't see the road and wondered if remedy affected depth perception." (This scared her. She felt like she was navigating through a sculpture.)

"Strangely detached from emotions…Wanted to talk with boyfriend over phone, but when he called, we were disconnected before I could say anything of depth, there was no way to reach him. I was upset, my emotional reaction time-always slow-seemed even slower."

"Dream last night. I was in a house in city or suburbs facing a large triangular piece of land like a commons, except that it was not developed into a park. It was as if someone plunked down a few

California hills inside a city block. Grass was very deep and 1 or 2 large oak trees. Someone from my house got lost in grass on way to a drug store. But he was only 15 inches high and it was very difficult to find him." (She thinks she found him.)

"Normal bowel movement upon getting up. None of acrid odor that I have had for last few months."

"Today feel sort of detached and spacey and not as affected by things like I usually am. Still detached but when something happens that upsets me I can deal with it, in a matter of fact way, without lots of emotions getting in the way."

"Ordinarily reticent about confronting people but now I deal clearly with son; confronted without anger. Today I say what I need to say simply and clearly, without beating around the bush, but also without being angry. I'm no longer willing to pretend everything's great while seething on the inside."

(Has lots of energy and is more methodical than usual. Usually when she goes away it takes her a day or two to get back in the swing of things. Today is as if she didn't go away.)

"Sensation of tickling or bubbles against sole of left foot at noon same time, as I had yesterday."

"Still feel very dreamy and relaxed physically but focused, busy and getting things done."

Day 5 - October 21, 1997

Dreams: "I dreamed I'd picked up some hitchhikers and took them out of their way and out of my way. I was trying to find my way back to the route we should have been on, but we were winding our way through the back streets of small country roads, trying to get our bearings on our location."

Day 6 - October 26, 1997

"Irritation on right buttocks, burning, painful to touch, itchy, want to scratch it but don't because I know it will hurt. Soreness. It is better cold water and worse heat, heat causing more burning, and it burns on urination. This is similar to a labial herpetic eruption that I tend to get but I have never had it in this location and usually get it after my menses, not at this time of the month."

Day 7 - October 27, 1997

(Soreness in irritated area continues today.)

"I feel like I have been injected with truth serum and must speak my mind, though not in an angry or confrontational way. Still feel emotionally detached."

"Able to joke around with my son without feeling offended or having my feelings hurt, which is new. I was too sensitive before to do this comfortably. I am less worried about offending others with my occasional sharp tongue."

Day 9 - October 29, 1997

"Still feel calm. Sad and blue about breaking up with boyfriend and a slight fear of being alone, but not nearly as intense as have normally experienced. Hugging boyfriend, I had a hard time getting the tears to flow, though I normally weep easily."

"Right elbow sore, aching on lifting. It feels like tendonitis, though for no apparent reason."

Day 10 - October 30, 1997

"Tearing pain in right elbow. Sharp pains if pick up anything, no matter how light."

"Rawness in perianal region. Feels like a diaper rash, vulva feels dry and itchy."

Day 11 - October 31, 1997

"Mind confused, unable to get motivated to start packing. Sad to be moving but anxious to get away from boyfriend's negative energy."

"Irritation of right buttocks is better today."

Dream: "I am asked to go from one classroom to another, I am causing disruptions and am apologizing as I am going through the room trying to tell them that I am going through under directions from others."

Day 12 - November 1, 1997

"Tingling in the ovarian area."

Day 14 - November 3, 1997

"Appetite good, crave peanut butter."

"Shooting pains in right elbow, tearing pains upon exertion burning sensations upon rest."

Prover #17

Prover #17 was a 26 year old woman who has many symptoms that look like Sepia, Ignatia, Nux vomica, Medorrhinum but especially Pulsatilla constitutionally. Her family history is very positive for alcoholism. She too mentioned the 'airplane taking off sensation of pressure.' Her proving produced many physical symptoms including the strong right sided complaints that you have read about in the other provers.

Day 1 - October 5, 1997

9:45 am P takes the remedy.

9:51 am P: "I feel increasing pressure inside the head, as if I am in an airplane that is taking off-the pressure is outward from the inside—with numbness behind my eyes."

10:02 am H: A warmth stays in the area behind the eyes and inside the top of the head. This is accompanied by a very face flushed.

H: The numbness behind her eyes fades.

P: "A heaviness moves down to my chest…It makes me want to take a deep breath…It is kind of a solid, massive feeling in the upper chest and head…This is definitely different from what I feel in the lower part of my body, which feels normal…The heaviness fades from my chest, but it comes back and stays in the head…The sensation of heaviness/pressure moves down to chest and back up to head."

10:16 am H: She experiences itchiness in the left axilla, in one specific point.

H: The cheeks and chin are red.

10:30 am H: The itchiness in left armpit returns to the same one point.

H: There is a hot sensation of the face. She usually feels somewhat warm in the face but this is much more.

H: Numbness at the top part of her head, "like a cap above the eyes."

P: "The outside sensations ameliorated, but I still feel some dizziness/numbness on top of my head."

11:10 am P: "The sight of my left eye changed, as if I see with this eye deeper or on a larger scale…Or I could say that that eye feels bigger, the eyeball itself." This lasts for 2 minutes.

H: There is an itchy point under her left breast, then 20 minutes later under her right breast, which is better by light scratching. The itch definitely moved left to right.

H: She generally feels stuffy and congested when inside. All her symptoms are worse inside.

12:15 pm P: "I feel a dull, stuffed-up feeling, with a kind of peaceful throbbing in the back of head, in occipital region for 1 minute."

H: A vaginal discharge, which is common for her to have, is much milder (less to no odor, less to no irritation on skin, and less in amount than usual).

2:00 pm P: "I have a hot flash with cold sweat. This is hotter than I usually am. The skin of my face feels cold and sticky on touching. This sensation of heat is better cool, fresh air."

Afternoon and evening H: She feels a small pointed pain in her left eye, coming and going quickly.

8:00 pm P: "I again feel stuffed in the back of my head, a kind of a solid feeling."

Day 2 - October 6, 1997

P: "I dreamt about my parents the day they are leaving my house after staying there for a week. They are about to catch their flight. The dream is about those hours when they are getting ready for leaving to the airport; leaving the house with suitcases."

H: The whole day: irritation of her labia and vagina from some previous discharge but the discharge is completely gone.

P: "There is a light, nice, good feeling to the whole day. I feel a kind of ease and energetic lightness especially in my head."

H: The whole day, especially in the evening, she was thirsty, mostly for cold water. She is usually thirstless.

H: She has an urge to take deep breaths; a kind of sighing that is sometimes better and sometimes worse during this day, but changed.

10:00 pm H: She feels a short pain in the right eye, followed by itchiness in left ear which extends down the eustachian tube to the throat. She develops an irritating itchiness in her throat, like a sore throat. It feels like a line moving between the eyes to the ear then to the throat.

11:00 pm P: "While sitting for a long time at the dinner table I felt a solid dizziness, from my forehead to the occiput in one wave for some seconds, then a shorter one a minute later."

Day 3 - October 7, 1997

The whole day P: "I was thirsty for cold water."

The whole day H: Generally, no new symptoms, but she feels unusually well.

The whole day H: The vaginal irritation became a burning sensation, with dryness.

Evening P: "In the evening I recognized an ulcer in the right side of my mouth."

8:00 pm H: P developed twitching in her right eye. Two hours later it moved to her left eye.

Day 4 - October 8, 1997

Upon arising and for 15 minutes H: Both ears itch, then it moves to the throat and then back to ears.

Upon arising and for 15 minutes H: She develops a toothache in her right bottom teeth. This pain then moves to the upper right teeth and then again down to the right bottom teeth and then ceases.

H: She was thirsty the whole day.

Early afternoon H: She had a bitter taste in her mouth for a while.

5:30 pm H: When something pushes or jars her stomach area, for a flash of time again there is a pinching pain.

H: She again develops, for a short time, twitching of her right eye.

10:30 pm P: "I am very chilly and tired."

All day P: "I recently desire sweets and salads and cold foods." (She usually likes warm foods.)

Day 5 - October 9, 1997

7:30 am H: Her nose felt full with pressure, but not stuffy. She then developed a left-sided stuffiness. In another 4 hours, both nostrils were stuffy, and then this sensation ceased.

The whole day P: "My feet were radiating heat. Usually I am warm but my feet stay cool. Now they are hot."

Noon P: "I feel a little bit of nausea. There is a slight heartburn after I snack (including after eating fatty foods like cheese and caviar). Twice in the morning I had a slight lower abdominal pain. This was mostly in the middle but then extended to the left side…The whole day I have had abdominal bloating from a gathering of gas."

H: She also still feels a dry smarting sensation in her vagina, though it is less than the previous days.

H: She is still thirsty all day.

P: "I am mentally more dull than in previous days, when I was more clear minded than usual. New is that it is not easy to concentrate. When reading, I get very sleepy."

The whole day H: She still has a desire for fresh air. She still has the urge to take deep breaths.

10:00 pm H: She feels a pain in the joints of her middle finger of the left hand. It lasts about 3 minutes.

11:00 pm P: "On going to bed, I felt in the stomach, a pinching, sensation, but this time on the surface, not deep where it was some days ago. It feels as if the area is bruised, or at least sensitive to touch. This lasted about 10 minutes. Before ceasing, it went back to its deep location for some seconds."

Day 6 - October 10, 1997

7:30 am P: "I woke up when I felt a strong discomfort in joint area of my index finger of my right hand and around it. This feels like it needs to be massaged and pressed at certain points which makes it feel better."

8:30 am P: "Eating some tahini with pita makes me feel sick for 40 minutes. It feels like it was too heavy and too fatty."

1:00 pm H: The left eye pain wanders to the ear in some seconds. The pain lasts all together less than a minute. It is a very slight pain and there is a kind of throbbing to it. Sometimes it feels to her like a wave-like pain. The pains are in different locations but are all of a similar nature. In half an hour there is a pressing sensation in the right eyeball, behind the eyelid, but longer lasting this time. With this pain comes a stuffiness in the right nostril.

1:30 pm H: P has a tremendous tiredness today.

All day P: "Generally, I feel calm and somewhat solemn in my behavior with people today."

Evening H: P is taking deep breaths at this time of the evening.

Day 7 - October 11, 1997

All morning until noon H: She has fullness in her nose.

All day H: She has a sensation of fullness in her breasts.

Day 8 - October 12, 1997

Several times today P: "…Especially around 10.00 am and 4.00 pm I had a slight nausea or better to say "nauseous discomfort," lasting for 10 to 15 minutes each time.

All day: H: "A bitter taste in mouth all day long."

All day H: P has a decreased appetite. She wants to eat less than usual. She is also having hot flashes on and off all day.

At night P: "I have a painful point between my thigh and abdomen (lower than my usual abdominal pains) the same radiating sensation which I feel with other pains in other parts of the body. It lasts for about 10 minutes."

Day 9 - October 13, 1997

H: She is still waking with full congested nose.

The whole day P: "There is a kind of impatience towards the flow of life, which feels too slow for me."

H: She experiences the same type of nausea as yesterday.

Day 10, October 14, 1997

7:30 am P: "On getting up, I felt a pain after urination, going upwards slowly, in the front of my abdomen. After that I passed a soft stool."

9:00 pm P: "I felt a strong but short (10 second) shooting pain in the area of the appendix (far right side of abdomen), which felt much better if I held my breath, or breathed shallowly."

H: P also noticed that she developed an ulcer in the front of her mouth.

Midnight P: "On going to bed, I had a sudden stuffiness in my nose. It was so sudden that I feel as if it will suffocate me."

Day 11 - October 15, 1997

6:20 am P: "My son wakes me up at 6.20 am. Within 5 minutes I have a fast onset of a cramp-like pain in my lower abdomen. It lasts for 15 seconds. In 3 minutes another comes and lasts 10 minutes. These are strong, cramp-like pains that stay even during an otherwise normal bowel movement. The pain radiates in the front and in the back. I am nauseous, with the urge to vomit. I then have a similar nauseous queasy spasmodic feeling in the now empty bowels. Finally these pains and sensations cease while sitting on the bathroom floor, one leg bent backward, pressing against the abdomen, while sitting on the other one underneath."

9:00 am P: "My left ear is throbbing with pain in an upward moving fashion, then, starting together with the ear, a crawling sensation in my nose, as just before sneezing. This lasts for 15 seconds, then again 2 more waves of the same sensation but weaker during the next few minutes. In 5 more minutes the pain is in the right ear, though only slight, and by 9:30 the pain is again in the left ear."

The whole day P: "The whole day I have had cold feet, which is usual for me. What I did not mention until now is that on previous days I had warm feet, which was new to me."

8:00 pm P: "I have a right sided throbbing pain in appendix area for 5 minutes, then for another 3 minutes it travels to become a left-sided pain in inner part of thigh."

P: "I just remembered that for the past week I have been chewing the inner wall of my cheeks, which I used to do as a teenager, but not since then."

Day 12 - October 16, 1997

P: "I was talking on the phone to some relatives about important issues, feeling the need to be able to explain myself clearly and persuade them about my being right. During the conversation, I felt my head becoming warm, and full, as if feeling my mind straining."

H: She is sighing today.

Day 13 - October 17, 1997

4:00 pm H: P experienced shooting, but not really too sharp, pain extending from her upper left teeth upwards to her left eye.

Day 14 - October 18, 1997

4:00 am P: "Crawling sand-like sensations moving upward in my left thigh, followed by twitching and a pulsating sensation, lasting for one minute, while lying next to my son who has problems falling asleep tonight."

P: "This is the second day of menstruation, which is a much weaker flow than usual, with no pain or other symptoms."

H: She is thirsty for cold water, which is new for her.

Day 15 - October 19, 1997

H: The ulcer in her mouth is still there.

H: She is still quite thirsty for cold water.

2:00 pm H: She has twitching of her right eye.

6:30 pm P: "I have a left earache, with pressing sensations in my ear, which is not usual for me. One minute later I have a mild earache and upper right eyeball pain, then in 2 minutes, twitching in the same eye."

10:00 pm P: "I have a mild right eye pain, somewhat pulsating, lasting some seconds, than a really slight pressing pain in my left eye."

H: What is marked is that all these symptoms take place indoors (pulsating, throbbing, twitching).

H: The menstrual flow is still much less than usual, with no pains or symptoms, which are usually related to her menses.

Day 16 - October 20, 1997

H: No symptoms experienced. She has the same generals; desires fresh air, thirst for cold water, and the ulcer in the mouth is still there.

H: She again experiences warm feet, noted in the evening.

Evening P: "I feel a very slight pressure behind my right eyeball (I am really tired), which feels like it is pressing outward and to the right."

Day 17 - October 21,1997

8:00 pm P: "I have pain in the left sole of my foot on the outer side. Then in 10 minutes it becomes a right-sided pain."

11:00 pm P: "I have a sharp pain for a short time in my right abdomen, over the appendix, then followed by a slight left-sided headache, then pain on the left side of abdomen, as a mirror image to the appendix and then for a longer time pain in left elbow, which is pulsating. At the same time, for a shorter duration, I have lower leg and right shoulder pains."

Day 19 - October 23, 1997

H: Her legs fall asleep easily while sitting.

Evening P: "I am bleeding somewhere in my mouth while brushing my teeth, as I had during pregnancy."

Day 22 - October 26, 1997

H: Menstrual bleeding lasted until today, which is the usual 6 days. However, there were an extra 4 days before these, with scanty bleeding, which was unusual.

Day 24 - October 28, 1997

5:00 pm P: "I had a strange sensation in the midline of the chest that if I took even a little breath, my chest would be torn apart. It was a very sharp, stabbing pain, which was better bending forward. It lasted maybe 30 seconds."

Day 26 - October 30, 1997

P: "For a much shorter time, and less intense, I experienced the same pain as yesterday, now more in the middle of the back rather then the chest."

Day 29 - November 2, 1997

P: "For some days, I have had short needle-like pricking sensations in different parts of the body, like the fingers, at various times of the day."

Evening P: "My right eyelid is very sensitive to slight pressure in one point in the middle of lower eyelid."

Day 30 - November 3, 1997

H: A stye developed in her right eyelid.

Day 31 - November 4, 1997

H: For the last week, she has developed pimples on forehead, yesterday on her right lower arm and today on left thigh and then the left wrist. They are small, pus-filled and red. The ones on the arms are somewhat itchy. She is also developed them today on her neck and upper chest.

Prover #18

Prover #18 was a 46 year old woman. Constitutionally she is most similar to Calcarea carbonica, Sulphur and Natrum muriaticum. Prover #18 produced a great deal of right-sided physical symptoms. Interestingly enough, she also had some of her chronic fatigue symptoms improve and a chronic rash cured during the proving. I end with this journal to point out that when a remedy is close, and when it produces a proving upon a person, while some symptoms become accentuated, others may go away completely. This is seen very often in practice, but it is seen in the provings as well. Towards the end of the proving, Prover #18 also had a delay in the onset of her menses which was also observed by other provers. What was interesting in her proving experience was, like the Alcoholus patients, there was a lot of dreaming before the menses and during menopause. The type of dreams is not as important as the sheer volume of dreams recalled. In practice, this symptom has led practitioners to Lachesis incorrectly.

This prover's journal is lengthy, and actually repeats symptoms several times, but it was left untouched. It shows how different provers and different homeopaths report symptoms differently. As I mentioned at the beginning of the reports, we did not try to give one "voice" to all the provers, as is sometimes done in recent provings. Rather, we left the language of the provers and their style stand as we received it. Length of report also varied from prover to prover. You read a proving of one page. This particular prover's report, was culled from an overall report that was three inches thick. The symptoms left are the ones that fit the proving.

Day 1 - JULY 26, 1997

10:35 am First dose taken with no effects at this time.

10:58 am (23 minutes after taking the dose.) Mild achy pain in the left eye at the front of the eyeball. Did not affect vision. Lasted about 2 minutes. Extending the corner of the eye back by pulling it, made the pain disappear but as soon as she released the skin, the pain returned. Pain was localized and intensity was mild to moderate.

11:19 am Moderate sharp localized pain at vertex of head. Lasted a few seconds. Sneezed immediately afterwards.

11:22 am Went from hot garage to air-conditioned house and the moderate sharp localized pain at vertex of head returned. Pain disappeared when she leaned over with her head down and as she raised the head, the pain returned as a dull ache which moved down toward the right temple. She walked around and the pain totally disappeared. The pain lasted two minutes.

11:30 am Mild irritation and chapping of right inner thigh. Red, mild burning, no itchiness. It was worse with perspiration and heat and gone by the next day.

11:54 am Momentary moderate cramping in right calf which abated about as soon as she could notice it. She rarely (2-3 times in her life) has had "charlie horses" in the past and if she did, they were at night while sleeping. The pain was similar to those "charlie horse" attacks.

11:55 am Outside right ear (earlobe to half way up the ear) was itchy and mildly burning. Scratching relieved it momentarily and then itching and burning returned. She applied a cold wet washcloth and it all went away in three minutes and did not return.

12:30 pm While sitting eating lunch, she experienced mild to moderate cramping of the ball of the right foot. It only lasted a couple of minutes. Wiggling her toes made it better.

1:20 pm New symptom from 12:30 pm returned. She put her socks and shoes on, stood up and the right foot cramped again. Cramping was slightly less than at 12:30 pm. She experienced the cramping on the ball of the right foot. She loosened her shoes and wiggled her foot and it made it better. The cramping only lasted a couple of minutes. Then she got in her car and as she drove, the cramping returned in the ball of the right foot. The cramping was intermittent and lasted a couple of minutes. This continued throughout the day (2:30 pm). The cramping on ball of foot is better with walking and worse when she sits down. The intermittent cramping is mild.

3:00 pm When she took her shoes and socks off, the cramping in the right foot stopped.

3:50 pm She was reaching up in the cupboard with the right hand and she experienced a momentary dull ache above the left eye over the eyebrow which lasted a few seconds.

4:03 pm While preparing supper, she experienced a momentary slight dull ache in the left temple.

5:00 pm As she left the chiropractic clinic in the heat of the day, she noticed a moderate sharp localized pain at the top of the head to the right (right parietal area). The location has changed from a central area to the right parietal area. While rubbing, the pain would cease. When she stopped, the pain returned. The pain lasted a couple of minutes. (This was a reoccurrence of the new symptom of Day 1, July 26th at 11:19am.)

5:05 pm A dull ache encircling her left eye lasted a couple of minutes while driving into the sunshine.

7:20 pm She sat down at the theatre and experienced a burning sensation the size of a quarter in the right chest next to the sternum (above right breast at 2 o'clock). This area is the rib head and was adjusted chiropractically at 4:30. This lasted about two minutes. This location and pain are chronic complaints. However, the burning symptom was an altered symptom. It usually is a localized dull ache without burning.

8:30 pm One inch above the right ear, a prickly sensation for a couple of minutes. When the sensation went away, she immediately experienced a moderately intense, sudden sharp pain in the left side just below the waist. This lasted about 30 seconds.

Day 2 - JULY 27, 1997

12:17 am Her son awoke her again. Stomach felt mildly crampy, menstrual type in the lower abdomen, with accompanying nausea. This is earlier than experienced before (altered symptom). This usually occurs when the period has already begun. Fell asleep and the symptom did not keep her awake.

4:30 am Sleep was restless and she was dreaming about walking across bridges across a deep river. Not all of them had railings and the bridges were at different heights. She was high up. This is a new symptom. She has never had this dream before. She was mildly concerned about walking across the bridge without a railing.

The left foot on top has a red rash on it which has increased in itchiness through the night. It is a moderate constant burning itch. Is worse when covered. Was worse with warm water. The rash has a white stripe through it.

6:55 am Left foot continues to burn and is worse when covered.

7:33 am Rash on top of left foot is in the same place but more intense in color and in burning. She would love to have scratched it.

7:52 am A warm shower irritated the left foot rash. The rash was slightly more intense after the shower. It burned more. It was also more itchy. It appeared redder.

10:00 am Sitting in Sunday School. A dull ache appeared behind the right eye (mild) which lasted about ten minutes. It was almost gone when it moved to the center of the forehead, was less intense and disappeared in a few seconds.

10:25 am A fleeting dull but focused pain in the right side, halfway between breast and waist lasted about one minute and then moved to the right lower back and lasted a few seconds before leaving. When it became back pain, it became milder and more widespread.

1:00 pm Focused moderate, sharp and sudden pain in the right side of the abdomen just above the pubic bone and groin. Was better when sitting. Lasted about 10 minutes. Walking and movement made it worse. It disappeared on its own.

End of Day General Observations Top of left foot continues to be red, mild itchy and mild burning when she thinks about it. The white stripe area is less distinct (size did not change).

11:00 pm (reoccurrence). The moderate sharp localized pain at vertex of the head returned momentarily as she looked into the bed light. (Same as Day 1).

Day 3 - JULY 28, 1997

6:00 am Woke up. Had restless sleep with dreams she cannot recall. (Doesn't usually have restless sleep with dreams.)

7:17 am The top of her left foot was burning and itching when she woke up and continues to do so. It's a constant mild to moderate burning and itching. The area and shape are the same as yesterday but the red color is not as bright, it is darker and muted. Open air makes it better, not wearing socks or shoes makes it better. Warm water makes it worse. Any rubbing of the area makes it worse. Motion doesn't affect it.

8:00 am Right heel is feeling better. Hardly bruised at all. Feels it occasionally when walking when applying pressure to the heel when walking. Was barefoot a lot last evening and this morning and did not bother the heel. (It usually does.)

5:23 pm Sudden dull mild ache front of left eyeball. Did not affect vision. Went away when she bent over. It lasted several seconds. (Same symptom of July 26th at 10:58 am except milder.)

7:00-8:00 pm Top of left foot rash felt good while swimming in the pool. Coolness of the water felt good on her foot. The rash began itching immediately when she got out of the pool at 8:00 pm. The rash was less red when she got out of the pool and gradually returned to its redness. The burning was less when she got out of the pool. The burning has stopped and the itching has remained the same. Continued to itch on and off throughout the evening.

10:00 pm She scratched the rash on the left foot and the rash got redder and puffy from scratching and became very itchy. Still no burning of the rash. Took a warm shower and it increased the itch even more.

Day 4 - JULY 29, 1997

6:00 am Rash on top of left foot does not itch. The area and shape of the rash remains the same however the color is much lighter. The white stripe is still obvious.

12:09 pm Dull mild ache widespread on top of head, left of center (parietal area). Lasted a few seconds. Not localized like Day 1, more widespread and to the left side.

5:15 pm While preparing dinner, she noticed a mild ache in her upper right arm on the outside just down from the shoulder. The arm felt heavy and weak on raising. It was a mild ache about the size of her hand in the outside muscle (lateral upper arm deltoid area). She remembers in high school having a severe ache there when she was sick in bed for 2-3 days. Had fever and muscle aches. Achiness left after about a minute and returned about 2 minutes later for a few moments. Returned again in the evening at about 7:00 pm on motion of the arm. Ache was milder than before (altered). Exact same area with feeling of weakness and heaviness.

End of Day General Observations: Her breasts are usually very sensitive prior to onset of menses and first day of menses. They have frequently in the past year or so been painful and tender to touch just prior to and at the beginning of her menses. With this menstrual cycle, the breast tenderness has been minimal and slightly more on the right. It only lasted less than a day and she wasn't aware of tenderness unless she bumped her breasts.

Top of left foot rash almost disappeared earlier today. Itchiness almost disappeared. It occasionally itches, no burning.

The right heel bruising pain is improving. This evening, walking on it caused a burning sensation on the inside of the heel. All day it has been occasionally tender to walk on the left bottom heel

Day 5 JULY 30, 1997

6:55 am When she put on her socks and shoes, she could feel a very mild itching on rash of top of left foot.

End of General Observations Top of left foot rash is barely visible to the eye. It has shrunk in size (half size of original rash) with small amount of color in the center (pink). Touching it brings on a slight itch. The itch is essentially gone.

The right heel is doing better. Only slightly sore (bruised feeling) when she walks. She had a short tennis practice this morning and the heel was slightly worse after tennis and improved throughout the day. She was not on it much during the day as she was sitting while teaching piano lessons.

10:38 pm While reading in bed, she had a vertical pain behind and in right eye running from eyebrow down through the eye straight down halfway the length of her nose along the eye socket Sudden sharp pain, like a line of pain was drawn there, of moderate intensity which did not affect the vision. Closing her eyes did not make any change. Pulling eye back at the corner did not change it. It went away after about one minute.

Day 6 - JULY 31, 1997

6:00 am Awakened from a dream (laying on her back). She dreamt that an unknown man was telling her how to put a tampon in. The tampon was huge. She woke up before she tried to put it in. Was not concerned about this man helping her at all during the dream; it was like a normal occurrence.

Three smallest toes on both feet were mildly crampy and achy when she woke up. Stretching toes did not help. Stretching heels (dorsiflexing) moderated the ache but did not make it disappear. The ache went away in 2-3 minutes while in bed. Changing positions from left side to right side did not change the ache.

9:00 am Warm shower water had no effect on rash on top of left foot. Warm water was bothering that area consistently since the beginning of the proving, making it itch, but not so this morning. In fact there was no itching. When she got out of the shower, the left foot has a red (1/4 inch) stripe on the inside of the rash area. No itching, no burning.

11:00 am Red stripe is totally gone. Rash area has shrunk more in size (1/4 size of original rash) and is lighter in color (light pink). No itching or burning.

Day 7 - AUGUST 1, 1997

5:00 am Woke up tired probably because she ate too many cookies the day before and went to bed late and woke up early for a trip.

5:45 am Tripped on porch step coming into the house while packing the car. Her body flew forward and her hand went through the window of the door, knocking the window out of the frame. The window did not break and came out of the door frame. Scraped both knees on the steps of the porch. Not badly hurt. The hand was fine.

6:00 am Her son told her she was crabby this morning.

6:35 am Left for a long car ride. Forgot the directions, drove back and couldn't find them.

Slept on and off on the way

10:30 am Arrived

1:30 pm Was walking watching the kids play hockey and noticed her right arm was heavy and hard to lift (like Day 4 at 5:15 pm, but not as intense). The muscles were moderately achy. The sensation went away after a few minutes. At first thought she was sore from too much tennis but 30 minutes later when she rechecked it, it was gone.

Day 8 - AUGUST 2, 1997

10:00 am Noticed some soreness on right arm very mild on upper underside muscle. (Location changed from outside upper arm to inside upper arm.) Also intensity changed to very mild. It did not last long, only a couple of minutes. Holding it still made it better, lifting the arm up made it worse.

Prover #18

10:30 am-4:00 pm Snacked on peppermint patty (offered to her) and diet coke. Mild stomach ache above the waist shortly afterward which was worse with driving. For several minutes while driving, the mild stomachache spread from the stomach to the back directly behind the stomach. Stomach and back pain lasted about 5 minutes. Then mild stomachache continued off and on for 1 to 1 1/2 hours. It felt bloated and gassy.

4:42 pm Experienced a sudden sharp moderate pain splitting her head slightly to the back in half. Touching her head made the pain worse. It lasted about a minute.

4:55 pm Dull mild ache behind the left eyebrow. Closing the eye did not change it. Disappeared gradually and lasted about one minute

End of Day General Observations: Right hand little finger has been achy on and off today, from the joint closest to the hand to the joint connecting the finger and hand. It is worse when writing and worse with bending it. Cold or hot do not affect it. Comes and goes with use. Had this several years ago in 1991.

Day 9 - AUGUST 3, 1997

6:45 am At the end of the walk, she had a pain at the top of the head which lasted several seconds and as it was disappearing, it moved a little bit above the left temple. Not as localized above the left temple, milder and lasted a few moments. (Day 1, 11:19 moderate, localized pain, this one is not as bad as day 1.)

10:00 am While standing in church, she experienced a sudden mild to moderate ache which followed her bra line from under her left arm and moved up the front up that line to where the arm meets your body. It disappeared shortly after sitting down; had lasted about one minute.

1:30 pm Same bra line pain while walking. Weather is hot. Pain not as intense as in the morning and only lasted a few moments.

Day 10 - AUGUST 4, 1997

6:30 am Woke up and went for 20 minute walk. Towards the end of the walk, she had a pain in the left eye and eye socket which only lasted a few moments. It was a sudden moderate achy pain. (Same pain as Day 1, 10:58 am with shorter duration and greater intensity.)

8:00 pm Took socks and shoes off and top of left foot began to itch slightly. She had worn shoes with socks most of the day, usually wore sandals. Itching is better with sandals or open shoe. Better with air.

Day 11 - AUGUST 5, 1997

4:30 am The alarm rudely awakened her and she packed the car and headed home from her road trip. The top of her left foot is slightly itchy this morning especially when something touches it. It is a very muted deep red color and only slightly visible and is getting smaller. Still no burning. Burning completely gone.

5:30 am Left for home. Did not sleep much in the car which is very, very unusual. She usually cannot keep herself awake in the car. She arrived home at 10:00 am.

1:15 pm In the afternoon while she was vacuuming, the push and pull motion with right arm, she felt a sudden bra line pain in her right armpit extending to upper portion of the bra above right breast. (On day 9, the pain was on the left side.) A mildly sharp, localized pain following the upper bra line occurred lasting a few moments.

Day 12 - AUGUST 6, 1997

8:00 am Rash on top left foot is even smaller. It is barely visible. The itch is more like a tickle and only occurs when touched or when in warm or hot water.

Right heel continues to improve. Very mild bruising feeling on the outer rim of the heel (medial to posterior area) only occurs when walking barefoot.

10:00-11:00 am Very sleepy, tired while teaching piano lessons. Kept yawning. Usually she feels tired only in the afternoon.

End of Day General observations Right chest area—dull ache localized fist size above right breast at 2 o'clock. Area has felt heavy on and off all evening. Pressing on it makes it worse, stretching both arms up makes it better. The aches come back when arms are down. Bending over makes it worse. Walking makes it better.

While doing laundry at about 8:00 pm, she noticed an ache at base of right hand, little finger (dorsal side). She had a moderate ache that came and went for 30 minutes. It was worse when bending the finger or using the finger. She was surprised it was totally gone by 9:00 pm. (Injured the finger about 7 years previous.)

Bottom of right foot is much improved and was able to walk barefooted this evening with only very mild discomfort (not pain, aware that her foot is there).

10:15 pm While lying in bed, she experienced a mild, crampy, achy feeling in the three little toes of both feet simultaneously. Wiggling did not affect it. Only lasted about 2 minutes. She then fell asleep. Same as Day 6, 6:00 am.

Day 13 - AUGUST 7, 1997

9:00 am-8:15 pm At about 9:00 am, she started to experience cramp-like, aches in both hands, at the base of the little fingers. (In the past it was only the right hand dorsal side.) Mild cramping, the size of a nickel at the base of the finger and lasted several minutes at a time, up to 15 minutes at a time. It was intermittent throughout the morning and early afternoon. Frequency increased as the day continued. Between 9:00 and 2:30, it happened 3 times. The frequency increased between 2:30 and 10:30 pm while on her long drive as a driver and as a passenger. It was worse when she drove. Opening and closing the hand ameliorated the cramping. Making a tight fist or stretching open her hand relieved the ache only while doing those motions. Immediately afterward, the ache would immediately return. At 8:15 pm, she stopped at a rest area and the warm water felt unusually good on her hands although she wasn't cold and her hands were not achy at that moment.

Early Evening Also experienced mild achy cramps in her feet around the three little toes, the left foot was worse than the right. While driving the achiness of the little toes moved to the back portion of right foot arch (before the heel) and only lasted a few moments. The left foot remained the same.

6:00 pm (similar to Day 4, 5:15 pm), while riding the car as a passenger, experienced the right upper arm ache. Much less severe than the past and lasted four minutes.

She did not sleep much traveling for 8 hours in the car today. This is very unusual for her. She was not sleepy at all while driving. As a passenger, she usually cannot stay awake in the car and sleeps more than 50% of any long trip. She slept about the last 20 minutes.

Day 14 - AUGUST 8, 1997

Noon She enjoyed the breeze off the lake, even waded in the water. Usually she is too hurried to do this; it was clear and beautiful weather.

1:30 pm Went down 231 steps and back up at the lake. She had no pain or discomfort doing this. Later on August 10th, she experiences pain doing the same thing.

10:00 am-8:00 pm Father drove the car for 3 hours and she did not sleep. She then drove for four hours and was not tired. He then drove from 5 to 6:00 pm and she drove from 6:00 to 8:00 pm and was never tired or sleepy throughout the trip. This is very unusual.

Day 15 - AUGUST 9, 1997

2:00 pm She felt a line of moderate, sharp pain under the right arm (armpit) and along the front of the shoulder joint. The same feeling as the bra line pain (DAY 9, 10:00am) except the location has changed. Moving the arm did not change the pain. Lasted about 2 minutes.

5:00 pm Sudden sharp moderate pain localized at top of head, intensified with touching it and lasted only a few moments. (Same as Day 1, 11:19 am.)

5:40 pm Pain in upper right arm is momentary and less intense (DAY 4, 5:15). Location same and pain same. Only change is intensity and did not last long at all. Fleeting pain.

End of day observations Left foot rash barely visible and itched mildly and momentarily while getting ready for bed.

Slight heartburn this evening after eating at the family reunion picnic at lunch and heavy dinner at 5:00 p.m. (had some heartburn with pregnancy).

Day 16 - AUGUST 10, 1997

1:15 pm Back on the road. Father is driving and is able to read without being sleepy.

2:30 pm She takes a turn driving and is not sleepy.

3:00 pm Went down 231 steps and up again at the lake (same as Day 14, 1:30 pm) and experienced a mild heavy ache in her chest on the way walking up. Disappeared before she got to the top. Weather was cloudy and it had rained.

4:00 pm Upper right arm is mildly achy, mostly heavy feeling. Lasted only a few moments.

During the driving, as the driver or passenger she was not tired.

9:35 pm Fleeting mild ache in left eye and socket, at front of the eyeball. Did not affect her vision. Lasted a few moments. Not as intense or as long as Day 1, 10:58 am.

Day 17 - AUGUST 11, 1997

1:00 pm Family drove 45 minutes and she was passenger in the car and could not stay awake. (This is what is typical for her as opposed to the wakefulness of the previous drives.) While sitting in the dental office for 30 minutes, she could hardly stay awake. She also had trouble staying awake during the ride home.

6:30 pm After dinner, while drying the dishes, she experienced a moderate, sharp localized pain at top of the head (same as Day 1). Shrugging shoulders made the pain worse and it gradually diminished and disappeared in 2 minutes.

Day 18 - AUGUST 12, 1997

Woke up at 6:00 am and went back to sleep and dreamed distorted dreams about buying houses. (Sister-in-law is presently looking for a house.)

7:15 am Got up feeling partially rested and head feels full like she's getting a cold. She has pressure around both eyes and above bridge of the nose. It's a rainy day today. She has a bad taste in mouth-sour. Her throat feels slightly clogged with phlegm and doesn't want to cough up.

8:45 pm As she was opening the back door of the station wagon, she experienced a sudden sharp pain in left foot, top outer side (anterior to lateral malleolus). Extremely painful when she put her weight on that foot. Every step she took, she experienced moderate to severe sharp pain. Got in the house and took her shoes and socks off and rotated the left ankle and heard some cracking sounds and foot was fine after that.

9:45 pm As she was laying on her back on her son's bed with her arms by her side, the pain in upper right arm returned, very mild. Stretching arms up to the ceiling made the pain disappear while she was stretching. The pain returned when she stopped stretching. Holding her knees and rocking made the pain disappear while doing that. But the pain was worse when she stopped holding her knees and rocking. She got up and was swinging her arms forward with elbows bent (same motion as speed walker) and went upstairs and it stopped. Pain lasted about 4 minutes.

End of Day General Observations Right heel is greatly improved. Has walked barefoot tonight with very little ache.

She has about twice per day for the last 2 days been uncomfortably warm for several minutes. It was not as intense or dramatic as hot flashes she had last winter but similar in feeling; warm all over and after a few minutes, the warmth disappears.

Day 19 - AUGUST 13, 1997

4:30 am The room was warm because it had rained and they did not open the windows. Awakened by husband and went back to bed and dreamed. She dreamed of being at a camp with lots of children. She was in charge of these children. She saw a friend that graduated from high school with her in her dream and the dream was all jumbled up.

End of Day General Observations Good energy level during the proving, more than usual. However tonight, she feels tired and is ready for bed.

Day 20 - AUGUST 14, 1997

2:00 am Husband woke her up because he was talking in his sleep. She was awakened from dreaming. She cannot remember the dream however she knows it was a fearful dream.

4:00 pm–midnight Traveled a far distance by car again.

4:30 pm Riding in the car as a passenger, she experienced pain at top of the head (mild sharp localized pain). Turning the head to each side did not affect the pain. Leaning forward and writing made the pain a bit more intense. The intensity not as bad as Day 1 and the pain disappeared in about 2 minutes.

10:20 pm While driving the car, she experienced a mild dull aching above her right breast at 2 o'clock which lasted almost 2 minutes.

10:30 pm While driving she experienced a mild sharp localized pain at the top of the head (same as 4:30 but a little milder, less intense) which lasted several seconds, a fleeting pain.

10:40 pm While driving, she had a dull mild ache in her right eye which only lasted a few seconds and which was similar to what she experienced with the left eye previously on Day 1, 10:58 am.

She was sleepier during this trip more than the other 2 trips during the proving but not nearly as much as she usually does.

Day 21 - AUGUST 15, 1997

End of Day General Observations Had an amazing amount of energy today after beginning so sluggishly.

Her abdomen feels mildly acidic tonight, right side, below the rib cage. Had blackberry cobbler at 9:00 pm. She felt very tired. Pressure over stomach made it worse. Applying pressure over the area or lateral to the area causes no change.

12:10 am Her son came in and woke up her husband. She slept through it. (Has never slept through this before.)

DAY 22 - AUGUST 16, 1997

Woke up, warm and sticky and dreaming. Her dream was about using wetlands and exchanging other wetlands in Spain. Dream was way out of proportion to a discussion she had had the night before with friends.

Day 24 - AUGUST 18, 1997

7:30 pm While reading in chaise lounge, she experienced a mild cramp-like ache in right foot, in the area at the base of the two little toes. She had not been in the swimming pool. It was a cool evening (67F). Moving her foot both by rotation of the ankle and wiggling the toes made it better. The pain lasted about one minute which was much less than before. (Same pain she had on Day 1 and Day 23 at 10:12 p.m.)

9:18 pm While standing brushing her teeth, she experienced the sudden pain at the top of her head (same as Day 1, 11:19). Moderate, not so localized, more widespread pain at the top of the head. Walking seemed to relieve it. It disappeared in about 30 seconds.

Day 25 - AUGUST 19, 1997

5:30 pm She was sitting in the car and her right heel felt bruised and achy. Simultaneously, she felt a mild cramp-like ache in the right ball of the foot and in the arch area. The heel ache persisted and the cramp-like pain in the ball and arch of the foot abated when she moved her foot around (rotation of the ankle). The cramp-like ache (ball and arch of right foot) lasted less than one minute while heel ache was intermittent for 15 minutes. (The cramp-like pain in the ball of the foot is new with the proving, however the bruised feeling is an old symptom and is not counted in the proving.)

Day 28 - FRIDAY, AUG 22, 1997

Her feet are feeling better. The left foot is close to normal-hardly any pain at all. The right foot is much improved. Her right foot hurt this evening when she walked on concrete when wearing thin soled beach sandals. Moderate bruised feeling of the heel area (edge of inside heel, does not include the arch). Walking on grass or in the house improved the pain while wearing the same thin-soled beach sandals.

Day 29 - SATURDAY AUG 23, 1997

7:45 am Got up and left foot rash has disappeared completely.

End of Day General Observations Early afternoon at about 1:15 pm She had an ache at the top of the head similar to what she has experienced before—mild dull pain at the top of the head more widespread than before (Day 1, 11:19 am). Lasted about 5 minutes (longer than before). Came on shortly after going outside (upper 80s clear sunny day) to explain instructions for a party game. Went away before going back inside.

Day 30 - AUGUST 24, 1997

No left foot rash. Still gone since yesterday.

Day 31 - AUGUST 25, 1997

Approaching menses and breasts are not sore at all. Unusual. They are usually mild/moderate sore to the touch, or when bumped.

Right foot heel has improved. The ache has changed to the back center of the heel, localized. Mild pain and pain was only occasionally when walking.

Day 32 - AUGUST 26, 1997

Her right heel has greatly improved. She can just feel it when walking tonight. It is not an ache or painful feeling—simply an awareness of having it.

No signs of menses beginning.

Day 34 - AUGUST 28, 1997

General Observations No sign of menses beginning. Late about two days. (She missed her period in December 1996 and January 1997.)

Day 35 - AUGUST 29, 1997

8:45-9:10 am While painting a set of shelves, her right hand and wrist were mildly crampy. It began shortly after she started to paint and continued while she would paint. The pain would stop when she stopped painting. (Yesterday she did about 30 minutes of painting and experienced the mild crampy towards the end of the painting.)

No sign of menses.

Day 36 - AUGUST 30, 1997

Woke up at 6:45 am Had dreams before waking up. Surprised she remembered so much. She dreamed about teaching one of her husband's music string classes at the elementary school. She was late and he made her go wearing only a brown haircutting cape and a sweatshirt — nothing else. (She had recently cut hair using a brown haircutting cape.) On the way to the school, she passed a field with many violinists including a few people she knows who do not play the violin. She got to the school—not the elementary school she thought she was going to—and passed ladies dressed immaculately in suits, and they were heading to a lecture given by the principal. She finally got to the rehearsal music room and she told the students "Never to take drugs because it would make them do strange things. I'm wearing an example so you know never to take drugs."

No signs of menses

Day 37 - AUGUST 31, 1997

6:30 pm Sitting in a chair, the ball of the right foot felt like a mild burning, not painful feeling. It lasted about 1 minute. The burning quality is an altered symptom.

That night, she had more distorted dreams. Cannot remember them.

Day 38 - SEPTEMBER 1, 1997

General Observations: Right foot is much better. No discomfort all day while wearing shoes. This evening has walked barefooted and can just barely feel she has a left heel. Her right heel is a dull mild ache in outer edge of inside heel while walking barefooted or dorsiflexion.

Day 39 - SEPTEMBER 2, 1997

10:30 to Noon Experienced the pain at the top of the head three times. Each was mild and not as localized, more fist size. The first one lasted 3 minutes, the second about 1 minute and the third was more mild than the other 2 and lasted about 10 seconds.

Day 42 - SEPTEMBER 5, 1997

Woke up dreaming a weird distorted dream. They had students in the house. A tornado came so they gathered in the very small bathroom in their home. The tornado took the house and spun it upside down (somersault fashion) a number of times and landed back perfectly in place (not even any stuff like furniture out of place-no mess at all). They were all frozen in their spots during the ride. She excitedly said to her husband, "That was better than the rides at the amusement part!" The weird part of the dream was the lack of concern about this tornado. *Her daughter had gone to an amusement about a month ago and went on numerous exciting rides. Also, in the spring she had piano students at her home and a tornado siren went off because a tornado had touched down in her county.*

No sign of menses

Day 43 - SEPTEMBER 6, 1997

Woke up dreaming. It was a crazy mixed-up dream. She was driving straight down (45 degree angle) a wide gravel mountain road with no caution signs. Somehow her friend was standing on the back bumper

Her breasts are mildly sore to touch in the nipple area, the right more than the left.

Day 47 - SEPTEMBER 10, 1997

Evening Taught piano from 3:00 pm-8:15 pm and she noticed her neck became stiff (the same stiffness from diving into the pool on day 37). Right side at the base of the neck is stiff; no pain, just stiffness.

End of Day General Observations Her breasts especially the right are more tender and sore to the touch, even touched lightly (before they were tender with firmer touch). Mild pain. Her breasts hurt with mild pain, especially right breast when pressed against her husband's body during sex.

Neck continues to be stiff on right, base of neck. Worse with motion, better at rest. Better when laying on back. Worse lying on her sides.

Day 48 - SEPTEMBER 11, 1997

Woke up dreaming a distorted dream. Her pastor and his wife were in her dream. *(She doesn't know which part they played in the dream.)* She was helping to organize a dinner. People had sent not only the food but the actual plates and tableware. These plates were all antique colored plates. They had green ones and brown ones and she broke a set of six brown plates.

6:00 am Woke up and feet were better. The ache when she first got up was more mild in the right foot. The left foot was normal.

She did not put on a bra this morning because her breasts were tender, mildly sore when touched. She experienced itchy breasts while teaching piano. Lasted a few minutes. It was mild in the nipple area.

End on Day General Observations Her breasts are not full heavy and tender tonight. No soreness when pressing firmly.

Her feet are much improved. Very mild soreness in right heel when walking barefooted. Left foot normal.

Neck continues to be mildly stiff, right side base of neck. No improvement. Better with rest, worse with motion. Better laying on back and worse lying on sides.

hanging on to her car with a frightened look on her face. Another person couldn't stop the car and it continued to accelerate. She was trying to apply the brakes and it didn't help. She was skidding on the gravel road and still continued to accelerate. Somehow she got to the bottom of the mountain and noticed that her friend was no longer on the back bumper so she went back to find her. In this dream, she was definitely concerned about her friend's welfare.

No signs of menses.

Day 44 - SEPTEMBER 7, 1997

Woke up dreaming about being up in another state. She was at her in-laws and they had a layer of hard pack snow that had turned into ice in the living room of their house. It was flat (not chunky) and her father-in-law was chopping at it and breaking it up and tossing it outside. Later in that room, there was a beautiful rose color carpet *(their carpet is ivory color)* and was like new. Also in that dream, her sister was telling her that they were to spend Christmas at her other sister's home and their parents were going to go along and see them there. *(Her sister would never, in reality, "tell" her what to do* and *would never leave her home for a Christmas holiday and also her father would never leave his home for a Christmas Holiday.)*

This evening her breasts are tender. She can feel a little bit of soreness when pressing firmly on them, the right more than the left but it's very mild.

Day 45 - SEPTEMBER 8, 1997

Feet are not 100% better but much improved over the last couple days.

Has felt warm today more so than usual (The weather has been hot and muggy.) She is wondering if she is beginning to experience menopause symptoms. (She missed 2 periods in December 1996 and January 1997 and had hot flashes at that time.)

Breasts feel heavy and full, very slightly tender to touch, especially the right and only sore if touched firmly. No other signs of menses.

Day 46 - SEPTEMBER 9, 1997

Evening general observations Her feet are better than yesterday. Her left heel has only a hint of ache at times when she is walking on it. Her right heel is mildly achy when she put weight on it.

Day 49 - SEPTEMBER 12, 1997

6:00 am Woke up dreaming. Doesn't remember the dream. However does remember a childhood friend was in the dream.

Day 50 - SEPTEMBER 13, 1997

No menses.

Her neck continues to be mildly stiff, right base of neck.

Day 51 - SEPTEMBER 14, 1997

Her right breast is mildly sore today when firmly touched.

Day 52 - SEPTEMBER 15, 1997

Her husband woke her up and she went back to sleep and dreamed. She was at her grandmother's house (grandmother moved out of her house 16 years ago and died 14 years ago). Her house was similar to her real memory of it but in her dream she had a bright purple telephone (the big old fashioned phone with the handle) hanging on her dining room wall. This purple phone was decorated with fake flowers which caught on fire through the wiring. They were trying to put this fire out.

She dreamed again another dream where another similar telephone was on fire. This one did not have any flowers on it. In her dream she remembers saying: "I must remember to tell the proving supervisor how I dreamed this experience and then it really happened." *(In her dream she thought this second event was reality.)*

Day 53 - SEPTEMBER 16, 1997

She went back to sleep around 3:30 am and dreamed. She dreamed that she got up and her husband had totally changed the living room furniture because he couldn't sleep. The furniture was totally different.

Day 54 - SEPTEMBER 17, 1997

She dreamed sometime during the night. She was going way up North to teach at a school. It was extremely rustic. A friend was there. *(He taught New Testament at a Bible College with her in the 1970s. He now teaches out of state and she recently met a former student of his during the summer.)* While there, a siren blew and everyone gathered for shelter in a huge entrance to a cave (half building and half cave). The siren was for a rock slide which was apparently common. A crew went out and gathered up the rocks with big equipment and then everybody went back to normal activities.

Day 55 - SEPTEMBER 18, 1997

Woke up dreaming that her period started in a big way. She was sitting on the toilet and a big clot the size of 2 grapefruits was expelled similar to a placenta after childbirth.

Day 56 - SEPTEMBER 19, 1997

Woke up dreaming. She dreamed she was selling a vacuum cleaner to an elderly woman a friend of the family. *(In real life, she died 2 weeks ago. She was in her late 80s when she died.)*

Day 57 - SEPTEMBER 20, 1997

Was crabby during the evening. (Menses started on Day 59)

Day 59 - SEPTEMBER 22, 1997

Got up, no dreams.

11:30 am Menses began. No symptoms before starting menses. (Sometimes that happens). The flow was slow to start.

6:00 pm Menses continue to flow slowly and lighter in color (more pinkish color) than usual. No cramps or discomforts (usually occurs when flow increases on day 2).

End of Day General Observations Menses continues slowly. Not using tampons, can still wear maxi pad.

Day 60 - SEPTEMBER 23, 1997

5:30 am Menses has continued. Flow is light in color and intensity. No discomfort.

End of Day Observations Menses remain steady, slow and light in color. Usually she has dark clots (none this time). Color more pink than red. (Has never had that before.) No cramps or discomfort. (Usually has abdominal cramps during the menses.) Much lighter flow, about 50% of what her flow is usually like. Duration was longer (almost twice as long). Did not get up in the night to change her pads. (Usually must do that for 2 nights because the flow is so heavy.)

Day 61 - SEPTEMBER 24, 1997

5:30 am Her menses were slightly heavier in the night (at the most maybe moderate flow). Did not need to change in the night, usually would need to change 1-3 times per night. Color is still light.

Noon Menses continue to be light in color and flow.

End of Day observations Menses remain steady, light in color and light in flow. Usually much heavier and with clotting.

Day 62 - SEPTEMBER 25, 1997

5:30 am Flow has continued to be slow. The color is a darker normal red and there are no clots.

End of Day Observation Her menses increased during the day to almost moderate. The color is the normal red. No clots. Usually her flow peaks on days 2&3 and then after 2 days of slowing down, the menses is complete. With this cycle, she is peaking at Day 4 which is not very common. Flow is much lighter. No cramps. (Usually has abdominal cramps during the period.)

Day 63 - SEPTEMBER 26, 1997

6:00 am Her right heel is improving. Only slightly bruised feeling.

Had very little menstrual flow during the night.

Noon Menses flow has been light but steady. A normal bright red color. No cramps.

End of Day Observations Menses continued light, no clots.

Day 64 - SEPTEMBER 27, 1997

7:15 am Menses flowed lightly during the night, flowed a little more the previous night.

End of Day Observations Menses continue but very slow.

Day 66 - SEPTEMBER 29, 1997

End of Day Observations   Menses light and intermittent (every 2 hours) This period never came to point of heavy flow and clotting and discomfort. Felt like it "never really came."

Day 67 - SEPTEMBER 30, 1997

Just spotted in the night, very little.

Menses only a few spots today.

Day 68 - OCTOBER 1, 1997

Menses has stopped. This cycle was unusual in lightness of flow and length of duration. It lasted about twice as long as usual but seemed to never reach a climax.

No left foot rash. Over the last week, she has experienced a lot of stress. Usually the chronic rash surfaces with stress. Usually rash surfaces with hot humid weather. Has not done so since it cleared (Day 29, 7:45 am when she got up). It appears to be cured.

The New England School of Homeopathy

The New England School of Homeopathy (NESH) was created in 1987 to translate homeopathic philosophy into the successful and predictable practice of medicine. Our goal is for practitioners of homeopathy to fulfill their potential role in health care—to help people attain freedom from illness on the mental, emotional, and physical planes so they may better realize their highest aspirations.

To fulfill this mission, the program and materials of NESH strive:

- To exemplify the highest purpose and achievement in the field of homeopathic medicine. NESH aims to inspire the greater homeopathic community to join in this endeavor, and to encourage and assist the non-homeopathic community in the exploration of and participation in homeopathy.
- To commit the full energies of NESH to provide each participant with the tools required for the successful practice of homeopathy in a thorough and expedient manner.
- To provide a philosophical foundation based on the principles of classical homeopathy.
- To establish a practical technical foundation essential to the successful practice of homeopathy.
- To transform homeopathic theory into predictable clinical results.
- To provide materials which are clinically significant and immediately applicable.
- To communicate actual experience. All materials bearing the NESH name have been clinically verified by the presenter.

The vehicles for accomplishment of these objectives are:

- Professional classes designed:
    - to educate the beginning practitioner in the effective application of homeopathy.
    - to enhance the practicing homeopath's knowledge, so that he or she may deliver consistently favorable results.
    - to foster the acquisition of techniques which will enable the practitioner to continue to learn from his/her own experience.
- A journal through which practitioners may learn and share their own discoveries with the homeopathic community. The journal serves to express a shared vision and create a resource for optimal learning by practitioners of all levels.
- A clinical setting for practitioners to support the transition from student to practicing clinician.
- An ongoing forum offering participants the opportunity to make the transition from clinician to teacher.
- Seminars presented by clinicians with expertise in a specialized area of homeopathy.
- Publication of reference texts which are relevant for the continuing education of homeopathic physicians and patients.
- Classes for the community at large which illuminate homeopathic theory and application, and encourage the growth of a patient population that is well-educated in the practice of homeopathy.

For more information write to:

New England School of Homeopathy
356 Middle Street
Amherst, Massachusetts 01002
www.nesh.com
email: nesh@nesh.com
tel: 413.256.5949
fax: 413.256.6223

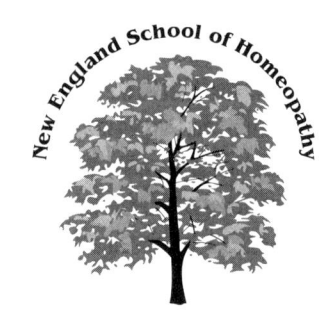

Index

Part One

Accidents, as spurious rubric, 75
Accurate prescriptions, x
Aconite
   masked proving of, 43
   proving acute remedies, 55
   temperature variations, 47
Acting *vs.* reacting, in political struggle, 39, 59
Acupuncture, 18–19
Acute complaints, 26–27
   in constitutional treatment, 31
   replaced by chronic ones, 99
   seemingly in sensitive provers, 99
Acute remedies, and chronic proved, 55
Advertising material, rights to, 125
Age of prover, 123
Aggravations in proving, 34–35
Agony, produced by plant tinctures, 97
Alcohol consumption, during proving, 119
Alcoholus proving, 17–19, 90
   alcoholism in family history, 92
   balance in, 115
   sensitives in proving, 113
   theory in application, x
Aletris farinosa, 47
Algebra to calculus compared, to proposed quantum leap in medicine, 61
Allen, T. F. MD, 46
Allopathic
   accusations, 39
   colleagues, vii
   discussions with homeopaths, 62–63
   latecomers to drug testing, 42
   materia medicas, specifics in, 24
   rhetoric believed by homeopaths, 44
Altered symptoms, in prover, 37, 112, 121
Amelioration, due to similarity of *Stress/Strain,* 26–27
American Institute of Homeopathy, 44, 47
Amorphousness, in choice of symptoms, 114–115
Analyzing, proving at web site, 131–132
Anatomy of a proving, 88–89
Animal experiments, 46
   disease states mimicking human, 60
Animals, as toxic remedies, 94
Anthropomorphysing, of objects, 78
Antidotal interference, 47
Antipsorics, and waiting time for symptoms, 55
Anxiety, from changing proving setting, 104–105
Archibel ProveIt program, 127, 132

Arnica
   assessing outside forces, 18
   for vicarious suffering?, 81, 102
Arsenicum, 47, 50
   example of dangerous engrafting, 56
   sensitivity to, 55
Art of refining symptoms, 114–115
Arthritis, 24–25
Articulate provers, as best provers, 109, 124
Assessing symptoms, 109
Assumptions, testing of, vii
Astronomy, scientific revolution in, 66
Attributes of objects, can they be proved, 76
Attribution, symptoms to remedy, ix, 18–19
Attuning the self, in proving, 67
Audio and visual rights to NESH, 125
Author's intention, 19

Background noise, 41, 59, 69, 82, 118
   see also Noise
   and threshold bar, 73
   too loud, 124
Bacteria, *Stress* as, 6, 138
Bar. see Threshold bar
Baseline model, 21–22
Belladonna, proving with placebo, 10
Benefits allopathy can gain,
   from homeopathy now, 60
Berlin Wall, proving a quality, 76–78
Beth Isreal Medical Center, N.Y., vii
Bias, regarding dose attenuation, 45
Biochemical individuality, not equality, 94
Biology and botany, scientific revolution in, 66
Blind spots, proving methodology's, 22
Blinded studies, 117, 124 see also Masking
   unblinding, 131–132
Bloodshed over objects, 77–78
Body parts, review of, 122
Body reaction, to *Stress,* 5
Books, homeopathic, last decade of, 40–41
Borderland, between health and disease, 42, 49
Bountifulness of nature, 95
Bowels griping with chilliness, 48
Brevity and elegance, of scientific discovery, 85
Bridges between
   constitutions in provings, 32
   new symptoms and remedy, 37
   remedies in practice, 31

Calcareas, proving substances from living beings, 93

Calcium, for functionality, 94
Cancer therapies, 24–25
Case-control studies, alternative proposed, 61
Case taking
  analysis and management, 9, 15–18, 23, 26–27, 36–38, 81
  of provers symptoms, 109–110
  rubric choices, 16
  skills improved, 14
Catalogue of symptoms, 113–114
Catastrophic drug reaction, minimized by sub-group selection, 61
Causation, separating potentized stress and daily strain, 137–138
Cavalier attitude, toward pre-trial phase, 102–103
Cerebral symptoms, *Lillium tigrinum* example, 48–50
Change brings change, rejected for proving mileux, 104–105
Change in food, changing proving baseline, 104–105
Characteristic symptoms, 137
Chemical analysis in provings, 45
Chemically sensitive, excluded from proving, 104
Chemotherapy, 24–25
China, 53–54
Chinese medicine, and polypharmacy, 86
Choosing provers, example of people with milk allergies, 93
Choosing proving substance, 92–95
Chronic effect of remedy, on human race, 54–55
Chronic *Stress/Strain* patterns
  removed, 6, 26–27
  symptoms partially removed, 37
Chronic symptoms
  cured or exaggerated, 54
  symptoms replaced by acutes, 99
Chronological symptom order, 47, 49–50
Clarifying prover's expression, 124
Clinical experience and new remedies, 80–81
Clinical phase, proving size of 15 to 40, 91
Cloistered seclusion, for proving, 104–105
Clumsiness, in *Arnica* proving, 18
Codifying medicines, by simillimum, 86
Coffee drinking, in proving, 119
Coherent provers, in self-description, 109

Cohort
  large, multi-centered and cultural, 91
  with PI design proving, 108
  and PI meet homeopaths, 110
  of provers small, 90
Collating information, viii
Collation tool, 127
Collective unconscious
  n=infinity proving, 68
  and placebo proving arm, 101
Committee of Drug Provings, 48–50
Common language, prover and supervisor, 119
Community of homeopaths, 59
  arguments within, 9
  disagreement on provings, 13, 20, 28
  documents offered to, 127–138
  fitting into scientific community, 43
  misconceptions within, 8
  publishing information for, 110
  as underclass, 39
Complete symptom, 124
Conceit and science, 52
Concept and perception, of attuning the self, 67
Concepts of homeopathy, logic and understanding of, 7
Concomitant symptoms, 120
Confusion
  as alienation from clinical experience, 10–11
  in choice of symptoms, 27
  and good intentions, 12
  and lack of results in practice, 22
Consent and release form, transfer rights, 125–126
Consent Forms, viii
Consenting adults, at least 18, 103
Constant feedback, to prover, 125
Constellation of changing symptoms, people with excluded from proving, 104
Constipation, from changing proving setting, 104–105
Constitutional nature
  acute state in, 31
  and complete symptom picture, 36–37
  number of, more important than number of provers, 92
  of provers noted, 33, 92, 111
  sensitive to remedy, 90
  shared by prover subset, 32, 90
  and size of proving, 90
  and *Stress* response, 29

Contracted pupils, 56
Convallaria majalis, 47
Cooperation, 48
Copyright interest, 125
Cosmology, 12 *see also* Rules
   to explain polypharmacy, 86
Creating a sensitivity to remedy, 55
Creating or disturbing order, using high or low potencies, 57
Criticism and analysis invited, 12
Criticism standard, 48
Cross-over trials, alternating placebo and verum, 102, 109
Culture, everyday language of, 120
Cumulative knowledge
   as good science, 12
   and journey of discovery, 72
Cured symptoms, 11
   coinciding constitution and medicine, 36–37
   focus of proving, 6, 117
   in individualized sensitives, 137
   materia medica basis in, 8
   proving category, 112, 121
   real basis of new remedies, 82
Current drug study design, 59–60
Cycles
   and incorrect prescription, 35
   matching to patient *Cycle*, 17–19
   in proving coalesce easily, 114
Cycles and Segments, 15
   contextualizing symptoms, 16–17
   model in provings and case analysis, 26–28, 30–38
   sequencing symptom flow, 112
   tree trunk and branches, 17
Cyclopedia of Drug Pathogenesy, 47, 49

Dance of Life, 28
Danger
   of engrafting remedy, 56
   of palliating pain, 57
   in repeating toxic substance, 110
   of wasting time and incorrect remedy, 85
Database for proving, 127
Databases, drowned by noise, 62
Death, from treatment, 24–25
Debating with allopaths, 39
Debriefing interviews, timing between, 112
Defamation claim release, 125
Defensive stance of homeopathy, 39
Demographic information, 127–135

Dental work, 123
Derivative works, of proving, 125–126
Designing proving, for who, 109
Diagnosis, in provings, 45
Differentiating symptoms, substance and other *Stresses*, 110
Digital photography, for documentation, 108
Dilute substances, as argument against homeopathy, 40
Direction symptom shifts, 120
Disappeared symptoms, recorded, 8
Discomfort of prover, 125
Discovery, of proving dynamics, 7
Discussion of concepts and ideas, not provers and personalities, 65, 69
Divine intervention, *vs.* simple evolution of an idea, 86
Divorce of proving and practice, of new remedies, 80–81
Doctor-patient privileges, and prover's disclosures, 125–126
Doctrine of Signatures, 66
   as a *lagging indicator*, 78–79
Documenting for posterity, 108, 113
Doing and being, of a proving, 13
Dollar bill, potentized, 80
Dose, 98–101
   repetition, 45, 49, 56, 98–101
   single, 47, 55
   small, non-toxic, not potentized, 60–61
Downloading database, 132
Drake, J. P. MD, 46
Drawing, symptom location, 120
Dream
   prescribing solely on, 70
   provings, 68
   recall, 71
   recording in proving, 122
   work and provings, 68–70
Driving force of homeopathic science, 59
Drooling in sleep, 122
Drug
   crude, in temporary experiment, 58
   defining of, 23
   reactionary effects, 45
   study design, 59
   uniformity of, 45
Drug researchers
   basically doing proving, 42
   hit or miss process, 60
   seek pathogenic effects, 48–49
   streamlining the process, 60–63

Index - Part One

Drug-testing pipeline, proposing a change, 63
Drug testing protocol, vii, 25–26
   began by Hahnemann, 42, 66
   drug trial standards, 100
   Herculean task, 44
   proposed non-random, 60–61
Dunham, Dr., 57
Duplication rights, of proving materials, 125
Duration of symptoms, 121
Dynamic action, of medicines on vital force, 26

Economy of vital force, beclouded, 57
Editorial control, and prover, 125
Educational material, rights to, 125
Effects of medicines, isolating, 41
Efficient response
   and non-random testing, 60–61
   remedy and, 6
Einstein, Albert, 85
Elegance, to scientific concepts and models, 85, 105
Eliciting symptoms, and dose repetition, 98–101
Emergent qualities, 77–79
Emotional
   excessive symptoms, 124
   functioning of volunteers, 117
Energy efficient method, of adapting to *Stress*, 27
English proving groups, two camps of, 65
Engrafting of remedy, danger of, 56
Environment, not filtered from proving, 73
Environmentally sensitive, excluded from proving, 104, 109
Epistemology of a proving, necessity of, 89
Equivalence of practice and provings, 8, 11, 15–16
Essence, defining proving, 23
European, popularity of seminar proving, 67–68
Everyday language, in proving, 120
Evolution of homeopathy, 39, 139
   vs. divine intervention, 86
   as leap or exaptation, 85
Evolving, due to *Stress*, 27
Exaptations, 85–106
Excessive *Stress*, adding more proving variables, 105–106
Excitement, over proving substance, 92, 95
Excluded from proving, people and situations, 103–104
Exercise and exertion, *Stress* as, 5
Experience, cannot be proved, 76

Experiment design
   eliminating noise, 41
   lack of, 138
   on sick of allopaths, 51
Experimental evidence, homeopathic *vs.* allopathic, 40
Experimental group, coalesced tightly, 72
Extraneous influences, 47
Extremities, neuralgic pains, 48

Fabric of life, provings connection, 80
Failure, as beginning of knowledge, 52
Falling out of favor, falling from forefront of medicine, 40–41
Fatal drug reactions, minimized by sub-group selection, 61
Fetus and proving, 123
Field work, current homeopathic, 40
Financial and political opponents, of homeopathy, 39
First few days of symptoms, 112
First proving dose, with supervisor present, 119
Five symptom categories
   abbreviations, 121–122
   of prover's symptoms, 112
Flow of drug influence, 57–58
Flow of symptoms, 112
Focus on cured symptoms, 9
Follow-up, 9
   proving analysis, 110, 112
   skills improved, 18–19
   theory and practice, 23
Foods
   as category 1 for provings, 93–95
   moderation in, 41
Forum for discussion, 65, 139
Framework, for proving methodology, 23
Frequently shifting symptoms, excludes prover, 111
Frothing at mouth, simulating *Opium*, 58
Future provings
   model of, 21–22, 74
   for sensitives, 123

Gasoline proved, and OPEC price rise, 74
Gender, of various constitutions, 29
General public opinion
   and homeopaths' self definition, 39–40
   tools to change, 40–41
General qualities, matching specific complaints, 7

General tendency of remedy, in toxicity literature, 108
General unspecified symptoms, 113–114
Gentleness, through extensive knowledge, 53
God, infallible, man as, 52
Governments possibly brought down, by proving, 74
Group dynamics, not influencing placebos, 101
Gruber, Frank MD, vi, 22
    iterative process with, 14

Hahnemann, Samuel, 9, 23, 34, 41–44, 103
    advice to young men, 56
    choosing medicines to prove, 93
    condemned human experiments, 51
    confronting science of the age, 66
    a constant experimenter, 95
    Doctrine of Signatures opposed, 79
    guidelines for provings, 26
    his love of truth, 59
    hope based on spirit of, 62–63
    hypothesis of, 20
    irony of nullifying his work, 24
    Materia Medica of Chronic Diseases, 54
    Materia Medica Pura, 16, 54
    methodology and discovery, 72
    observing minor *Sepia* poisoning, 92–93
    potency of provings, 95–96
    revolutionary thought, 43
    and streamlining current drug tests, 61
    translating medical texts, 86
Hall, Graham, viii
    tech wizard and homeopath, 127
Handouts
    to homeopaths and provers, 111
    to provers and supervisors, 117–135
Hatred, of those knowing more, 53
Hawthorne Effect
    as additional variable, 71–72
    embracing it to diminish it, 102–103, 111
    of encouraging attention, 71
    limited by cross-over trials, 102
    limiting, 109
Health and disease
    defined, 20
    greater model of, 22
    murky realm between, 42, 49
Health emergency, of provers, 117
Healthy people
    are not asymptomatic, 103
    eliminating noise, 41–42
    and provings, 25, 29, 53, 103

used same as single drug, 87
volunteers, 60–61
Herbs, 18–19
Herscu, Paul ND
    Stramonium with an Introduction to Analysis Using Cycles and Segments, 9
    The Homeopathic Treatment of Children: Pediatric Constitutional Types, 9, 69
History
    forgotten, 44
    of Hahnemann's discovery, 85
    and Herscu's model, 139
    materia medicas, 24–25
    misconceptions corrected, 39–44
    and polypharmacy, 85–86
    of provings, 23–24, 66
    recapturing moral highground, 63
Homeopathic
    basis in *Stress/Strain*, 6
    contributions, 41–44
    forum for debate needed, 65
    institutional memory lacking, 44
    practice with unknown substance, 8
    resurgence, 65
    scientific or not, 39
    self-definition, 65
    similar and *Stress/Strain*, 26–27
    successful strategies in practice, 19
Homeopathic history
    biology and science, 5
    history and heritage, 39–44
    relating to provings, x
Homeopaths
    lacking agreement, 20
    linchpins in proving, 109
    present when remedy given, 112
Homeopathy
    at crossroads, 93–94
    fragmentation of, 23
    logic and understanding in, 7
    understanding its process, 20
Hoover, Todd MD, vi, vii, 24
Hot-tubbing, in proving, 119
Human substances to prove, 93
Humility, and an open mind, 52
Hyperfocus on prover, to limit Hawthorne Effect, 102–103
Hypothesis
    Hahnemann's, 20
    testing of, vii
Hysterical people, excluded from proving, 104

Ideal proving, perfect outcome, 7–8
Idiosyncrasies, 47
    safeguards against, 44
Ignorance, of homeopathic history, 40, 65
Immune system, efficiency, 6
Inaccuracy in provings, 10
Including and excluding symptoms, aggravated in proving, 34
Incomplete improvement, in proving, 35
Incomplete proving, *Cycles* not complete, 114
Individual characteristics
    vs. general features, 96
    out of general population, 61
Individual predisposition
    as basis of homeopathy, 81, 87
    and response, 118
Individualize information, 123, 137
Infections, attributing, 138
Infighting, over provings, 14
Influence, strong, to prover eliminated, 42, 47
Influenza, 24–25
Informed consent, viii
    disclaimer form, 116
Initial proving interactions, supplies dispensed and PI's instructions, 110
Innocence, state of physician, 52–53
Innovation and dialogue, 12
Insects, as toxic remedies, 94
Institutional memory
    lacking, 44
    result of ignorance of, 59
Insufficiently self aware, excluded from proving, 104
Integrity of remedies, 10–11
Intensify the effect of remedy, how to, 56
Intensity of symptoms, 121
Interconnectedness
    all areas of homeopathy, 22
    and isolating variables, 80
    of provers, 72–73
Interdisciplinary discussion, allopaths and homeopaths, 62–63
Interference to predisposition, as *Stress*, 26
Intermittent fevers, and *China,* 54
Intermitting symptoms, 121
Internet
    proving site instructions, 132–135
    use of proving, 125–126
Interpersonal phase, step 1, proving, 108–110
Interpretation of dreams, by patient, 70
Interpretation of provings, encouraged, 22

Intervention, second after remedy, the proving itself, 72
Interview, 14–15*see also* Case taking
Invasion of privacy, claim release, 125
Irregular heart, 56
Isolating one variable, 76*see also* Variable
Isopathy, difference with homeopathy, 79
Issues deflected, in homeopathic books of last decade, 40–41
Iterative process, 14, 24, 60

Jerking in sleep, 122
Journals, x
Judgment, new basis, 49–50
Jumbling of primary and secondary symptoms, 45
Jung, Carl, justifying n=infinity proving, 68

Kent, James Tyler MD
    Lecture XXVIII The Study of Provings, 51–58
    Repertory, 10
    on *Stress/Strain,* 27
Keynotes
    trap of matching poor, 17
    what are they, 137
Knowledge
    cumulative, 72, 85
    lack of as lethal, 61
    little *vs.* extensive, 53

Laboratory work, current homeopathic, 40
Lac defloratum and milk allergies, 93
Lack of sex or company, changing baseline, 104–105
Lagging indicator, 78–79
Language
    of nature, 51
    of repertory, 16
    of *Stress/Strain,* 6
Laundry list of symptoms, 16–17, 19
Lawton, Jeenet, viii
Lawyer, Jack, viii, ix
Learning, from all sources, 53

Lectures on Homeopathic Philosophy, Kent, J.T., 50–59
Legal Advice, viii, 116
Legal requirements, 103, 125–126
Legislative bodies, and homeopathy, 39–40
Level playing field, of homeopathic substances, 94

Lifelike drug picture, 45
Lifestyle during proving, 104–106
Lillium tigrinum, 47–48
Literature search, on toxicology, 101, 108
Liver complaints, and yellow flowers, 79
Liver symptoms and remedies, in *Alcoholus* proving, 92
Location of symptom, specifying or drawing, 120
Loose stools from, changing proving setting, 104–105
Losing things, a symptom, from prover losing remedy, 74
Low potency provings, gives general features, 96
Lycopodium, 17
   in *Alcoholus* proving, 92
Lying down, as spurious rubric, 75

Mainstream medicine, to include homeopathy, 63
Mapping drug side effects, 86
Marchand, Jonathan MD, ix
Masking, 44–45
   current homeopathic thinking, 42, 66
   diminishing preconceptions, 69, 109, 118
   homeopathy's contribution, 59
   substance known to 3 maximum, 101
Master prover, 54–55 *see also* Principle investigator (PI)
Materia Medica, ix, x
   allopathic specifics in, 24–25
   based on practice, 9
   becoming warped, 88
   cured cases methodology, 69
   describing proving symptom, 125
   dreams in, 69–70
   full potential of, 32
   Hahnemannian, 44, 51–57
   inaccuracies entering, 24–25
   incomplete data in, 34
   on-line web site, 130–131
   organizing a not user friendly, 17
   provings and practice in, 116
   pure, by honest testing, 41
   use skills, 19, 51
Mawn-Mahlau, Sam, viii
McGuire, Kim, viii
Meaning of proving results, conflict over, 9
Mechanics of proving, and improved case taking, 14–15

Medical community. *see* Allopathic
Medical intervention, in proving, 117, 125
Medical Safety, consent forms and, viii
Medical students, as provers, 46
Medical thought, homeopaths in forefront, 40–41
Medications, 123
   new, during proving, 123
   and provers, 109
Medicines
   as category 1 for proving, 93–95
   as external force, 29
   as unique *Stress and Strain* response, 29
Meditation proving, 67
   lowering threshold bar, 76
   participants coalesced tightly, 72
   in proving and case taking, 139
Memory, 122
Menstrual cycle, and proving completion, 123
Mental/emotional symptoms
   and dreams, 69–70
   excessive, 124
Mental faculty, 122
Mental functioning, of volunteers, 117
Mercurius, human interaction lengthly, 94
Metabolization of substances, by body, 42
Methodology, viii
   to be set forth, 22
   clung to superstitiously, 137
   and conflict over provings, 9
   cross-over trials, 102
   diagnosis and chemical analysis, 45
   of including and excluding, 88
   many and one model, 15
   testing it, 90
   towards a purer truth, 59
Miasms
   in parody provings, 77
   prodromal period, 55
Microsoft Access 97, 127, 132
Mind symptoms, database selection, 127
Minerals, and polypharmacy, 86
Minutia, burying important symptoms, 114–115
Mirror images
   fussy provings and fuzzy practices, 138
   proving and practice as, 8–9, 11, 70, 78, 81, 105, 137, 139
Mirroring, other provers, ix
Misconceptions on provings, 65–83
Modalities, 121

Model
   elegance of, 85, 106
   explaining proving needed, 13, 138
   of future provings, 21
   of health and disease, 20
   of homeopathy, health and disease, 5 to 12
   and intent in using healthy people, 103
   one workable, 22, 29–38
   of provers' constitutions included, 32–33, 91
   proving, simplified figure, 30
   of proving, complex figure, 33
   proving's philosophical, 22–63, 89
   of strategic decision making, 19
Moral higher ground, homeopathy to recapture, 63
Motif feeling, of dream, 122
Mottled face, 56
Movies, proved, 67
Multi-cultural, large cohort, 91
Muscle building, *Strain* as, 6
Myriad of symptoms, 85

Name withheld, of prover, 125–126
Natrum muriaticum, 102
   proving substance from living being, 93
   reproving of, 57
Natural and synthetic compounds, trillions to choose from, 60
Natural medicine
   allopathic viewpoint, 40
   irony of allopathic dependency on, 60, 62
Natural things of prover, eliminated, 54
Neuralgic pain with languor, 48
New England School of Homeopathy (NESH), ix
   online proving web site, 127–135
New remedies, cures not repertory for use, 82
New symptoms
   remedy *Strain vs.* outside *Stress*, 6
   which provers develop, 37, 112, 122
New York City, 30c isopathic remedy, 80
Newton, Sir Issac, 85
Noise, background
   and databases, 62
   eliminating, so pure event is seen, 41, 59, 66, 82
   entering repertories, 82
Non-homeopaths as provers, importance of, 104
Non-interference, with single dose, 55
Non-random drug testing, proposed, 60–61
Non-verbalizers, excluded from proving, 104

Noxious dose, 7–8
Nullification of homeopathy, rejected in placebo symptoms arising, 101–102
Number of provers
   15 to 45 suggested, 89
   vs. constitutional types, 92
   lose many at 1m potency, 97
   minimum number, 46
Nux Vomica, in *Alcoholus* proving, 92

Object of proving, in handout, 117
Objects attributes
   anthropomorphized, 78
   bloodshed over objects, 77–78
   proving studies of, 76
Old school
   Hahnemann on, 52
   view of illness, 51
Old symptoms, unchanged in proving, 112, 121
Onset time of symptoms, 121
Open ended *vs.* close ended questions, as provings *vs.* current drug testing, 61
Open minded, 52
Opium
   Alumina, dynamic antidote, 58
   in apoplexy, 58
   suspending vital force, 57
   in toxic doses, 56
Opponents, powerful, of homeopathy, 40
Order of the economy, of vital force, 27
Organic derangements, remedy characteristics, 48–49
Organism
   change of vitality, 29
   vitality of, 26
Organon of Medicine, Hahnemann, 32, 66, 87
   Aphorism 105-145, 38, 51
   Aphorism 107-112, 57
   Aphorism 108, 25
   Aphorism 134, 29
   Aphorism 135, 29
   Aphorism 136, 29, 36–37
   Aphorism 142, 34
Orme F.H. MD, 46
Ossified cerebral convolutions, 57
Outside forces, 18–19
Ovarian pain, 48
Over-prescribing a remedy, confirming symptoms eventually, 85
Overdosing in allopathy, 24–25

Paralyzed, one side, in *Alumina,* 58
Parents, prescribing skills, 14
Parody provings, refrigerator, vacuum cleaner, etc., 77
Partial hold of chronic picture, a few symptoms created, 54–55
Past symptoms, distant past, return in proving, 112, 121
Pathogenic drug effects, 48–50
Pathology, clinically defined by *Strain,* 28
Patients as teachers, x
Perceptions heightened, in proving, noting constitutions, 33
Periodic table of elements, polycrests among, 94
Perspiration, 122
Peruvian bark, 53–54
Perverted vital force, slightly by medicine, 27, 57
Pharmacist
    attenuation known by, 45, 101
    and placebos, 124
Pharmacopoeia, x
    consulting, 108–109
    and publishing provings, 115
Phase 1 Drug Studies, 26
    close to proving, 42
    Hahnemannian invention, 59
    removing confounding symptoms, 87
    seminar provings as, 68
    streamlining proposed, 60
Phase 1 proving, toxic and poisonous symptoms, 97, 100
Phase 1, 2, 3 and 4 drug trials, natural homeopathic drift, 61
Phase 2 proving, finding general characteristics, 97, 100
Phase 3 proving, reproving using sensitives and high potencies trials, 97, 100
Philosophical model of provings
    angels on pin analogy, 27
    consistency in, 23
    proving's, 22–63
Philosophy, viii
    confusion of well intentioned homeopaths, 12–14
    encouraged to set fourth, 22
    harmless speculation, 74
    reasoning will improve allopathy, 41–42
    theoretical rules and principles, 51
Phosphorous, proving substance from living being, 93
Photographic rights, 125
Physical functioning, of volunteers, 117

Physical state, general, 122
Physicians, as provers, 46
Physiologic drug testing, homeopathy's contribution, 59
Physiologic tolerance, drug researchers seek, 42
Picture of drug
    coincides in constitutional similar, 36–37, 90
    fragmented in toxic dose, 27
Pilot studies, testing placebo effect, 10–12
PI's (primary investigator)
    catalogues symptoms, 113–114, 124
    instructions, 110
Placebo, 9–12
    arm, unblinding, 131–132
    arm and proving size, 89
    current homeopathic thinking, 42, 65
    diminishing preconceptions, 69, 101–102
    effect *not* interconnectedness, 73–74
    group developing best symptoms, 72–73
    as homeopathy's contribution, 59, 101–102
    imagination and idiosyncrasies, 45
    number of in proving, 101, 109, 124
    pilot and multi-center study, vii
    political boards and, 12
    used in cross-over trials, 102, 109
    vs. verum, vii, 43, 100
Plant species
    events to them before potentization, 78
    polypharmacy of, 86
Poisoning record, for phase 1 proving, 97
Poisonous
    drugs led to provings, 66
    influence of drug, 27, 96
    substance predisposed as remedy, 94
Political historical aspects, 39–40
Polycrests
    not coincidental, 93–94
    proved by Hahnemann, 57
    view that all remedies are, 82
Polypharmacy, 41, 86, 104
    Hahnemann confronts, 66
Potency choice
    for phases of proving, 97
    for reproving, 123
Potentized medicines, as subset of all medicines, 26
Practice
    as basis for *materia medica,* 9
    complicated by incomplete *materia medica,* 34
    enjoyment enhanced, 13

misconceptions in, 8, 12
   proving symptoms choice and, 14
   Strange, Rare, or Peculiars in, 37
Pre-trial phase, 102–103
Preclinical trials, streamlining, 61
Predicting, appearance of symptoms, 17
Predicting indicator, 78–79
Predisposition
   interference to, 26
   and meditative *Stress/Strain*, 76
   and response to world, 91
   with shared remedy *bridges*, 31
   as strain response, 91–92, 137
   Stress, and, 5, 28
   and susceptibility, 29, 81
Pregnant women, not to be provers, 103–104, 109, 123, 125
Prescriptions
   incorrect, symptoms distinguished, 34–35
   initial to followup, x
   no apparent effect, 36
   as provings, 23, 34
   side effects as basis, 42
   single drug, 59
   solely on dreams, incorrect, 70
Primary investigator, viii *see also* Master prover
   selection of, 108
Primary symptoms
   incomplete picture of the whole, 28
   requiring different remedy, 58
   and secondary symptoms jumbled, 45
   and secondary undiscriminated, 37
   Stress produced, 27
   toxic, minimized in potency, 35
   value of, 50
Principle investigator (PI), 92–93
Prodrome period, before symptoms produced, 55–56
Progressively ill people, excluded from proving, 104
ProveIt program, 127, 132
Provers
   300 to 500 in first stage, 91
   environmental sensitivity not substance, 99
   gender, age, temperament, and residence, 46
   Lac defloratum and milk allergies, 93
   on medications eliminated, 103–104
   minimum number, 46
   needed of many constitutions, 32
   no remedy in three months, 123
   non-homeopaths as provers, 104
   not in proving for 3 months, 109
   one person only, 89
   as own experimental control, 118
   pregnancy and, 103–104, 109
   regular lives of, 109
   regular symptoms and noise, 98
   sensitives sought, 137
   sensitivity and remedy description, 96
   small cohort of, 90
   strengthened by proving, 34
   supervisor contact, 118–119, 123
   thought to be proving another remedy, 69
   untraumatized lifestyle of, 105–106
   who are they?, 103–104
   who made their medicine, 42
Proving Web Site, how to use, 127–135
Provings
   1940 to 1970, 65
   assessing symptoms, 109
   attuning the self in, 67
   basic concepts, 5–12, 60
   benefits to practitioners, 138
   conflict about how to do, 9
   conflict and lack of theory base, 24, 137
   criticism standard, 48–50, 60
   cross-cultural experience of, 104
   dream, 68
   English groups, 65
   first phase to find sensitives, 91
   fragmented image of, 13, 27
   of grossest character, 56
   Hahnemann's guidelines, 26
   Hahnemann's polycrests, 21
   importance of, 13–38
   incomplete, 114
   initial interactions, 110
   interpersonal phase 1, 108–110
   lifestyle during, 104–106
   living, organized, unmangled, 47
   medical history of, 41–50
   meditation based, 67
   movies, 67
   negated by seamless interconnectedness, 80
   new symptoms, 6–7
   n=infinity, 68
   non-traditional, plethora of, 68
   or etiology, 79
   perfection to be sought in, 82–83
   placebos in, 10–11
   practice using unknowns, 8–9

primary investigator's instructions, 110
proving themselves, 72
proximity based, 67
quality *vs.* quantity, 46
redefined, 6–8
refining and redefining, 69
related to case taking, 34
renaissance of, 13
reprovings, value of, 57, 90
seminar occurring, 67–68
settings, 104–105
sign of successful, ix
size, 89
songs, 67
symptom choice, 10
symptoms in theory and practice, 29–33
ten steps of, 107–108
by thinking of remedy, 68
uniqueness in individual susceptibility, 81
web site, 127–135
what they are, 13–14
what they are not, 65–83
when officially over, 123
without boundaries, 74
words, 67
Proximity of provers, 10–11
Proximity of remedies, 10–11
Proximity of substance, 67
Pruefung *see also Provings,* 25
Psyche
   Hahnemann quoted, 25
   in various constitutions, 29
Psychology, and dreams, 68
Public opinion wants to know, our standards, how we cure, and allied healer relations, 39–40
Publicity rights, 125
Publishing provings
   encouraged, 21, 115
   rights, 125–126
Pulsatilla, 78
Purity, physician's state of, 52
Pushing murky realm
   of health/disease symptomology, 42
   using sub-toxic doses, 61

Qualifying symptom changes, 109
Qualities
   can they be proved?, 76–78
   use determined, 79
Quality *vs.* quantity, of symptoms in proving, 46, 113–114
Quantum leap in medicine, interfacing clinical trials and practice, 61
Question declining, by prover, 125
Question posing
   and dose repetition, 124
   helping define proving, 22, 138
   by supervisor, 119

Radiation therapy, 24–25
Randomized clinical trials, alternative proposed, 61
Rare symptoms appear, in sick not healthy, 36–37
Rarely used remedies, frequently coming up, 21
Ratio, of sensitive people, 55–56
Rational map, of drugs and side effects, 86
Raw data, into *Segments* and *Cycles,* 17
Reaching out to a substance, through meditation, 76
Recorded products, rights to, 125
Recording symptoms, essential aspects, 120–121
Recreational drugs, 41, 109
Refinement of symptoms, 114–115, 123
   internet site tool for, 127
Refining and redefining, proving thinking or process, 68, 138
Reflecting reality, in provings, 139
Remedies
   have similar *Segments,* 17–18
   introduction of new, x
   rare and common differentiating, 21
   sickness in image of, 53
Remedy
   best study is proving, 54
   causes symptoms without stopping vital force, 27
   Cycle matched to patient *Cycle,* 17–19
   no effect and case analysis, 36, 81
   not working yet not injuring, 100–101
   as Stress producing substance, 14–15
   wait, repeat, or change, 18
   wrong prescription as proving, 23
Renaissance in homeopathy, vi, 14
Repertorizing skills, 18–19
Repertory
   balance in, 138
   becoming warped, 88
   proving method omitted, 82

as proving/practice interface, 61
rapidity of changes in, 20–21
symptoms included before proving, 74
Repetition of dose
incorrect, 109
maximum of 3 in toxic substance, 110
in proving, 98, 100, 119–120, 124
Repetitive proving symptoms, as *Segments* of remedy, 113
Report of the Directors of Provings 1885, 44–50
Reproducibility of remedy, 108
Reproducible results, 38
Reproducing rights, of proving, 125
Reproving, using sensitives, 90, 115
Resolved symptoms, in proving, 35
Resonance of dream emotion, with rest of case, 70
Resonance with medicine, 34
Respiratory symptoms, *Lillium tigrinum* example, 48–50
Response patterns, to medicines as *Stress*, 26
Resurgence of homeopathy, 65
Return of past symptoms, belong to needed and proven remedy, 38
Rhetoric, of allopaths believed by homeopaths, 44
Rhus toxicodendron, 55
Right to end further interviews, 125
Rothenberg, Amy, ND, vi
Rothenberg, Joan, viii
Rubrics
added coincidental to proving, 75
choosing, 16
experimental haphazard choice, 11
fewer before yet more cures, 88
impact of expanding, 21, 67
Rules of provings
published 1885, 44–50
same as daily practice, x, 11
Ryan, Christopher MD, vii
collaboration with, 60–63
Ryan, Jane, viii

Sacred ritual objects potentized, 76–77
Safeguards, against idiosyncrasies and imagination, 45
Safety of prover, 125
Salt, for human functionality, 94
Sawyer, A.I. MD, 46

Science
conceit and, vii, 23
cumulative knowledge in, 12
dialogue and innovation in, 12
homeopathy in center of, 5
jealousy in, 53
recapturing moral high ground, 63
rhetoric *vs.* pure, x
Scientific method
Hahnemann's, 25–26, 85
homeopathy's contribution to, 59
single variable in, 66
Scientist, Hahnemann as consummate, 86
Second class citizen status, of homeopaths, 39
Secondary symptoms
common to drug and simillimum, 35
and primary undiscriminated, 37
requiring different remedies, 58
Strain produced, 27
Segments in a *Cycle*
importance of *Segment* order, 17
overlapping of two medicine cycles, 35, 38
repetitive symptoms in provers, 113
as rubrics exemplifying etiology, 79
shared by provers, 33–36
shared with simillimum, 37
and unique remedy features, 114
Seminar provings, 67–68
excessive variables, 105
Sensation, describing, 120
Sensitivity
lack of, 120
levels explained, 98–101
to potentized substances, 6–7, 37, 55, 87, 90, 96, 113–114, 137
Sepia poisoning observed, 92–93
Sequence of events, recording symptom circumstances, 121
Sequence of symptoms, 49, 112
Lillium tigrinum example, 49–50
Serenity, from changing proving setting, 104–105

Set theory representation
of explaining unexplainable symptom distribution, 32
of potential symptoms and predispositions, 30
Setting of proving, 104–105
Sexual organs, example in *Lillium Tigrinum*, 49
Sexy substances, proving of, 93
Shalts, Ed MD, vii, 10

Sheldrake Dr., justifying n=infinity proving, 68
Side effects
    drug researchers minimize, 42
    minimized by sub-group selection, 61
    rational map of, 86
Sifting symptom process, at end of proving, 113
Silica, 102
Silicate of Alumina, prodromal period before symptoms, 55
Similarity, and level of response, 7
Similars, elegance of concept, 85
Simillimum, 78, 86, 101
Simplicity, state of, 52
Single drug effect, 41
Size of proving
    to match purpose, 89
Sleep symptoms
    placement in *materia medicas*, 69–70
    in proving, 122
Sloppy technique, yet valuable information, 42
Smith, Linda, viii
Songs proved, 67
Spasms in sleep, 122
Species
    interaction with medicine, 37
    not individual plant proved, 78
    toxic dose and predisposition, 29
Specific characteristics, *vs.* general characteristics, 96
Specific complaints, matching generalities, 7
Spinal phenomena, *Lillium tigrinum* example, 48, 49–50
Stannum metallicum, 47
Staphysagria, 21
Steady state, 99–100, 103
    see also Threshold bar line
    ability to *see* changes, 109–110, 112
    elusive in pregnancy, 104
    establishing provers, 110–111, 118–119
    hysterical people lacking, 104
    and placebo use, 124
Step 1 of proving, interpersonal phase, 108–110
Step 2 of proving, beginning interactions, 110
Step 3 of proving, establishing steady state, 111
Step 4 of proving, eliciting and reporting symptoms, 111–112
Step 5 of proving, agreeing on threshold bar, 113

Step 6 of proving, catalogue of symptoms, 113–114
Step 7 of proving, refining symptoms, 114–115
Step 8 of proving, retesting sensitive provers, 115
Step 9 of proving, publishing proving, 115
Step 10 of proving, *materia medica*, 116
Stertorus breathing, 56, 58
Strain
    clinical pathology, 28
    creating symptoms, 14
    explaining return of old symptoms, 38
    fever, 6
    majority of new symptoms, 35
    muscle building, 6
    return to healthy state, 27
    before *Stress*, in meditative proving, 76
    vigorous in sensitives, 115
Stramonium, 26
Strange, Rare, or Peculiar symptoms, in very sensitive provers, 36–37
Stream of Providence, Hahnemann's view, 52
Stream of vital action, 27 *see also* Vital Force
    disturbed yet not suspended, 57
Streamlining current drug tests, 72
Stress and Strain, 6
    chronic symptoms partially cured, 37
    as cycle of existence, 28
    homeopathy redefined by, 6
    meditation and, 76
    model in provings and case analysis, 26–29
    predisposition, and, 5 to 7
    proving theory, and, vi, vii, 137
    risk/benefit in potency, 137
    Straining defined, 5
    unique to a medicine, 29
Stress as
    bacteria, 6
    exercise and exertion, 5
    provided by potentized medicine, 26
    proving substance, 14–15
    similar to environment of prover, 73, 112
    strong to sensitive provers, 96
    as toxic drug, 27
    unique to individual constitution, 29
Sub-group selection, efficacy to allopathic studies, 14, 60
Sub-toxic symptomology, obtained without prover injury, 97
Substance
    of cellular interaction for millennium, 93

how its qualities are impregnated, 77
how tolerated and absorbed, 42
as interesting and exciting, 92
as isopathic also homeopathic, 79
of living being to prove, 93
masking known to 3 maximum, 101
as noxious *Stress*, 6
preparing for proving, 108
from sacred rituals, 76–77
species related, 37
symptoms and provers separated, 125
Successful proving, by exclusion of symptoms, ix, 48
Suffering, in Hahnemann's view, 52
Suggestibility
limited by cross-over trials, 102
limited by placebos, 69, 101–102
of provers, 109
Sulfur, for human functionality, 94
Sulphur, 55, 102
Supervisors, viii
as prescribing homeopaths, 124
provers consult with, 118–119, 125
view web site, 129–130
Supplies dispensed, 110
Suppressing parts of truth, as self limiting, 40
Surgery, 123
Susceptibility, 29
and eliciting symptoms, 98–99
importance in placebo/verum trials, 100
to impressions proved, 67
precise to substance at high potency, 97
Suspended action, of vital force by *Opium*, 27
Symptoms
accepted by placebo prover pre-trial, 103
altered by constitution, 37
antipsorics, 55
arising from incorrect remedy, 81
attributing incorrectly, 110
as *bridges* between remedies, 31–32
change due to herbs or acupuncture, 18–19
choice of, 14, 16, 27
chronological order of, 47
circumstances surrounding, 121
common and unique, 29–34
common in shared constitutions, 34
common to human experience, 81
complete, 124
concomitant, 120
connectedness of, 22
from constitutional subsets, 32

cured, 6, 8, 11, 36–37, 82, 112
developed before proving, 74
differentiating symptoms, 110
direction of, 120
discerning disease and remedy, 34–35
duplication of, and group size, 90
duration of, 121
experienced by single prover, 34
five categories, 112
general unspecified, 113–114
Hahnemann's polycrests and number of, 21
imagination conceived, 50
individual and totality of, 29
intensity of, 121
limiting confounding, 87–88
list and proving method, 67, 72
location of, 120
many *vs.* few or none, 65, 74, 138
mental/emotional and dreams, 69–70
mind, 128
modalities of, 121
of morbid character, 48
new in provings, 18, 112
new remedies, number of, 21
none reported, ix, 38, 46, 56
number of: 100's or 1,000's, 11
number of: 1,000 to 2,000, 88
old symptoms, 112
onset time, 121
original, appearing, 54
pathognomonic, 49
placebo cutoff time for, 10
placebo group develops, 72–73
plethora of dream, 70
predicting appearance of, 17
primary and secondary undiscriminated, 37
primary as *Stress* produced, 27–28, 34
prodromal period, 55
produced by low potencies, 96
prover to be aware of, 121–123
in provers, not disease, 118
provers not sharing, 118
qualifying changes, 109
quality *vs.* quantity, 46, 113–114
rarely developed in the healthy, 36–37
real and imaginary, 47
reappearing from distant past, 112
recording disappeared, 8
refining, 114
from remedy *Strain vs.* outside *Stress*, 6

repetitive in provers, 113
resolved or dissipated, 34
return of past, 38
rubrics from placebo group, 73
secondary *Strain* produced, 27–28
sensation of, 120
sequence varies with prover, 49
serious later stage, 50
shared *Segments*, different *Cycles*, 17
as side effects, 42
sleep, 69–70
Staphysagria and new remedy, 21
Strange, Rare or Peculiar, 37
sub-toxic, 97
threshold bar of, 71, 73, 81
totality perceived, 28
true ones buried, 73
typifying *Segments*, 114–115
who develops new, 37
Synagogue scroll, can its attributes be proved, 77
Synchronicity, in n=infinity provings, 68
Synthesizing, physician experience, x
Synthetic compounds, from natural, 60

Talbot, I.T., MD, 46
Technique, *vs. why* it happens, 24
Teeth grinding, 122
Temporary improvement, in proving, 35
Ten steps of a proving, 107–108
Theory *see also* Philosophy
  argues against methodology, 83
  into practice, 107–135
  of sensitivity, 119
Thermometer, 45, 47
Thirtieth potency in provings, 54–55, 57, 123–124
  in phase two provings, 97
Three proving categories of substances, 93–95
Three proving phases, 97
Three times daily, prover self review, 122
Threshold bar of symptoms, 71, 73, 82–83, 88, 99
  clarifying symptoms above, 113
  set in pre-trial phase, 103
  triangle figure, those above and below bar, 98–101
Thuja, reproving of, 57
Time-consuming aspect, of provings, 95, 127
Tinctures, 54
  in provings, 95

Tomato effect, in homeopathic history, 40
Tongue coated, 48
Totality of symptoms, 28–29, 34, 51
Toxic effects, 42
  data in provings, 117
  in less than lethal dose, 87
  minimized in potentized medicine, 35
Toxic substances
  crude doses, 56
  gross *Stress* of, 27, 29
  learning effects of, 86
  at material doses, 96
  proving origins in, 7–8, 137
  repetition in proving, 110, 112
Transactions of the Thirty-Eighth Session of the American Institute of Homeopathy, 44–48
Translating symptoms, to repertory, 16
Trauma, as spurious rubric, 75
Truth as goal, 63, 87
Tuning, treatment as untuning and retuning, 28
Type face in repertory explained, 61

Unblinding proving, on web site, 131
Unconsciousness, 56
Uniformity of drug effects, 45
  Arsenicum example, 50
Unique features of remedy, outshine non-unique, 114
United States, popularity of seminar proving, 67–68
Unreliability, of toxic primary symptoms, 27
Untraumatized lifestyle, for provers, 104–105
URL, 127–135
Use of substance, determines qualities and attributes, 79
User friendly symptoms, 16–17

Variables
  isolating one, 41, 66, 80
  removing, 26
Verification, from other provers, 50
Verum *vs.* placebo, vii, 131–132
Videotape rights, 125
Vienna Society, 57
Vital force or influx
  positive medical action on, 26
  stream of disturbed, 27
Voice and speech, example of exaptation, 85–106
Volunteers, 46, 60

Waiting
   after prescribing, 124
   for effect of single dose, 54–55
Water and its constituents, emergent qualities
   example, 79–80
Web site
   documentation, viii, 127–135
   double-blind provings, 131–132
Western Electric Co., 1920's experiment, 71
Why placebo provers get symptoms, 10–11
Win/win situation with allopaths, *vs.*
   win/lose or lose/lose, 41–42
Woodward A.W. MD, 48–50
Word, finding write, 122
Words proved, 67
Wright, A.R. MD, 46
Writing information, about symptoms, 111
Writing symptoms, 123
   defines homeopathy, 7
   four days before proving, 119
   of remedy's general sphere, 8
www.nesh.com, 127

Young people, professing and turning from
   homeopathy, 52

Index

Part Two

Abdomen, 178
Aberrant great vessels, 164
Abstraction deficit, 163
Accidents
    and blood alcohol levels, 158
    and gross motor incoordination, 171
Accommodation, visual, poor at night, 175
Acting out, 176
Acuity of senses, 167, 169–70
    revelry or rage, 170
    of vision, 175
Acute
    and chronic states, 159
    as if severe in proving, 231
Addiction to alcohol and stimulants, 165
Agenesis of the corpus callosum, 163
Alcohol
    agony and pain causing, 149
    direct toxic effects, 160
    drug plague on humanity, 158
    and energy needs, 160
    in human history, 144
    neurologic arena, 160
    overlooked as remedy, 150–51
    percentage in drinks, 157
    and pregnancy, 161–65
    relation to homeopathy, 149–52
    studied extensively, 159
    as water of life, 157–58
    why prove?, 147
Alcohol dehydrogenase (ADH), in different cultures, 156
Alcohol-related birth defect (ARBD), 162, 164
Alcohol-related neurodevelopmental disorder (ARND), 162, 164–65
Alcoholism
    addiction in America, 159
    family history, 181
    and nutrition, 160
    in patient history, 144
    red flags of, 160
    and rubric Alcoholism, 151
Alcoholus
    and alcoholism remedies, 151
    anger compared with *Cannabis indica*, 185
    and *Carbo vegetalis*, 160
    case, 183–85
    Cycle, diagram, 166
    in *Encyclopedia of Pure Materia Medica,* 144, 149–50
    figure of remedy relationships, 150
    five distinct groups, 152
    food cravings, 178
    frequency of use, 144
    and *Lycopodium,* 178–79
    many sensitive to, 148
    mirrored in *Ferrum Metalicum,* 160
    name change needed, 152
    as needed children's remedy, 148–49
    and *Nux Vomica,* 178
    symptomology under other remedies, 149
Allen, T.F., 145, 149
Allergies
    flare-up in wrong season, 283
    involving ears, 176, 266
    involving nose, 175
    respiratory tract, 180
Anacardium children, resembling *Alcoholus,* 168
Anger
    sudden, 185
    unpremeditated, 169
Anhalonium, 205
Animal dander, 180
Antisocial behavior, 160
Anxiety lowered, 160
Appetite, diminished or binges, 172, 178
Apprehended or caught, no worry of, 168
Aqua Vitae, 157
Arnica, 184
Arrhythmias, 160
Arthritis, 180, 266
Asphyxiation, and blood alcohol levels, 158
Asthma, 180, 245
Atrial septal defects, 164
Attention problems, 170
    and strong shock, 173
Auditory problems, 164
    processing and understanding, 170
Autistic patients
    beauty disturbing, 169
    confused by sensory cues, 170
    and crowd stimuli, 171–72
    rage and aggression in, 169
Awkward in sports, 171

Balance, and blood alcohol levels, 158
Beauty, disturbing, 169
Beer, 151, 157–58
Belligerance, aggression, and blood alcohol levels, 158
Benzene, 151
Birth control, 160

Index - Part Two

Birth defects, 148, 161
Birth weight low, 162
Blackouts, and blood alcohol levels, 158, 160
Blame others, 184
Blatant behavior, 183
Blinded by lights, at night, 175
Bloating and gas, 159–60
Bloodstream, shared by fetus and mother, 161
Body warmth, and blood alcohol levels, 158
Brain functioning, 148
    alcohol damage, 160
    and blood alcohol levels, 158
Breaking things, 171
Breasts swell and ache, premenstrual, 179
Bronchitis, 180

Calcarea carbonica, constitution, 298
Calling names, 184
Camptodactyly, 164
Cannabis indica, 205
    Alcoholus and anger, 185
    Alcoholus children like, 168
    Alcoholus related remedy, 181
    Alcoholus used as often, 144
    entranced like *Alcoholus*, 169
    like *Alcoholus* with possessions, 171
    out of body feeling, 167
    and *Sulphur* client, 150–51
    symptomology, 149
Car accidents, 171
Car accidents and alcohol, 157
Carbo vegetablis, 213
Carcinosinum
    Alcoholus related remedy, 181
    chronic symptoms, 273
Cardiac defects, 164
Cardiac syndromes, 159
Cardiomyopathy, 160
Case of *Alcoholus*, 183–85
Central nervous system
    depressant, 160
    neurodevelopemental abnormalities, 163
Cerebellar degeneration, 160
Cerebellar hypoplasia, 163
Chastisement, intolerance of, 184
Chemical impacts, concern of clinician, 144
Chest symptoms, 179
Chest to head, hot flashes, 179
Children, in choosing *Alcoholus* proving, 148
Choking, vomiting, and blood alcohol levels, 158

Choosing, useful remedy to prove, 147–48
Chromosomal problems, 148
Chronic fatigue symptoms, 298
Cirrhosis of liver, 159
Clarity in dreaming, confusion while awake, 174
Cleft palate, 161
Clinician's perspective, 144
Clinodactyly, 164
Close up and close in, 184
Clothes textures, heightened awareness of, 169
Cocculus indica, 283
Coffee, 173, 178
Coffee, tea and alcohol, in religion and culture, 156–57
Cognitive abnormalities, unexplained by family or environment, 164
Colors, vibrant, 169
Comatose state, and blood alcohol levels, 158
Concentration difficulties, with unique attitudes, 183–85
Conception
    and abstinence, 165
    while parents drinking, 181
Conductive hearing loss, 164
Confusion, 167, 170–72
Congenital abnormalities, including dysplasias and abnormalities, 164
Congestive heart failure, 160
Conjecture, 144
Constipation, 178
Contradicting parents, 167
Contradiction, intolerance of, 184
Coordination and judgment, and blood alcohol levels, 158
Corpus callosum, 163
Cranial size decreased, 163
Crimes and alcohol, 157
Criteria of proving substance, 148
Cycles and Segments, model tested, 147
Cycles and Segments of *Alcoholus*, 205, 213

Daily interaction, as basis of *Alcoholus* proving, 148–49
Death, and blood alcohol levels, 158
Deception, 168, 185
Dementia, 160
Depression, 167, 172
    and desire for stimulation, 172
Diarrhea, 178
Discharges, 167
Disorientation, and blood alcohol levels, 158

Disruptive nature, of questions and answers, 167
Distillation, 157
   and body and soul destruction, 157
Dreams
   of airplanes, 266
   of being lost, 174
   of car accidents and mishaps, 171, 173
   of destruction, 173
   fear of drowning, 174
   increased menopause, 298
   increased premenstrual, 179, 298
   of large bodies of water, 173–74
   noisy causing restlessness, 173
   of suspense and deception, 174
   of throwing all out window, 174
Drinking water, dangers of, 155
Driving really fast, 173
Drug of choice, 159
Dryness of skin, 180
Dullness while studying, 183

Ears
   as in flying, 265
   otitis media, 176
Eating disorder, feeling unloved, 172
Eating with hands, 171
ECG abnormalities, 160
Egging people on, 168
Elbows arthritic, 180
Emotions intensified, and blood alcohol levels, 158
Emperor with No Clothes, story of, 150
Encyclopedia of Pure Materia Medica , Allen T.F., 145, 149–50, 174, 205, 213
Entranced by sensory stimulation, 169
Environmental, toxic water supplies, 155
Enzymes, and alcohol metabolizing, 156
Epidemic disease, and water supply, 155
Erections difficult, and blood alcohol levels, 158
Erethism, 179
Esophageal veins engorged, 159
Ethanol content, 151–52
Euphoria, and blood alcohol levels, 158
Excessive joy, 167
Exhilaration, 167
Explorers, conquests, aristocracies and capitalization, religion and alcohol, 156–57
Extremities, 180
Eye-hand coordination, 163
Eyes, 175

Face, 176–77
Facial anomalies, 162
Facial features lacking, in Fetal Alcohol Syndrome, 161
Falling, 171
Family and friends, lost to alcohol, 157
Family history, of alcoholism, 181, 184
Fatty liver, 159
Feeling good, 167
Female, 179
Fermentation
   and the advent of refrigeration, 155
   and aseptic and antiseptics, 156
Ferrum Metalicum and *Alcoholus*, 160, 176–77
Fetal Alcohol Effects (FAE), 162
Fetal Alcohol Syndrome, Diagnosis, Epidemiology, Prevention, and Treatment, 1966, 165
Fetal Alcohol Syndrome (FAS), 148, 161, 164–65
   from multi-generational drinkers, 164
   in multi-generational drinkers, 165
   severity of, 162
Fibrocystic breast disease, 179
First born, with dominant disposition, 183
Flailing arms and legs, 171
Flatus which relieves, 178
Flexion contractures, 164
Floating feeling, 167
Flushing
   and heat of face, 176–77
   of skin, 180
Focus lessened, and blood alcohol levels, 158
Folic acid, 161
Foods
   absorption poor, 159
   child averse to, 177
   pleasantness of and success mechanisms, 155
   in system with alcohol, 159
Forethought or afterthought, acting without, 169
Fork and spoon incoordination, 171
Freedom, sense of, 167

Gag reflex, and blood alcohol levels, 158
Gagging, of autistic children, 169
Gait disoriented, 171
Gas and bloating, 178
Gastritis, 159
Gastrointestinal system, 159
Generals, 181

Index - Part Two

Generational toxic interaction, of *Alcoholus*, 148
Genetic problems, 148
Genetics, sweets and fermentation, 155
Germ theory, and boiling water, 155
Glucose stores, 160
Grabbing, 183
Growth retardation, 162

Hahnemann Pharmacy, 151
Hands, arthritic and stiff, 180
Happiness happier, and blood alcohol levels, 158
Hard and mean, 184
Hay fever, 177
Head feels fluid filled, 175
Headaches, 175
Hearing acute, slight noise bothers, 176
Hearing muffled, 163
 and blood alcohol levels, 158
Heart failure, and blood alcohol levels, 158
Heartburn, 159–60
Heat sensation
 and dryness in eyes, 175
 stomach to head, 173
Helleborus, 184
Hemivertebrae, 164
Herpes like, 175, 177
Herpes simplex, 179–80
 proving flare-up, 231, 277, 283
Higher feeling, then energy fails, 172
History, of alcohol in human species, 144
Hitting siblings, 168
Homicide, 160
Horseshoe kidneys, 164
Hot flash feeling, in headache, 175
Hot flashes, chest to head, 179
Human species use of alcohol, 148–49, 155
Hurtful things, told without hesitation, 169
Hydronephrosis, 164
Hyoscyamus
 Alcoholus related remedy, 181
 children resembling *Alcoholus*, 168
Hyperactivity, 148, 170
Hypercritical, 184
Hypoglycemia, 160
Hypoplastic kidneys, 164
Hypoplastic nails, 164

Ignatia
 chronic symptoms, 273
 symptoms like, 289

Immature emotionally, 168, 183
Impaired fine motor skills, 163
Impulsivity, 148, 163, 169–70, 183
Inhibition lowered, 160, 167–68
 and blood alcohol levels, 158
Intelligence lowered, 148
Interference, intolerance of, 184
Interrupting parents, 167
Intoxication, 157
 as side effect, 157
Introversion, in adults, 172
Iron stores increased, 160
Irrelevant symptoms, screening of, 144–45
Irritability premenstrual, 179
Isolating behavior, 160

Jesting, as if drunk, 185
Jokester, immature, 168
Journals of provers, 143

Klippel-Feil syndrome, 164
Korsakoff's psychosis, 160

Lachesis
 Alcoholus related remedy, 181, 217
 relation to alcohol, 149, 151
Language reception and expression, deficit in, 163
Laughing excessive, 167
Learning difficulties, 148, 164
Levitation feeling, 167
Light irritates, 167
Lightheadedness, and blood alcohol levels, 158
Liver symptoms and disease, 178–79
Loquacious and loud, 168
Loss of consciousness, and blood alcohol levels, 158
Loudness
 of music, 173
 of speech, 167
Low alcohol drinks, 157
Low IQ, 165
Lycopodium
 Alcoholus bloating similar, 178
 Alcoholus related remedy, 181, 213, 231
 Alcoholus sensitivity to, 151
 constitution, 283
Lying, 184
Lying for fun, 168

Made fun of, then confusion and
   withdrawal, 171–72
Male, 179
Malformation, virtually every, 164
Malnourished, 160
Manic-depressive, 172
Materia medica
   challenging writing, 147
   reflecting practice, 153
   reflecting substance process, 151
   symptoms to repertory, 144
Maternal alcohol exposure, alcohol related
   effects, 164–65
Mathematical skills deficit, 163
Maturing after *Alcoholus*, 184
Meat craving, 178
Medorrhinum
   as *Alcoholus* related remedy, 181, 217
   and *Alcoholus* sensitivity to, 151
   chronic symptoms, 273, 289
   constitution, 245, 277
Melancholic longing, 174
Memory impairment, and blood alcohol
   levels, 158
Memory problems, 163, 171
Menopause, 176–77, 298
   hot flashes, 179
Menses delayed, 179, 229, 298
Mental and emotional problems, 148
Mental retardation, 161, 170
Micro nutrients, and fetus, 161
Microbes, 155
Microcephaly, 163
Mid face flat, 162
Midline birth anomalies, 161
Mind wandering, 183
Model and methodology, testing of, 145
Mood altering drug of choice, 159
Mood disorder, 148
Mood swings, 160
   and blood alcohol levels, 158
Morality, no sense of, 168
Morphinum
   as *Alcoholus* related remedy, 181
   children resembling *Alcoholus*, 168
Mouth, 177
Mucous discharge, clear with sneezing, 176
Multi-generational drinkers, 165
Musculoskeletal, 180
Mythology eschewed, 144

Narcolepsy, 172
Nasal congestion, in warm room, 176
National Clearinghouse for Alcohol and Drug
   Information, 162
Natrum muriaticum, as constitution, 298
Nausea and vomiting, and blood alcohol
   levels, 158
Neck too weak, to hold head, 175
Neurologic problems, 148
Neurologic systems, 159
Neuropsychiatric effects, 160
Neurosensory hearing loss, 164
Ninth Special Report to the U.S. Congress on
   Alcohol and Health 1997, 162
Noise, overload causing aggression, 169–70
Nose, 176
Nosode like quality, *of Alcoholus,* 144, 181
Nothing works, 172
Numbness and tingling, 160
Nutrition, sacrificed, 160
Nux Vomica, 184, 231
and Alcoholus sensitivity to, 151
constitution, 245, 253
Nux vomica
   Alcoholus related, 181, 289
   constitution, 231
   relation to alcohol, 149
Nux vomica, Calcarea carbonica
   constitution, 231

Occam's razor, and human alcohol
   interface, 155
Ocular problems, 164
Olympic medalist, coordination lost, 231
Opium
   as *Alcoholus* related remedy, 181
   narcolepsy like *Alcoholus,* 172
   symptomology, 149
   used as often as *Alcoholus,* 144
Optic neuropathy, 160
Otitis media, with sharp pains, 176
Out of body feeling, 167, 171–72
Outside of themselves, unemotional
   seeming, 169
Overpowering sleep, 173–74

Pain awareness, and blood alcohol
   levels, 158
Palpebral fissures, 162
Pancreatitis, 159
Pandemic disease, and water supplies, 155

Index - Part Two

Partying, 157–58
Pasteurization, 155
Paucity of symptoms, and brilliant cures, 144
Pectus excavatum and carinatum, 164
Peptic ulcer, 159
Peripheral nerve damage, 160
Peristaltic waves, type 3, in acute alcohol ingestion, 178
Philtrum flattened, 162
Phosphorous, 205
    with *Sulphur* constitution, 252
Physically harassed, 172
Pinpoint sharp pain, 180
Placebo
    arm of proving, 152
    group, no symptoms, 153
    and verum vials, 151
Pleasantness
    and blood alcohol level, 158
    and distorted reality, 156
    in foods and genetics, 155
Poetry eschewed, 144
Polite boy, after *Alcoholus*, 184
Pollen, 180
Polyneuropathies, 160
Poor attention, 148
Popularity of alcohol, 159
Potentization process, alcohol and, 150–52
Practical jokes, annoying and destructive, 168
Pregnancy and alcohol, 161–65, 181
Premaxillary zone abnormalities, 162
Premenstrual symptoms, 179
Prohibition, 158
Prostate swelling, 179
Provers, not all one "voice," 298
Proving
    antidoted, 269
    having symptoms of severe acute ailments, 213
    included old symptoms for context only, 204
    mirroring practice in *Alcoholus* model, 150–51
Public bathroom, smells, 176
Pulsatilla
    contains *Alcoholus*, 151
    symptoms, 289
Pyramid diagram, of symptom sensitivity sets, 153

Questions and responds disruptively, 167
Quinn, Michael, 151

Radioulnar synostosis, 164
Rage, 167
    as autonomic response, 169–70
Rash, chronic, cured, 298
Reaction time slowed, and blood alcohol levels, 158
Reality, heightened and distorted, 156
Reclusivity, 171–72
Recreational alcohol, 158
Recreational drug experience, like *Alcoholus* dream, 174
Rectum, 178
Refractive problems, secondary to small eyes, 164
Regurgitation, 178
Religious tolerance and intolerance, of alcohol, 156–57
Remedies seem to fail, and consideration of *Alcoholus*, 181
Remedy close, then symptoms cured and/or accentuated, 298
Remorse, no sense of, 168
Renal aplastic or dysplastic, 163–64
Repertory, balance in, 187
Repetition of dose, in proving, 152
Respiration and heart rate, slowed, 160
Respiratory arrest, and blood alcohol levels, 158
Respiratory tract, 180
Restaurant smells, sensitivity to, 176
Restless sleep, 173–74
Restlessness, 183–85
Retinal vascular anomalies, 164
Right side, 175–81
Right-sided headaches, 175
Rubrics
    of *Alcoholus* added cautiously, 187
    in repertory for alcohol, 149
Rush from stimuli, 173

Sadness becomes sadder, and blood alcohol levels, 158
Sadness premenstrual, 179
Safe sex practices, 160
Salt craving, 178
School performance, 160, 163
Science, 145
Scoliosis, 164
Scotch, warmth of, 173
Scratchy sore throat, 177
Seasonal allergies, 176
Segment of Heightened Senses, 213

Segment of Weakness, 213
Self-isolation, 160
Sensitivity to *Alcoholus,* and symptom production, 204, 213
Sensory stimulation, entranced by, 169
Sepia, 231, 289
Severe processing problems, 170
Sex drive increases, 170, 179
Sexual intercourse painful, 179
Shame, lack of, 168
Sharp shooting pains
   in headaches, 175
   in right eye, 175
Shoplifting, 168
Shortened fifth digit, 164
Shy people, blushing, 176–77
Side effects, of alcohol studied, 159
Silly behavior, 183
Sinusitis, acute or chronic, 176
Skeletal defects, 164
Skin, 180
Skin eruptions, with or without tingling, 175
Skull fracture, 184
Sleep, 173–74
Smell, sense of, more accentuated, 176
Smoke as allergen, 180
Sneezing with, clear mucous discharge, 176
Social perception, 163
Soul is leaving feeling, 167
Sound irritates, 167
Species use of alcohol, 148–49
   discovery and uses, 155
Speech
   mistakes in, 170
   slurred and blood alcohol levels, 158
Spelling mistakes, 170
Spicy food, craving, 178
Spina bifida, 161
Spirit drinks, 151
   shock of, 173
Stable center, lacking, 169
Statistics
   of alcohol addiction, 159
   of alcohol and birth defects, 161
   of alcohol and society, 157
Stealing
   money, 168
   as stimulation, 173
Sternum joining ribs, sharp pains, 179
Stimulation, 167, 171–73
Stomach, 178

Stomach, bleeding, 159
Strabismus, 164
Striking and scratching, if approached from side, 170
Striking out, when reigned in, 169
Structural brain abnormalities, 163
Stuffiness, 176
Stumbling, 171
Succession of alcohol, 152
Suicide, 160
Sulphur
   constitution, 245, 253, 277, 298
   relation to alcohol, 149
   relation to *Alcoholus,* 151, 181, 213, 217
Sulphur diarrhea, in acute alcohol ingestion, 178
Surgery, 157
Susceptibility, of drinker, 159
Swallowing pains, throat to ears, 177
Sweets, craving for, 178
Swelling sensation, or fullness in throat, 177
Sycotic miasm, 181
Sympathetic, as if, 169
Symptoms
   Alcoholus rare ones, 149
   as context dependent, 143, 204
   left out purposely, 187
   none in placebo group, 153
   as vitamin and micronutrient related, 159
Syphilitic miasm, 181

Tastes, strong sense of, 169, 177
Taunted, 172
Tearing in eyes, 175
Teens, 168–69
Teratogenesis, 148, 161, 164
Tetralogy of Fallot, 164
Thiamin deficiency, 160
Thirst, for cold water, 177
Thirtieth potency dilution, 152
Threshold bar of symptoms, 153
Throat, 177
Tingling and itching in nose, 176
   and itching mouth, throat, and palate, 177
   with or without skin eruptions, 175
Tingling, facial, and viral skin outbreaks, 177
Toluene, 151
Torticollis right-sided, 180
Toxic environment
   and alcohol's daily contact, 149
   and water supply, 155
Tuberculinum, 213

Unpleasant dreams of water, 173–74
Upper lip, flat, thin, 162
Ureteral duplicators, 164
Urinary tract, frequent urging, 178

Vacation from life, 172
Vaginal tract dry, 179
Vasodilation, fascial, 173
Ventricular septal defects, 164
Violent acts, 160
Viral infection
   in eyes, 175
   flare-up, 180
   in mouth, 177
Visual distortions at night, 175
Vivid dreams, 174
Voiding urine incompletely, 179
Voluminous provings, 145
Vomiting, of autistic children, 169

Warm-blooded, 181
Watch television, 172
Water of life, alcohol as, 157–58
Water supply safety, 155–56
Weakness, 167
Weepiness premenstrual, 179
Weight loss, 160
Well indicated remedies fail, and *Alcoholus,* 144
Wine, 151, 157–58
Withdrawal, 167, 171–72
Withdrawn feeling premenstrual, 179
Wound cleaning, 157
Writing mistakes, 170

Yeast and sugars, 155

About the Author

Paul Herscu ND, a native of Rumania, is a graduate of the National College of Naturopathic Medicine in Portland, Oregon. With his wife and partner, Amy Rothenberg ND, and their children Sophie, Misha and Jonah, he resides in Amherst, Massachusetts from where he practices, teaches and writes about homeopathy.

Dr. Herscu has taught widely throughout the Europe and the United States. He is the founder and director of the New England School of Homeopathy and was the long time editor of the *New England Journal of Homeopathy*. His first book, *The Homeopathic Treatment of Children, Pediatric Constitutional Types* has been acclaimed as an exceptional description of eight well known remedies as they relate specifically to children. His next book, *Stramonium with an Introduction to Analysis Using Cycles and Segments* lays out his philosophical foundation for the study and practice of homeopathy. Dr. Herscu publishes the twice monthly *Herscu Letter* which is available via email. Further information can be found at The New England School's web site: www.nesh.com.

–Notes–